Public Health
NUTRITION
From principles to practice

Edited by

MARK LAWRENCE & TONY WORSLEY

Open University Press

This edition published by:

Open University Press
McGraw-Hill Education
McGraw-Hill House
Shoppenhangers Road
Maidenhead, Berkshire
England, SL6 2QL

email: enquires@openup.co.uk
world wide web: www.openup.co.uk

and Two Penn Plaza, New York, NY 10121-2289, USA

First published in Australia and New Zealand in 2007 by Allen & Unwin Pty Ltd

A catalogue record of this book is available from the British Library

ISBN-10: 033522320-6 (pb); 033522309-5 (hb)
ISBN-13: 978 033522320 6 (pb); 978-033522309-1 (hb)

Library of Congress Cataloging-in-Publication Data
CiP data applied for

Typeset in Baskerville 11/13 by Midland Typesetters, Australia
Printed by Southwood Press, Australia

10 9 8 7 6 5 4 3 2 1

The McGraw·Hill Companies

Foreword

I am pleased to comment on this book because it is a ground-breaking text in the developing field of public health nutrition. In their introductory chapter the editors, Mark Lawrence and Tony Worsley, define public health nutrition as 'the promotion and maintenance of nutrition-related health and wellbeing of populations through the organised efforts and informed choices of society'. Indeed, this book has been written in the belief that the most important issues confronting food and nutrition scientists in the twenty-first century are beyond the scope of conventionally defined human biology. As Uauy (2005), the current president of the International Union of Nutritional Sciences (IUNS), has said 'we must be willing to encompass the social, economic, political and human rights dimension of nutrition'.

This book comprises eighteen chapters grouped into four sections under the titles 'Principles', 'Populations', 'Priorities' and 'Practice'. These provide a notable comprehensive discussion of the issues. In relation to 'Priorities', Margetts argues that 'priorities need to be viewed in a context that includes ideology about responsibilities and solutions. This is the challenge to public health nutrition'. He further states that 'the way we currently operate is not good enough — if this book is to make any difference it has to enable public health nutritionists to be better informed, more critical and less naive about the causes and therefore the solutions to major international public health problems'.

In the chapter on 'Policy and Politics', Lawrence refers to an Australian Broadcasting Corporation (ABC) television programme which asked the question 'do parents need government help to control what their children eat?' The answer was that parents needed and wanted help but the present government would not help and neither would the food industry. This problem has been around for quite a long time. It could be said that the situation is at an impasse, so what can be done?

My answer is 'people power led by public health nutrition scientists'. Parents have to band together in increasing numbers in voluntary organisations to oppose the TV advertising of foods of high sugar and fat content. The situation cannot be met by individuals. It requires an organisation as has occurred in the past with other public health problems.

Public health nutritionists have an obligation to take the opportunity of participating and leading in such organisations — in this book it is called 'public health practice'. As Lawrence points out some form of political lobbying will be necessary. A choice may need to be made between 'working from within' or making a public stand to challenge the policy process as has occurred successfully with smoking.

Over the past 20 years my personal 'policy and political' experience has been mainly in the field of international public health nutrition with the problem of brain damage due to iodine deficiency. I was involved in field research (Papua New Guinea) and research with animal models over a 20-year period (1964–85), both of which established that iodine deficiency in pregnancy was a cause of brain damage to the foetus and that this could be prevented by correction of the iodine deficiency before pregnancy.

Over the period 1976–84 I visited India, Thailand, Indonesia and China and became aware of the massive problem in these countries. It seemed to me that concerted international action was required and that the United Nations (UN) agencies needed to be involved. In 1984 I was invited by the UN Subcommittee on Nutrition (SCN) to prepare a report on the global situation. In my report I proposed that an international non-government organisation (NGO) in the form of a multidisciplinary network of professionals with expertise on iodine deficiency be established to work with national governments, World Health Organization (WHO) and United Nations Children's Fund (UNICEF) to assist in the development of national programs based on the distribution of iodized salt.

This recommendation was approved by the SCN and a Steering Committee was set up at a WHO/UNICEF Intercountry Meeting in Delhi in March 1985. Initial funding support was provided by UNICEF and the Australian government. The International Council for Control of Iodine Deficiency Disorders (ICCIDD) was formally inaugurated with WHO and UNICEF support in Kathmandu, Nepal, in March 1986. The ICCIDD now comprises more than 700 multidisciplinary professionals from 100 countries. Over the period 1987–97 the ICCIDD held a series of Regional Meetings throughout the world with WHO and UNICEF support, attended by professionals from countries of the region to discuss the practical details of implementing national programs using iodized salt.

Over the period 1990–98 the number of countries with IDD elimination programs had increased from 46 to 93. By 2000 two-thirds of the global population (now estimated by WHO to be in excess of 2 billion from 130 countries at risk of brain damage) had been covered by iodized salt.*

This is an example of an initiative taken by nutrition scientists that led to the establishment of a global programme for the elimination of iodine deficiency, now accepted by WHO as the most common preventable cause of brain damage. This strategy of an NGO involving public health nutrition scientists could be appropriate for other international and national nutrition problems.

I commend this book as it breaks new ground for the twenty-first century, where substantial challenges await public health nutrition scientists. The opportunities have been outlined and we, as public health nutrition scientists, are called upon to decide about our involvement.

This book, with its great wealth of expertise, will be an essential companion for the journey.

BASIL S. HETZEL, MD
International Council for the Control of Iodine Deficiency Diseases
Women's and Children's Hospital, Adelaide, Australia

---

* Hetzel B.S., 'Eliminating Iodine Deficiency Disorders: The role of the International Council in the Global Partnership Round Table Discussion', *Bulletin of World Health Organization*, vol. 80, no. 5, pp. 410–17.

Contents

Referees

KAREN CAMPBELL
Deakin University, Melbourne, Australia

GEOFFREY CANNON
World Health Policy Forum, Juiz de Fora, Brazil

CLARE COLLINS
University of Newcastle, Newcastle, Australia

SIMONE FRENCH
University of Minnesota, Minneapolis, United States of America

OSMAN GALAL
University of California, Los Angeles, United States of America

TIM GILL
University of Sydney, Sydney, Australia

VERONICA GRAHAM
Department of Human Services, Melbourne, Australia

ROGER HUGHES
Griffith University, Gold Coast, Australia

ROBERT JEFFERY
University of Minnesota, Minneapolis, United States of America

SHARON LAURENCE
National Aboriginal and Torres Strait Islander Nutrition Strategy and Action Plan, Melbourne, Australia

CLAUS LEITZMANN
Justus Liebig University, Giessen, Germany

BARRIE MARGETTS
University of Southampton, Southampton, United Kingdom

SINEAD MCELHONE
Leeds Metropolitan University, Leeds, United Kingdom

SUE MILNER
Department of Human Services, Melbourne, Australia

CARYL NOWSON
Deakin University, Melbourne, Australia

JANE POTTER
VicHealth, Melbourne, Australia

LAUREN WILLIAMS
University of Newcastle, Newcastle, Australia

AGNETA YNGVE
Karolinska Institute, Stockholm, Sweden

Contributors

KYLIE BALL, School of Exercise and Nutrition Sciences, Deakin University, Melbourne, Australia

ANDREA BEGLEY, School of Public Health, Curtin University of Technology, Perth, Australia

COLIN BELL, School of Exercise and Nutrition Sciences, Deakin University, Melbourne, Australia

JOHANNES BRUG, Department of Public Health, Erasmus University Medical Centre, Rotterdam, The Netherlands.

CATE BURNS, School of Exercise and Nutrition Sciences, Deakin University, Melbourne, Australia

DORIS CAMPBELL, Department of Obstetrics and Gynecology, University of Aberdeen, Aberdeen, United Kingdom

MARTIN CARAHER, Department of Health Management and Food Policy, City University, London, United Kingdom

MICKEY CHOPRA, Department of Dietetics, University of Western Cape, Bellville, South Africa

JOHN COVENEY, Department of Public Health, Flinders University, Adelaide, Australia

GILL COWBURN, Division of Public Health and Primary Health Care, Oxford University, Oxford, United Kingdom

DAVID CRAWFORD, School of Exercise and Nutrition Sciences, Deakin University, Melbourne, Australia

STEVEN CUMMINS, Department of Geography, Queen Mary College, University of London, London, United Kingdom

IAN DARNTON-HILL, UNICEF, New York, United States of America

MICHAEL DAVIES, Department of Medicine, University of Adelaide, Adelaide, Australia

SIMONE FRENCH, School of Public Health, University of Minnesota, Minneapolis, United States of America

SHARON FRIEL, National Centre for Epidemiology and Population Health, Australian National University, Canberra, Australia

BASIL S. HETZEL, International Council for the Control of Iodine Deficiency Diseases, Women's and Children's Hospital, Adelaide, Australia

ROGER HUGHES, School of Public Health, Griffith University, Gold Coast Campus, Australia

CLARE HUME, School of Exercise and Nutrition Sciences, Deakin University, Melbourne, Australia

WENDY HUNTER, School of Exercise and Nutrition Sciences, Deakin University, Melbourne, Australia

KNUT-INGE KLEPP, Department of Nutrition, University of Oslo, Oslo, Norway

MARK LAWRENCE, School of Exercise and Nutrition Sciences, Deakin University, Melbourne, Australia

MARGARET LUMBERS, School of Management, University of Surrey, Guildford, United Kingdom

JIM MANN, Department of Human Nutrition, University of Otago, Dunedin, New Zealand

BARRIE MARGETTS, Institute of Human Nutrition, University of Southampton, Southampton, United Kingdom

GEOFFREY MARKS, School of Population Health, University of Queensland, Brisbane, Australia

LEISA MCCARTHY, Chronic Diseases Research Division, Menzies School of Health Research, Darwin, Australia

PHILIP MCMICHAEL, Department of Development Sociology, Cornell University, New York, United States of America

SARAH MCNAUGHTON, School of Exercise and Nutrition Sciences, Deakin University, Melbourne, Australia

MONIQUE RAATS, School of Management, University of Surrey, Guildford, United Kingdom

MALCOLM RILEY, Baker Heart Research Institute, Melbourne, Australia

AILEEN ROBERTSON, Suhr's University College, Copenhagen, Denmark

INGRID RUTISHAUSER, School of Exercise and Nutrition Sciences, Deakin University, Melbourne, Australia

JO SALMON, School of Exercise and Nutrition Sciences, Deakin University, Melbourne, Australia

JULIE SAUNDERS, School of Exercise and Nutrition Sciences, Deakin University, Melbourne, Australia

JANE SCOTT, Division of Development Medicine, University of Glasgow, United Kingdom

CHRISTINA STUBBS, Queensland Health, Brisbane, Australia

BOYD SWINBURN, School of Exercise and Nutrition Sciences, Deakin University, Melbourne, Australia

ANNA TIMPERIO, School of Exercise and Nutrition Sciences, Deakin University, Melbourne, Australia

MARK L. WAHLQVIST, Asian Pacific Institute, Monash University, Melbourne, Australia

KAREN WEBB, Department of Public Health, University of Sydney, Sydney, Australia

TONY WORSLEY, School of Exercise and Nutrition Sciences, Deakin University, Melbourne, Australia

HEATHER YEATMAN, Graduate School of Public Health, University of Woolongong, Woolongong, Australia

AGNETA YNGVE, Department of Biosciences and Nutrition, Karolinska Institute, Stockholm, Sweden

Preface

MARK LAWRENCE
TONY WORSLEY

Public health nutrition is concerned with promoting and maintaining the nutritional health of populations. The population's nutritional health is a fundamental resource for the social, cultural and economic wellbeing of local, national and global communities. Historically, the nutritional health of populations was essential to the survival of communities and their capacity to thrive. In contemporary times, hundreds of millions of people globally struggle to gain sufficient food for health. Meanwhile, in many countries, over-consumption and dietary imbalances are contributing to epidemics of obesity and diet-related chronic diseases, such as diabetes, cancers and cardiovascular disease, as well as stressing the carrying capacity of food and nutrition systems. These are complex public health nutrition challenges. Their solutions are found in a population-wide perspective to food and health relationships.

The early years of the twenty-first century are an exciting period of growth and development for public health nutrition as a profession. Initiatives that are invigorating current public health nutrition research, training, policy and practice agendas include the:

- World Public Health Nutrition Association
- World Health Organization's Global Strategy on Diet, Physical Activity and Health
- journal, *Public Health Nutrition*
- New Nutrition Science project

- First World Congress of Public Health Nutrition in Barcelona
- development of professional registration schemes and special interest groups for public health nutritionists
- preparation of competency standards and increased availability of courses for advanced level training and practice in public health nutrition.

Promoting and maintaining the nutritional health of populations requires a workforce with specialised knowledge, skills and competencies. Public health nutritionists are involved with multifaceted and multidisciplinary strategies at the local, national and international levels. They contribute effectively to a wide range of employment areas, including government departments, non-government organisations, the private sector and academic research and teaching. Conventional nutrition science provides an important knowledge contribution, but it is not sufficient to address fully the social and ecological dimension underlying public health dynamics. Similarly, a public health perspective requires a nutrition science dimension to fully appreciate the interactions of food with social, biological and environmental systems.

Traditionally, books on nutrition have examined the relationships between food and health in terms of individual nutrients, an individual's food choices and an individual's physiology. There is much available knowledge for these nutrition perspectives. Yet, the causes of, and solutions to, malnutrition, obesity and social and environmental concerns cannot be explained by such perspectives alone. For instance, why is it that distinct patterns of nutritional health can be observed within communities and across populations? And why has the proliferation in the availability of low-fat and low-energy food products coincided with increasing obesity rates among many populations? Also lacking is a book that provides a focus on practical skills and competencies to act on knowledge.

The aim of this book is to provide an up-to-date, research-based and peer-reviewed scholarly reference that spans the theoretical and applied nature of public health nutrition. It is particularly suitable for public health practitioners, researchers and administrators, as well as students of nutrition, dietetics and/or public health wishing to obtain advanced and specialised competencies in public health nutrition at upper undergraduate and introductory postgraduate level. We have subtitled this public health nutrition reference book 'from principles to practice' to reflect that its scope extends from an exploration of core public health nutrition principles to a coverage of particular knowledge, competencies and skills that are recognised widely as critical for professional practice.

Public Health Nutrition brings together leading researchers and practitioners from a diversity of professional backgrounds. Consistent with the collaborative theme of public health nutrition activities, many chapters in this reference book are the product of collaborative teamwork among authors with multidisciplinary expertise and/or multinational experience and knowledge. Authors were asked to promote an analytical approach that would challenge the reader to think critically and gain deeper insights into topics to help identify and work towards practical solutions for public health nutrition challenges. The book is designed in a user-friendly format, with frequent reference to topical case studies and new perspectives gained from cutting-edge research to build understanding of concepts and skills for applying knowledge to practice.

With this in mind, the book covers a diverse range of topics, set out in eighteen chapters. Each of the chapters can stand alone as a self-contained analysis of a particular topic; however, inevitably there are recurring principles and themes running across chapters and throughout the book, for example the role of evidence-based practice and ethical considerations. During the design of the book and the editing of the individual chapters, attempts were made to link common themes across topic areas to present an integrated approach to public health nutrition. Therefore, the chapters are grouped into four sections, with each section reflecting a coherent theme of public health nutrition. Each section is introduced by an expert in the thematic area who provides an overview of the common threads across the chapters in the section.

The opening section outlines key public health nutrition 'Principles' that are woven throughout the book. The section begins with a chapter that proposes a conceptual framework and guiding principles for thinking about public health nutrition problems, solutions, responsibilities and outcome measures. This is followed by chapters that analyse the philosophical and evidential dimensions that inform public health nutrition knowledge, and provide an overview of public health nutrition reference standards and dietary goals and guidelines.

The 'Population' focus of public health nutrition is explored in the second section of the book. This section presents a series of chapters on those population groups defined by life stage, for whom nutrition is especially relevant: mothers and infants, children and adolescents, and older adults. The emphasis of each chapter is on analysing the food and health relationship for each of these population groups from a physiological, social, cultural, political and economic perspective.

The third section examines those issues that are 'Priorities' for public health nutrition. Although the judgement of what might be considered a priority issue inevitably is subjective, the chapters in this section reflect those issues that are prominent in the initiatives identified above as stimulating contemporary public health nutrition research, training, policy and practice agendas. These priority issues are: economically, geographically and socially disadvantaged populations; indigenous communities; obesity prevention; international nutrition; and global developments in the food system.

The final section of the book focuses on the 'Practice' of public health nutrition. This section deliberately is the largest part of the book, in recognition of the lack of reference books that provide practical skills in public health nutrition, and in deference to the breadth and scope of competencies in this applied area. Each of the chapters in this section describes a core practice for public health nutrition. Strategies are provided for acting on each of the practices at either a local or national level. The specific practices that are analysed are: monitoring the food and nutrition situation of populations, physical activity, research skills, project management, professional practice, promotion and communication, and policy and politics.

Public health nutritionists face a range of social, biological and environmental challenges in promoting and maintaining the nutritional health of populations. We believe that this book will provide readers with inspiration, insights and competencies to be better equipped to meet the challenges that lie ahead.

MARK LAWRENCE
TONY WORSLEY
Melbourne, January 2007

SECTION 1: PRINCIPLES

Overview

AGNETA YNGVE

The opening section of this reference book contains three chapters that capture the definition of public health nutrition, discussions regarding the integration of public health concepts in nutrition, and recommendations and guidelines in nutrition. Collectively, these outline principles intended to assist public health nutritionists in thinking about how and why they might address the complex challenges with which they are confronted in their professional roles. Therefore, this 'Principles' section provides a foundation for the following 'Populations', 'Priorities' and 'Practices' sections of the book.

As with any young discipline, public health nutrition has evolved gradually and slowly as a merged entity of the areas of public health and nutrition. Skills and competencies needed for the public health nutritionist have changed from the classical nutritionist's strict biomedical perspective to having a public health focus. We therefore have had to develop a whole new concept of public health nutrition as a basis for the training of a public health nutrition workforce as well as for developing correct useful recommendations and guidelines in the area of nutrition.

The chapters in this first section point to the importance of working on an *upstream* level, the area that involves policy issues, agricultural sustainability and environmental factors, rather than working on lifestyle approaches or secondary prevention when signs of illness are already apparent. The need for introducing issues regarding sustainability of production/transportation systems clearly points at the need for introducing aspects of politics and ethics in food production, import/export and land use into training programmes. *Macro*-level issues need to be solved by use of macro-level skills and we need to understand the politics, lobbying systems and power games that are ongoing on global, international and national levels. This involves skills in politics rather than policy formulation, and demands another addition to training.

The public health nutritionist needs to have a clear view of the multinational food industry's dual role as bad guy–good guy in partnerships. Ethical considerations regarding collaboration with the industry and retail sectors are tricky and require special skills. The development of beneficial products by a particular food industry is for example often counterbalanced by the development of other products of a more questionable nature; for example, high-fibre breakfast cereals and the simultaneous and constant introduction of new high-sugar breakfast cereals of different shapes aimed at children; or the development of 'snack products' for children or ice-cream that resembles sweets more than anything else. Suddenly what was previously considered 'sweets' is now to be found in the ice-cream counter, the breakfast cereal shelf and among the biscuits.

This is not rocket science. In public health nutrition we do fully understand the need of the food industry to develop new products and to market these in novel manners. We can also see retail chains developing their own healthy lines and at the same time providing weekly leaflets of offers containing mostly what we would not consider healthy options. The use of store space for different products is obviously decided by profit, not by health gains. Restaurants and fast-food outlets are obviously also selling for profit, not for the public good. So, as public health nutritionists we can understand food industry, retail and catering but we cannot be expected to collaborate without setting firm conditions on our collaboration. This requires training in ethics and how to collaborate with the private sector.

The environmental aspects range from the global perspective of sustainability of crops, water and land use to the more local perspective of building local environments that work from an individual perspective, providing access to good foods and environments suitable for walking and cycling. City planning aspects of nutrition and health have only to a limited extent been considered a part of public health nutrition and therefore need to be ensured a more prominent position in public health nutrition research and training.

Food-based dietary guidelines are certainly culturally sensitive, and need to be based on what we understand about the needs and the perception of dietary guidelines in the population. Practice and research on these issues requires an understanding of underlying marketing principles and marketing research, which should already be sufficiently covered in today's public health nutrition training. However, as professionals involved in health-monitoring systems, we need to identify simple dietary goals that can be used for assessing the adequacy of a population's diet; for example, how much fruit and vegetables should children eat per day on average in different age groups? Population goals exist but not for specific age groups. As mentioned in chapter 3, evidence-based practice is a key issue for the success of any communication of food-based dietary guidelines. We are not there yet.

What we also need to understand more fully is how paradigm shifts in the public's view of food choice or nutrition related behaviour can be achieved. The shift in breastfeeding rates in Sweden during the 1970s, for example. Do we fully understand how that really happened? Sweden had really low breastfeeding rates during the 1960s and rates may have started to pick up as a part of the environmental, naturalistic, feministic, green wave movements, or as a result of discussions regarding the routines surrounding delivery involving the French obstetrician Frederick Leboyer. Combined with this there was a strong midwifery profession pushing for change, peer-support groups being formed, and maternity leave being prolonged. Can histories of change provide future public health nutritionists with blueprints for future possibilities for change?

As explained in chapters 1 and 2, the future public health nutrition should include aspects of ecology, agricultural science, political science, city planning, marketing, monitoring, ethics, health economics and philosophy. It also clearly points to the importance of public health nutritionists collaborating with other disciplines. Certainly an exciting future. The chapters in this first section of this book provide an interesting and promising introduction to the new public health nutrition. These three chapters point at the past and the future, how public health nutrition has evolved from classical nutrition science, and what public health nutrition will need to encompass in order to stand up to the new challenges which we will face. The chapters also describe in an elegant way how dietary recommendations and guidelines have been constructed over the years.

Public health nutrition continues to be an area where networking with other professionals is essential, as well as building our own professional bodies for strengthening of the evidence base for practice, creating a solid workforce and providing good leadership.

1

Concepts and guiding principles

MARK LAWRENCE
TONY WORSLEY

What is public health nutrition? For the purposes of this book, the following definition of public health nutrition, as proposed in the draft constitution of the World Public Health Nutrition Association, has been adopted:

> The promotion and maintenance of nutrition-related health and wellbeing of populations through the organised efforts and informed choices of society (The Barcelona Declaration 2006).

The scope of public health nutrition is multifaceted. It extends to political, cultural, social and economic factors insofar as these are determinants that affect the adequacy and sustainability of food systems, people's food and physical activity related behaviours, and their health and ecological consequences.

From its principles to its practice, public health nutrition draws from the rich heritage of its nutrition science parent discipline and a public health orientation. The 'marriage' of nutrition science and public health shapes how we think about, or conceptualise, public health nutrition and its application to policy, research, training and practice. Public health nutrition is concerned with the nutritional health of populations. The emphasis around this area is a point of divergence between the professional practice of public health nutrition and that of clinical nutrition science and dietetics.

This chapter presents an analysis of core concepts that underpin ways of thinking about public health nutrition as an introduction for the chapters that follow. We start with an overview of modern nutrition science that serves to locate the scientific foundations of public health nutrition. This overview is followed by an examination of three public health approaches that represent different ways of framing and responding to public health issues. Central to the chapter is a conceptual framework that integrates the nutrition science and public health dimensions of public health nutrition. This conceptual framework provides a coherent basis for thinking about public health nutrition problems, interventions and outcome measures in order to help inform policy, research, training and practice agendas. Then we review, briefly, guiding principles that relate to public health nutrition as now taught and practised.

The nutrition science basis to public health nutrition

Here we provide a brief overview of modern nutrition science. This perspective serves to locate the emergence of public health nutrition agendas, and to identify the scientific origins of the reference standards and guidelines used for current public health nutrition policy and practice.

The origins of modern nutrition science

The foundations of modern nutrition as a biological science, including the demonstration of respiratory processes, calorimetry, and that, from the chemical point of view, living things are composed predominantly of carbon, hydrogen, oxygen and nitrogen, were first laid in Europe in the late eighteenth century (Carpenter 2003). Over the next 100 years, nutrition as an academic science was pursued particularly within biochemistry as a sub-branch of medicine, and advances occurred in the areas of macronutrient metabolism and understandings of the energy content of foods and the notion of energy expenditure.

One crucial nutrition intervention was undertaken before the beginnings of nutrition as a formal science, in the mid-eighteenth century. Lind conducted controlled trials demonstrating that citrus juice could help prevent and cure scurvy in British sailors. Though it took more than 40 years, this evidence was translated into what was to be one of the first documented public health nutrition interventions when the Lords of the British Admiralty agreed to the inclusion of citrus fruits in the rations of sailors, resulting in the virtual disappearance of scurvy from the Royal Navy. This episode is insightful also for illustrating an early example of nutrition being used by a government for utilitarian means, in this case to increase the capacity of its naval forces to undertake military and exploration duties.

Later, in many nations, the industrial revolution was manifesting itself in the crowding of cities, hunger, poor sanitation and widespread prevalence of communicable diseases. These poor living conditions were the impetus for major legislative activity to improve sanitary conditions and general hygiene practices in cities around the world. At this time, nutrition science was also applied to public health activities in many countries in the form of regulations to address food adulteration and safety, and feeding programmes for mothers, children and families (Rosen 1993; Egan 1994).

Discovery of nutrients

Throughout the late 1800s and into the early twentieth century, hunger and nutrient deficiency diseases were common in industrialised countries. Following Pasteur's promotion of the concept that diseases are caused by micro-organisms – the 'germ theory of disease' – it was a challenge for scientists to think that diseases could also be diet-related, let alone caused by the absence, or a deficiency, of specific nutrients. But so it proved. In 1912, Funk coined the term 'vitamine', combining the Latin word for life, *vita*, with the class of chemical compounds called 'amines' (Funk 1912). The term referred to a chemical substance he had isolated, which previously had been demonstrated to be essential in the diet. As more vitamins were identified and found not to be amines, the spelling was amended to the present vitamins. Throughout the first half of the twentieth century, the structures and functions of many vitamins were identified and elucidated.

The advances in nutrition science knowledge were put into practice through the introduction of the concepts of 'protective foods' and a 'balanced diet' into public health campaigns. With the outbreak of the Second World War came actual or potential food shortages, and government policies in affected countries focused on food rationing and ensuring an adequate level of nutrition, as then understood, for their populations. In Britain, margarine and flour were fortified with vitamins A and D, and calcium, respectively. In the United States, white bread was enriched by the addition of niacin, riboflavin, thiamin and iron.

Progressively, methods were developed to determine the vitamin content of foods and for quantifying human requirements for nutrients. The nutrition science research into human nutrient requirements culminated in the establishment of the first reference standards for nutrient intakes in North America in the late 1930s and early 1940s (IOM 2000). These reference standards were used in the planning of food supplies in a variety of institutions, including hospitals, prisons, schools and the armed forces. Reference standards for nutrient intakes now have been developed by United Nations' (UN) agencies and many national authorities.

The nutrition science knowledge was also used for the development of food selection guides – a nutrition education tool that can be used in translating relatively abstract nutrition science principles into practical advice about the number and types of food serves to be selected in accordance with nutrient requirements and recommendations. An explanation of the rationale, underlying principles, current developments and application of these reference standards for nutrient intakes and food selection guides is provided in greater detail in chapter 3.

Dietary imbalances and chronic diseases

In the second half of the twentieth century in industrialised countries, the focus of nutrition science shifted from diseases caused by hunger and malnutrition, to diseases caused by over-consumption and obesity. Nutrition research that had been investigating nutrition deficiency problems was supplanted by studies into the role of diet in the aetiology of certain chronic diseases such as coronary heart disease (Keys 1957). In middle- and low-income countries, endemic hunger and malnutrition began to co-exist with diet-related chronic diseases, a dynamic referred to as the 'demographic–nutritional–epidemiological transition' (Popkin 2004). This transition is closely associated with the influence of social changes on dietary patterns, such as increasing urbanisation and the globalisation of food systems (Hawkes 2006).

Towards the end of the twentieth century, nutrition research produced increasingly strong evidence that the nutritional status and health of the mother was a critical predictor of foetal nutrition, which in turn has consequences for nutritional health throughout the life span. The research pointed to a 'new paradigm of public health nutrition' (Scrimshaw 1995). It indicated that the role of public health nutrition interventions should extend beyond helping to prevent chronic disease among certain 'vulnerable' population groups at set points in time, to the provision of a strong nutrition foundation at the very beginning of life for longer-term health promotion and chronic disease prevention for all. The public health nutrition of mothers and infants, and the possible role of nutrition in influencing health inter-generationally is considered in chapter 4.

The emerging evidence about the relationship between dietary patterns and chronic disease at this time was translated into recommendations for dietary patterns, foods and nutrients associated with wellbeing and protection against disease. These dietary profiles have been quantified and presented by UN bodies, governments and their agencies, and authoritative organisations, as dietary goals and targets for population diets. Advice in the form of dietary guidelines has been provided for government policy and consumer messages to assist policymakers, shapers of institutional and other food supplies, and consumers, to shift patterns of food production and consumption towards the dietary goals and targets. With the promulgation of dietary goals and dietary guidelines, food selection guides became increasingly sophisticated in the concepts they portrayed. The rationale, application, scientific derivation and practical examples of the dietary guidelines and goals are described in greater detail in chapter 3.

Nutrition science into the twenty-first century

At the start of the twenty-first century, nutrition science continues to evolve. Curiously, this evolution is occurring in two contrasting directions: the reductionist paradigm of so-called 'molecular nutrition', and the holistic paradigm of what is termed the 'New Nutrition Science'. We use the notion of a 'paradigm' in the sense of meaning a conceptual worldview to explain relevant observed phenomena. Lang and Heasman (2004) have undertaken a similar analysis of these latest developments, albeit with the use of the terms 'Life Sciences Integrated Paradigm' and 'Ecologically Integrated Paradigm', respectively. These latest nutrition science developments are reviewed briefly below.

Molecular nutrition paradigm

Molecular nutrition is a generic term that broadly refers to the science that is extending our knowledge of nutrition-related molecular, cellular and genomic mechanisms. With the development of sophisticated technologies and methods, and the mapping of the human genome, scientists are increasing their research capacity to investigate interactions between nutrients and the genome. The term 'nutrigenomics' has been coined to refer to the integration of genetic principles and technologies with food and nutrition science (Afman & Müller 2006).

As diagnostic tools and knowledge of the effects of nutrients and food components on the regulation of gene expression and subsequent metabolic profile develops, it has been predicted that there will be a need for dietary guidelines tailored for specific individuals and/or genetic groups within populations. For example, according to Go and colleagues (2005):

> (molecular nutrition) will enable the tailoring of nutritional advice based on a person's specific metabolic profile, i.e. personalised dietary recommendations and guidance.

Molecular nutrition is referred to as a reductionist paradigm because it is informed by an analytical approach based on dissecting the food and health relationship into constituent parts. This approach assumes that the relationship between food and health can be explained by summing the knowledge gained from these separate analyses. Research methods strive to control confounding factors such as individual, social and environmental circumstances so as to isolate precise linear relationships between single food components; for example, a specific nutrient, and metabolic pathways. One challenge for this approach is that people do not eat single food components in isolation; they eat a range of foods that comprise a mixed diet.

New Nutrition Science paradigm

Since its development in the late eighteenth century, nutrition science, seen as a biological discipline, has combined basic sciences such as chemistry with allied sciences including medicine. In spite of this breadth of biological scientific inputs, a growing number of people working in nutrition and food, and nutrition policy and practice believe that the conventional theories, principles and practice of nutrition science are not sufficient to address the major nutritional challenges of the twenty-first century. Their view is that, whereas nutrition science has provided valuable insights into increasingly specific mechanistic relationships within the human and animal body, it has tended to pay less attention to social and environmental contexts. According to the 2005–09 President of the International Union of Nutritional Sciences (IUNS):

> The most important and urgent issues that confront food and nutrition scientists in the twenty-first century are beyond the scope of conventionally defined human biology. We must be willing to encompass the social, economic, political and human rights dimensions of nutrition (Uauy 2005).

In 2005, a workshop was held at the University of Giessen, Germany, to agree principles, definitions and dimensions of the New Nutrition Science. The location was apt, for it was at the University of Giessen that Justus von Liebig developed nutrition as a biochemical discipline. This workshop was a joint initiative of the IUNS and the World Health Policy Forum. The papers prepared for the workshop have been published as a special issue of the journal, *Public Health Nutrition* (Leitzmann & Cannon 2005). Emerging from the workshop was The Giessen Declaration, which proposes a foundation for a new general theory of nutrition science as a whole, and defines nutrition science as:

> . . . the study of food systems, foods and drinks and their nutrients and other constituents; and of their interactions within and between all relevant biological, social and environmental systems . . . [with the purpose to] . . . contribute to a world in which present and future generations fulfil their human potential, live in the best of health, and develop, sustain and enjoy an increasingly diverse human, living and physical environment (The Giessen Declaration 2005).

The New Nutrition Science is referred to here as a holistic paradigm because it is informed by an analysis of the food and health relationship based on integrating social (including cultural, economic and political) and environmental (including ecological) dimensions, with the 'classical' biological (biochemical, physiological, medical) dimension.

Hence, whereas the reductionist approach seeks to control for the potential confounding effect of these broader dimensions, the New Nutrition Science regards them as integral to explaining the relationship between food and health. The assumption made in this approach is that, for the food and health relationship, food's contribution is more than the sum of its chemical components, and health outcomes are more than functional indicators of metabolic pathways.

Evidence for the holistic nature of the food and health relationship is available from several perspectives that illustrate more complex interactions than might otherwise be anticipated from conducting mechanistic studies. The food matrix has been shown to mediate physiological processes; for example, randomised controlled trials have demonstrated that consuming the same amount of saturated fat from two different foods can have different effects on plasma cholesterol responses (Nestel et al. 2005). It has also been highlighted that there are synergies between food components and health outcomes that are greater than would be expected from the sum of the individual dietary components (Jacobs and Steffen 2003). From the ecological, food culture and lifestyle perspective, studies have reported both an inverse relationship between diets comprising foods from a diverse biological base and mortality in men and women (Kant et al. 1993), and positive associations between various cuisines, such as the Mediterranean diet, and public health outcomes (Trichopoulou & Lagiou 1997).

The public health context to public health nutrition

The World Health Organization (WHO) describes public health as:

> a social and political concept aimed at improving health, prolonging life and improving the quality of life among whole populations through health promotion, disease prevention and other forms of health intervention (WHO 1998).

This description highlights the broad meaning of public health and the diversity of interventions important to its achievement.

In this section, we set out to examine the breadth of public health and its diversity of interventions, which form the public health context for public health nutrition. This examination is based on an adaptation of a public health schema, originally developed for health promotion (Labonte 1998). The three public health approaches within the adapted schema are the:

1. socio-ecological approach
2. lifestyle approach
3. biological approach

These three approaches differ in terms of how public health problems are defined, the focus of their interventions in addressing these problems, responsibility for the interventions, and their outcome measures. Here we briefly review the characteristics of each of the approaches, and provide some nutrition examples.

Socio-ecological approach

The socio-ecological approach to public health, also referred to as the 'upstream' approach, operates from the premise that health opportunities are not distributed randomly within populations. Instead, the determinants of public health are regarded as being embedded in the social, economic, cultural, ecological and other circumstances in which people live (Marmot 2005); for example, patterns of food insecurity and the prevalence of obesity generally are distributed inequitably towards lower socio-economic status communities in society. According to McMichael (1999):

> If epidemiologists are to understand the determinants of population health in terms that extend beyond proximate, individual-level risk factors (and their biologic mediators), they must learn to apply a social-ecologic systems perspective when conducting public health research.

The socio-ecological approach reflects a 'communitarian' perspective to the analysis of public health problems and the targeting of interventions. Interventions focus on promoting food security for all and food system sustainability. Responsibility for interventions aligned with this approach is taken primarily by government together with civil society, industry, health professional organisations and the media. Outcomes are measured in terms of social equity in nutritional health profiles and secure and sustainable food systems.

The conceptual and scientific basis of the socio-ecological approach closely aligns with the integrated biological, social and environmental focus of the New Nutrition Science paradigm. As Nestle (2006) a leading food policy analyst, comments: '. . . the New Nutrition restates well known ecological models of public health nutrition'.

Lifestyle approach

The lifestyle approach to public health, also referred to as the 'disease prevention' or 'midstream' approach, represents the view that the population's health is defined by risk-factor profiles that are the consequence of inappropriate lifestyle behaviours. The conceptual foundation to this approach draws heavily on the population strategy to preventive medicine espoused by Rose (1992). Rose argued that the incidence of morbidity and premature mortality can be reduced for an entire population only by changing risk-factor distributions at the population level, not by concentrating on individuals in the upper end of the risk distribution; that is the causes of individual cases are not necessarily the determinants of incidence among populations. Rose's explanation quite reasonably assumes that most disease within a population occurs in individuals at moderate risk. Interventions that aim to shift the mean exposure to risk factors of the whole population are therefore likely to achieve a greater impact on public health than those restricted to high-risk individuals. However, equity considerations still demand special attention for these high-risk people.

In accordance with this approach, interventions are targeted at changing individuals' lifestyle behaviours in the hope that this may add up to changed exposure patterns to risk factors at the population level. Interventions frequently are focused on education and campaigns directed at individuals. Responsibility for interventions aligned with this approach rests with government campaigns, health professional organisations and individuals to change their behaviour. Such interventions have been criticised as a form of victim-blaming, as they place the onus for change onto individuals, and imply that individuals are free to choose whether or not to modify their risk of chronic disease. It is relevant to note that Rose always argued for interventions in which politicians accepted that the state has a responsibility to make policy changes that have the effect of making healthy choices easy choices.

The application of Rose's logic to public health nutrition is illustrated by the concept of population dietary goals that represent '. . . the population average intake that is judged to be consistent with the maintenance of health in a population' (WHO 2003). Dietary guidelines are promulgated in many countries to encourage dietary behaviours among the population consistent with the concepts of variety, balance and moderation, to support the achievement of national dietary goals. Also, food supply interventions, such as the development of fat-, sugar- and/or salt-reduced food products, are undertaken to support dietary behaviours consistent with the dietary guidelines. Outcome measures focus on the population groups' dietary behaviour patterns in accordance with dietary recommendations.

Biological approach

The biological approach to public health, also referred to as the 'downstream' or 'medical' approach, reflects a view of health as being an asymptomatic state and defined as the absence of biological abnormalities and symptoms of individuals that might lead to disease and disability (Labonte 1998). This biological approach emanates from a view of public health in which the individual and/or an individual's biology is the unit of analysis for planning, implementing and evaluating an intervention. Inasmuch as it acknowledges public health at all, it conceives of public health as the sum of the health of an aggregate of individuals rather than the health of populations as integrated wholes. Which is to say, it is informed by an ideology of 'individualism'.

Health problems experienced by individuals are explained by deviations from biological norms. These deviations may be detected in individuals as pathological disturbances or by screening for clinical indicators of specific causal agents; for example, raised levels of risk factors for a disease or genetic abnormalities. The focus of interventions aligned with this approach is to control potential disease exposure and genetic predispositions to disease, restore 'abnormal' risk factor levels to normal, or treat disease symptoms. Responsibility for such interventions rests primarily with health professionals and the manufacturers of products and technologies that might help restore an individual's biology to a 'normal' state. Outcomes are measured in terms of the biological health of an aggregate of individuals.

The conceptual and scientific basis of the biological approach closely aligns with the reductionist focus of the molecular nutrition paradigm. Proponents of nutrigenomics suggest that nutrition activities within the biological approach will progress beyond so-called 'functional foods' and into the realm of integrating molecular nutrition principles and technologies into food and nutrition sciences. As an example, Gillies (2003) argues there is a new era that will see the merging of medicine and nutrition into a 'unifying paradigm of molecular nutrition', which focuses on nutrient and gene interactions that will eventually be applied at the community level as an approach to public health nutrition.

Integrating nutrition science and public health

In the previous two sections, the characteristics of the nutrition science and the public health dimensions to public health nutrition were examined separately. These two dimensions need to be integrated if we are to have a coherent basis to inform public health nutrition training, research, policy and practice agendas. Table 1.1 outlines a conceptual framework for thinking about the relationships between public health nutrition problems, interventions responsibilities and outcome measures. Although there is an attempt to delineate the approaches on the basis of these characteristics, in practice the approaches are not necessarily mutually exclusive; that is, the boundaries between the approaches are 'permeable' (Labonte 1998). The framework provides a strategic tool for public health nutritionists to align a public health nutrition problem with an appropriate solution and relevant outcome measure.

As Nutbeam and Harris (1998) state:

> One of the greatest challenges for practitioners is to identify how best to achieve a fit between the issues of interest and established theories or models which could improve the effectiveness of a program or intervention.

Nevertheless, there may be times when a public health nutrition problem is best tackled by a combination of interventions derived from each of the three approaches, implemented in such a way as to complement each other. For example, in order to prevent coronary heart disease among populations, Jackson et al. (2006) recommend the adoption of a multifaceted approach that offers immediate treatment approaches for high-risk individuals at the same time as investing in longer-term health-promotion interventions for the population as a whole.

The identification of the public health nutrition problem, the choice of intervention, responsibilities and outcome measures are not always straightforward. The different ways that the aetiology of a public health issue can be conceptualised is illustrated in Table 1.2. This figure highlights the different ways that the endemic appearance of pellagra in the south of the United States during 1906–40

Table 1.1 A conceptual framework for thinking about the relationships between public health nutrition problems, interventions, responsibilities and outcome measures

	Different public health nutrition approaches		
	Socio-ecological	Lifestyle	Biological
Problem definition	Poor social and environmental circumstances (food insecurity, inequity), non-sustainable food systems	Population's lifestyle behaviour patterns not consistent with recommendations	An individual's nutrition-related risk factor profile exceeds normative limits, genetic predisposition to diet-related disease, disease symptoms
Focus of interventions	Promote food security for all and food system sustainability	Education and campaigns to shift the population's lifestyle behaviour(s), policy changes to help make healthy choices easier. Development of fat-, sugar- and/or salt-reduced food products	Production and consumption of functional food products directed at abnormal risk factor or nutrient–gene screening profiles
Responsibility for the intervention	Governments taking the lead together with civil society organisations, food industry, health professional organisations and media	Health professionals, governments, food industry, and individuals within the population	Health professionals and the manufacturers of special products and technologies
Outcome measures	Social equity in nutritional health profiles and secure and sustainable food systems	Population's dietary behaviour patterns in accordance with recommendations	Individual's nutrition risk-factor levels, dietary control of an individual's genetic predispositions to disease, and treatment of disease symptoms

might be defined, interventions selected, responsibilities allocated and outcomes measured (Bollett 1992).

Guiding principles

We propose that public health nutrition should be based on and guided by a set of principles that affect its approach to problem identification and problem solving. This has a direct bearing on the practical application of the conceptual framework outlined in the previous section. In this section of the chapter, we begin with a brief analysis of evidence-based practice from a public health nutrition perspective. Then we explain that public health nutrition subscribes to the same guiding principles, or traditional values, that promote civic virtue and the public good. This explanation is based on a review of the key public health values of equity, efficacy, democracy, good governance and participation, and ethics that are used to judge the outcomes of public health programmes.

Evidence-based practice

The concept of evidence-based practice in the profession of public health nutrition relates to the fundamental role of what is accepted as high-quality scientific evidence, assembled and organised according to agreed principles and methods, for informing policy and programme decisions. This should offer an objective, transparent and rational basis for decision-making. That said, respect should be given to tradition, culture and custom, which, while they may not have a basis in current scientific method, have contributed immeasurably to our knowledge and understanding of food and dietary practices that are consistent with health and wellbeing.

The field of medicine has pioneered the application of evidence-based practice in the health arena. The term 'evidence-based medicine' refers to '. . . the conscientious, explicit, and judicious use of current best evidence in making decisions about the care of individual patients' (Sackett et al. 1996). There are well-established rules and procedures for conducting evidence-based medicine. In particular, there is a hierarchy of evidence levels for ranking the quality of evidence based on the capacity of the research design to control for potential bias, and in which the randomised controlled trial is positioned as the gold standard for scientific investigation.

Margetts et al. (2001) propose a rationale for an evidence-based approach to public health nutrition. The proposal builds on the concept of an evidence-based nutrition that has been defined as, 'the application of the best available

Table 1.2 Different ways the 1906–40 US pellagra endemic might be defined, interventions selected, responsibilities allocated and outcomes measured

| | Different public health nutrition approaches | | |
	Socio-ecological	Lifestyle	Biological
Problem definition	Socioeconomic conditions (Mertz, 1997)	Reduced niacin availability in the population's food supply resulting from the removal of niacin from maize as a consequence of the manufacturing process (Park et al. 2000)	Niacin deficiency in individuals (Goldberger et al. 1918)
Focus of interventions	Economic recovery	Niacin restoration of maize to replace processing losses; education on food and meal preparation involving maize	Mandatory fortification of food products with niacin so individuals would be exposed to increased amounts of niacin
Responsibility for the intervention	The US government in the context of broad changes outside political control, but not with public health as a main motive	Health professionals and maize producers and processors	Manufacturers of niacin-fortified foods
Outcome measures	The incidence of pellagra was declining well before the introduction of mandatory niacin fortification in the US (Nestle 1994)	Maize's niacin content was restored so as to qualify as an inherent source of niacin in the diet	Increased dietary niacin intake of individuals

systematically assembled evidence in setting nutrition policy and practice' (Brunner et al. 2001). Throughout its history, nutrition knowledge has been derived from a rich research method toolbox, including epidemiology, dietary surveys, animal studies and metabolic diet studies. The spectrum of public health nutrition knowledge is discussed in chapter 2, and research methods and monitoring in public health nutrition (and physical activity) are examined in chapters 12 to 14 of the present book.

Nevertheless, there are challenges in applying evidence-based practice to public health nutrition. The previous section highlighted the existence of public health nutrition paradigms that capture the different ways of framing public health nutrition problems, interventions, responsibilities and outcome measures. As Daly and Lumley (2005) argue, '. . . when a given problem is studied, different approaches to research will ask different questions, collect different data and use different frames of analysis'. For example, in the context of substantiating health claims for use on food labels, Truswell has commented, 'Agreement to apply appropriate principles of evidence-based medicine to public-health nutrition will bring welcome objectivity and the opportunity to have rules of evidence for claims and disputes' (Truswell 2001). An evidence-based medicine approach may be well-suited to inform those interventions where the context involves investigating a linear causal relationship between a nutrient and human physiology. Conversely, for those public health nutrition issues where social, cultural, political and economic contexts are critical, the ability of a randomised controlled trial to capture the complexity of the relationship between foods and/or diets and nutritional health outcomes is strongly questioned (Brunner et al. 2001; Mann 2002; Heaney 2006).

Methodologically, there is a need for innovative research designs, methods and indicators to support an evidence-based practice approach that is relevant to a broad view of public health nutrition. This approach needs to be sensitive to outcomes that are inclusive of parameters such as the wellbeing of the population and the sustainability of food systems. Similar challenges have been recognised in the health-promotion literature. There is a call to expand decision-making frameworks to consider: empirical data derived from a range of social science methods; innovative measures of health outcomes; and investigations that increase understanding of the complex interrelationships of systems (Rychetnik et al. 2002).

This discussion has asserted that evidence-based practice is fundamental to decision-making in public health nutrition. Although there are rules and procedures for evidence-based practice in many disciplines, in public health nutrition the concept is still in its infancy. Because public health nutrition is based on contested views about how problems are defined, interventions selected, and outcomes measured, inevitably evidence-based public health nutrition is a political concept. There may be contested views over what counts as evidence, what research should be funded, and how the findings should be interpreted and applied. Public health nutrition policy and politics are explored in chapter 18.

Equity

Equity is the idea that everyone in society should be given access to sufficient resources needed to attain optimal health. This is not the same as equality, which often means that we treat everyone in the same way (for example, that everyone receives identical levels of health care). Instead, equity refers to the idea that people are not all the same, that some have greater needs than others, and that they should have as much help from society as they require. It is much easier for well-off people to attain good health (and access to health resources like medical care) than poor people. Equity suggests that these poorer, less well-resourced people should have more help than their better-off peers. There is much debate in many countries about the affordability and prioritisation of equity goals; some societies are more willing to remedy social inequalities than others. Right- and left-wing politicians differ not only in their acceptance of the equity principle but also in the ways in which equity may be achieved. For example, conservative thinkers see small business as an excellent way to spread wealth around the community, thus increasing equity, whilst left-wing proponents see greater roles for the state; for example, through taxation policies that redistribute wealth.

Efficacy

Efficacy is related to concepts of efficiency and effectiveness. Resources for public health nutrition promotion are usually very limited, so we have to make sure that the work we do actually has meaningful positive outcomes for the population groups that are involved. For example, we can talk of an intervention being efficient, meaning that resources were spent in ways that did not involve much wasted money and time. The notion of effectiveness adds on the idea that interventions (or other nutrition-promotion projects) also need to deal with problems that are important to the population group. To take an extreme example, the production of handguns can be highly efficient, but would not normally be regarded in peacetime as a particularly effective way to achieve public good. Effectiveness is about efficiency in reaching public good goals. Finally, efficacy is about the effectiveness of programmes in attaining desirable goals within a normally operating system. To illustrate the difference, one can cite many school nutrition-promotion interventions conducted by university researchers, which are effective in increasing children's consumption of fruit. However, once the intervention stops (because the monies supporting the intervention are spent) the children's eating soon worsens. In contrast, an efficacious programme would be one that was able to be implemented as a normal part of school life. The normal situation in Japanese primary schools, in which children are not allowed to eat high-energy snacks in the morning before a highly nutritious lunch is served, is likely to be an efficacious nutrition-promotion programme — it is straightforward to operate, and has been sustainable in that culture for many years.

The equity effectiveness loop brings the two concepts together in a six-part action cycle as seen in Figure 1.1 to ensure that programmes reach all parts of the population (Tugwell et al. 2006). Programme efficacy is modified by at least four modifiers: access, diagnostic accuracy, provider compliance (in health service applications), and consumer adherence.

The high value placed on equity leads naturally to a focus on marginalised groups, such as the financially disadvantaged, and those with poorer access to resources that promote health and wellbeing. This can be quite a controversial viewpoint, which is certainly not shared by everyone in today's 'individualist' society. It proposes that, in addition to individual interests and goals, we should also be interested in community goals (such as protection of the environment, care of sick people, and children) in which everyone has a stake. Consequently, it proposes that government and good governance are important for the maintenance of the population's health and wellbeing.

Democracy, good governance and participation

While the public's health might be promoted by benign despots, current public health has a strong democratic flavour that emphasises respect for individuals and community groups, and encourages their voluntary participation in decisions that affect their lives. Public health emphasises cooperation among community groups and efficacy. It supports notions of 'good governance', whether local, national or international. This means that governments should be agencies that promote the health of all groups in the population, 'without fear or favour' (Wahlqvist et al. 1999). The orientation of public health is very much towards the communitarian values (guiding principles in people's lives), especially the values of harmony, universalism and benevolence, but also security.

One challenge for public health nutritionists is to engage with and include groups of people who do not value public health values as highly as they do. This means that they should attempt to develop positive responses to individualist philosophies (such as neoliberalism) in order to find ways to use their positive qualities in the promotion of the public good.

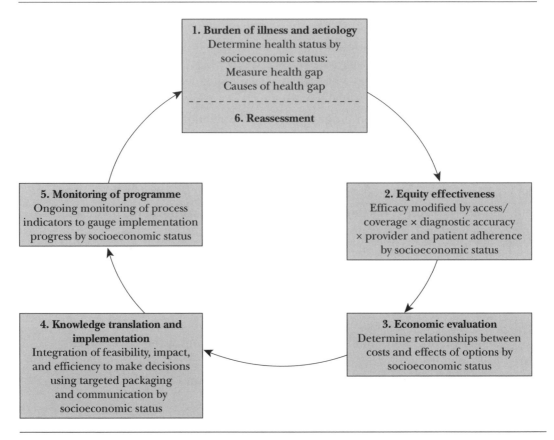

Figure 1.1 The equity effectiveness loop

Source: Tugwell et al. 2006

Ethics

Public health nutrition practice, even when based on agreed principles, has moral underpinnings, and frequently encounters ethical dilemmas. When formulating decisions that have public health outcomes, policymakers often need to balance the interests of the individual and the interests of society (the public good). The public good may be best achieved by protecting individual rights within the society or by protecting the collective rights of the society as a whole.

Consider the dilemma associated with Case study 1.1 about selecting the best policy to respond to epidemiological evidence that increasing a woman's folate consumption during the peri-conceptional period can help reduce the risk of having a neural tube defect-affected conception.

CASE STUDY 1.1

THE ETHICAL DILEMMA OF PROTECTING
THE HEALTH OF INDIVIDUALS AND POPULATIONS

Mandatory fortification of a food product(s) with a nutrient(s) is a powerful public health nutrition policy intervention. The Codex Alimentarius Commission (Codex) recommends such a policy approach when there exists evidence of a population-wide deficiency of a nutrient(s) (Codex 1987). For instance, mandatory folic acid fortification of a staple food may be recommended to protect a population's health where there exists endemic anaemia due to inadequate folate reserves in the food supply. However, in this case study we ask whether there might be circumstances where mandatory folic acid fortification of a staple food(s) may be recommended despite a lack of evidence of a population-wide folate deficiency.

Neural tube defects (NTDs) are a group of malformations that in severe form are incompatible with life, but more commonly take the form of handicaps such as spina bifida that disable people throughout life, and which have substantial emotional, social and economic costs for affected families, as well as being a burden on society. Fortunately, the incidence of NTDs is relatively low, affecting approximately one to two per 1000 births in many countries. Although the biological mechanism for folate's protective role is uncertain, it is believed that, when consumed in high doses, it compensates for a congenital defect in folate metabolism in at-risk individuals. In this context, the additional folate is acting more as a therapeutic agent than as a conventional nutrient. National authorities have available several policy options to promote an increased folate intake among the target group (women of child-bearing age). These options include promoting increased folate from dietary sources (though it is difficult to obtain a therapeutic dose of folate from dietary sources alone), folic acid supplement intake, and/or either voluntary or mandatory folic acid fortification of certain foods.

With reference to the different approaches shown in Figure 1.1 previously, the promotion of folic acid supplementation represents the policy option that matches the biological nature of the problem – it can be targeted to those individuals with the genetic defect responsible for poor folate metabolism, and the dose can be controlled. The limitation with this approach is that it is not possible to identify those individuals who are predisposed to the congenital defect and require the folic acid supplement. Also, the neural tube closes by the 28th day after conception, a period when many women may be unaware they are pregnant. This lack of awareness is especially relevant, given that it is estimated that approximately 40 per cent of pregnancies are unplanned.

Many national authorities are attracted to a population approach in the form of mandatory fortification of certain foods with folic acid. This increases the target group's exposure to folic acid passively, without the need to promote behaviour change. However, this means that all children, teenagers, adults and older people who consume folic acid-fortified foods would have a raised exposure to synthetic folic acid. This is important to consider, as concerns have been raised about potential risks associated with elevated levels of unmetabolised folic acid in the blood, which may promote carcinogenesis (Van Guelpen et al. 2006; Stolzenberg-Solomon et al. 2006).

Hence, there is an ethical dilemma confronting policymakers (Lawrence 2005). Mandatory fortification with folic acid will increase the exposure to folic acid of the target group and reduce incidence of NTDs; yet it also will raise exposure to synthetic folic acid of the population as a whole, which may be risky. On the other hand, approving an alternative targeted policy option avoids risk among the population as a whole, but it may not expose all individuals in the target group to sufficient additional folic acid, and this would lessen the potential extent of the reduction in NTDs.

This case study illustrates why ethics is a core concept within public health nutrition. Professionals are frequently challenged to exercise both scientific and ethical judgement in choosing from among available policy and programme options. Presented with the contrasting scenarios for the above case study, how would you act to balance protecting the health of individuals and the population as a whole?

In the public health nutritionist's daily practice, a key ethical guideline to consider is the *precautionary principle*, which is often expressed as *first do no harm*. The precautionary principle encourages detailed assessment of the likely effects of any health programme. This is particularly relevant to policymaking in response to the folate–NIDs relationship (Lawrence & Riddell 2007). Here the potential risks and benefits associated with mandatory folic acid fortification need to be assessed in their own right, as well as in comparison with potential risks and benefits associated with policy alternatives.

Conclusion

Public health nutrition has developed its own special field of theory and practice, which has evolved along with advances in nutrition science and prevailing public health ideologies. The conceptual framework presented in this chapter integrates the nutrition science and public health context dimensions. The application of the framework to public health nutrition research, training, policy and practice agendas is shaped by guiding principles, notably equity, efficacy, democracy, good governance and participation, evidence-based practice, and ethics.

This introduction to public health nutrition sets the scene for the remainder of this book. In the following two chapters, knowledge, reference standards and guidelines are explored in greater depth. In the three following sections of the book, the emphasis shifts towards putting principles into practice, first with populations, then in addressing priorities, and finally with practical skills.

REFERENCES

Afman, L. and Müller, M. 2006, 'Nutrigenomics: From molecular nutrition to prevention of disease' in *Journal of the American Dietetic Association*, vol. 106, pp. 569–76.

Barcelona (draft) Declaration on the Formation of the World Public Health Nutrition Association, The, 2006, Inaugural Planning Meeting, 30 September, Barcelona.

Bollett, A.J. 1992, 'Politics and pellagra: The epidemic of pellagra in the US in the early twentieth century' in *Yale Journal of Biological Medicine*, vol. 65, pp. 211–21.

Brunner, E., Rayner, M., Thorogood, M., Margetts, B., Hooper, L., Summerbell, C., Dowler, E., Hewitt, G., Robertson, A. and Wiseman, M. 2001, 'Making public health nutrition relevant to evidence-based action' in *Public Health Nutrition*, vol. 4, no. 6, pp. 1297–99.

Carpenter, K.J. 2003, 'A short history of nutritional science: Part 1 (1785–1885)' in *Journal of Nutrition*, vol. 133, pp. 638–45.

Codex Alimenterius Commission (Codex) 1987, 'General principles for the addition of essential nutrients to foods', CAC/GL, September (amended 1989, 1991).

Daly, J. and Lumley, J. 2005, 'Editorial: Evidence and context' in *Australian and New Zealand Journal of Public Health*, vol. 29, no. 6, pp. 503–04.

Egan, M.C. 1994, 'Public health nutrition: A historical perspective' in *Journal of American Dietetic Association*, vol. 94, no. 3, pp. 298–304.

Funk, C. 1912, 'The etiology of the deficiency diseases' in *Journal of State Medicine*, vol. 20, pp. 341–68.

Giessen Declaration, The, 2005, printed in *Public Health Nutrition*, vol. 8, no. 6A, pp. 783–86.

Gillies, P.J. 2003, 'Nutrigenomics: The Rubicon of molecular nutrition' in *Journal of American Dietetic Association*, vol. 103, no. 12. pp. S50–55.

Go, V.L.W., Nguyen, C.T.H., Harris, D.M. and Lee, W-NP. 2005, 'Nutrient-gene interaction: Metabolic genotype-phenotype relationship in *Journal of Nutrition*, vol. 135, pp. S3016–20.

Goldberger, J., Wheeler, G.A. and Sydenstricker, E. 1918, 'A study of the diet of nonpellagorous and of pellagorous households in textile mill communities in South Carolina in 1916' in *American Medical Association Journal,* vol. 71, pp. 944–49.

Hawkes, C. 2006, 'Uneven dietary development: Linking the policies and processes of globalization with the nutrition transition, obesity and diet-related chronic diseases' in *Globalization and Health*, vol. 2, no. 4, cited at <http://www.globalizationandhealth.com/contents/2/1/4> on 10 December 2006.

Heaney, R.P. 2006, 'Nutrition, chronic disease, and the problem of proof' in *American Journal of Clinical Nutrition*, vol. 84, pp. 471–72.

Institute of Medicine (IOM) 2000, *Dietary Reference Intakes: Applications in dietary assessment*, National Academy Press, Washington, D.C.

Jackson, R., Lynch, J. and Harper, S. 2006, 'Preventing coronary heart disease: Does Rose's population prevention axiom still apply in the twenty-first century?' in *British Medical Journal*, vol. 332, pp. 617–18.

Jacobs, D.R. and Steffen, L.M. 2003, 'Nutrients, foods, and dietary patterns as exposures in research: A framework for food synergy' in *American Journal of Clinical Nutrition*, vol. 78, pp. S508–13.

Kant, A.K., Schatzkin, A., Harris, T.B., Ziegler, R.G. and Block, G. 1993, 'Dietary diversity and subsequent mortality in the First National Health and Nutrition Examination Survey Epidemiologic Follow-up Study' in *American Journal of Clinical Nutrition*, vol. 57, pp. 434–40.

Keys, A. 1957, 'Diet and the epidemiology of coronary heart disease' in *Journal of American Medical Association*, vol. 164, no. 17, pp. 1912–19.

Labonte, R. 1998, 'Health promotion and the common good: Towards a politics of practice' in *Critical Public Health*, vol. 8, no. 2, pp. 107–29.

Lang, T. and Heasman, M. 2004, *Food Wars: The global battle for mouths, minds and markets*, Earthscan, London.

Lawrence, M. 2005, 'Challenges in translating scientific evidence into mandatory food fortification policy: An antipodean case study of the folate-neural tube defect relationship' in *Public Health Nutrition*, vol. 8, pp. 1235–41.

Lawrence, M. and Riddell, L. 2007, 'Mandatory folic acid fortification: What would Hippocrates say?' in *Australian Family Physician*, vol. 36, pp. 1–4.

Leitzmann, C. and Cannon, G. (eds), 'The New Nutrition Science project' in *Public Health Nutrition*, vol. 8, no. 6A, pp. 667–804.

Mann, J. 2002, 'Discrepancies in nutritional recommendations: The need for evidence based nutrition' in *Asia Pacific Journal of Clinical Nutrition*, vol. 11, S510–15.

Margetts, B., Warm, D., Yngve, A. and Sjostrom, M. 2001, 'Developing an evidence-based approach to Public Health Nutrition: Translating evidence into policy' in *Public Health Nutrition*, vol. 4, no. 6A, pp. 1393–97.

Marmot, M. 2005, 'Social determinants of health inequalities' in *Lancet*, vol. 365, pp. 1099–104.

McMichael, A.J. 1999, 'Prisoners of the proximate: Loosening the constraints on epidemiology in an age of change' in *American Journal of Epidemiology*, vol. 149, no. 10, pp. 887–97.

Mertz, W. 1997, 'Food fortification in the United States' in *Nutrition Reviews*, vol. 55, no. 2, pp. 44–9.

Nestel, P.J., Chronopulos, A. and Cehen, M. 2005, 'Dairy fat in cheese raises LDL cholesterol less than that in butter in mildly hypercholesterolaemic subjects' in *European Journal of Clinical Nutrition*, vol. 59, pp. 1059–63.

Nestle, M. 1994, 'Cultural models for healthy eating: Alternatives to "techno-food"' in *Journal of Nutrition Education*, vol. 26, pp. 241–45.

—— 2006, 'Comment on New Nutrition Science project' in *Public Health Nutrition*, vol. 9, no. 1, pp. 94–95.

Nutbeam, D. and Harris, E. 1998, *Theory in a nutshell*, National Centre for Health Promotion, Sydney.

Park, Y.K., Sempos, C.T., Barton, C.N., Vanderveen, J.E. and Yetley, E.A. 2000, 'Effectiveness of food fortification in the United States: The case of pellagra' in *American Journal of Public Health*, vol. 90, no. 5, pp. 727–38.

Popkin, B.M. 2004, 'The nutrition transition: An overview of world patterns of change' in *Nutrition Reviews*, vol. 62, no. 7, S140–3.

Rose, G. 1992, *The Strategy of Preventive Medicine*, Oxford University Press, New York.

Rosen, G.A. 1993, *History of public health: Expanded edition*, The Johns Hopkins University Press, Baltimore.

Rychetnik, L., Frommer, M., Hawe, P. and Shiell, A. 2002, 'Criteria for evaluating evidence on public health interventions' in *Journal of Epidemiology and Community Health*, vol. 56, pp. 119–27.

Sackett, D.L., Rosenberg, W.M., Gray, J.A., Haynes, R.B. and Richardson, W.S. 1996, 'Evidence-based medicine: What it is and what it isn't' in *British Medical Journal*, vol. 312, pp. 71–72.

Scrimshaw, N.S. 1995, 'The new paradigm of public health nutrition' in *American Journal of Public Health*, vol. 85, no. 5, pp. 622–24.

Stolzenberg-Solomon, R.Z., Chang, S.C., Leitzmann, M.F., Johnson, K.A., Johnson, C., Buys, S.S., Hoover, R.N. and Ziegler, R.G. 2006, 'Folate intake, alcohol use, and postmenopausal breast cancer risk in the Prostate, Lung, Colorectal, and Ovarian Cancer Screening Trial' in *American Journal of Clinical Nutrition*, vol. 83, pp. 895–904.

Trichopoulou, A. and Lagiou, P. 1997, 'Healthy traditional Mediterranean diet: An expression of culture, history and lifestyle' in *Nutrition Reviews*, vol. 55, no. 11, pp. 383–89.

Truswell, A.S. 2001, 'Levels and kinds of evidence for public-health nutrition' in *Lancet*, vol. 357, pp. 1061–62.

Tugwell, P., de Sabigny, D., Hawker, G. and Robinson, V. 2006, 'Applying clinical epidemiological methods to health equity: The equity effectiveness loop' in *British Medical Journal*, vol. 332, pp. 358–61.

Uauy, R. 2005, 'Defining and addressing the nutritional needs of populations' in *Public Health Nutrition*, vol. 8, no. 6A, pp. 107–14.

Van Guelpen, B., Hultdin, J., Johansson, I., Hallmans, G., Stenling, R., Riboli, E., Winkvist, A. and Palmqvist, R. 2006, 'Low folate levels may protect against colorectal cancer' in *Gut*, vol. 55, pp. 1461–66.

Wahlqvist, M.L., Kouris-Blazos, A. and Savige, G.S. 1999, 'Food security and the Aged' in Ogunrinade, A., Oniang'o, R. and May, J. (eds) 1999, *Not by Bread Alone*, Food Security and Governance in Africa, Toda Institute for Global Peace and Policy Research, Witwatersrand University Press, South Africa, pp. 206–21.

World Health Organization 1998, *Health Promotion Glossary*, WHO, Geneva.

—— 2003, 'Diet, nutrition and the prevention of chronic diseases' in *Report of a Joint WHO/FAO Expert Consultation*, Technical Report Series 916, WHO, Geneva.

2

Knowledge

MARK L. WAHLQVIST

This chapter builds upon concepts and guiding principles introduced in chapter 1, particularly ethics, values and evidence-based practice, in order to focus on the question, 'What is public health nutrition knowledge, and how should it be applied? In answering this question, the philosophy of public health is examined. After discussion of evidence-based public health nutrition, consideration is given to various research designs and their usefulness in providing answers. Finally, some of the emerging themes in public health nutrition research are discussed.

Philosophy of public health nutrition

To understand the philosophy of public health nutrition, it is first necessary to expound *the descriptor*, namely, 'this field of scholarship and practice seeks to establish broad public benefit for nutrition science in human health, irrespective of age, gender, ethnicity, belief or location'. In so doing, 'nutritional science' is defined as the study of the 'assimilation of and function dependent on molecules derived from any organism's environment' (Solomons 2006; Wahlqvist 2006). More than this, the New Nutrition Science project of the International Union of Nutritional Sciences (IUNS) (Cannon & Leitzmann 2006; Leitzmann & Cannon 2005) in The Giessen Declaration (2005) requires 'biological social and environmental dimensions' to address 'personal, population and planetary health' through a 'comprehensive under-standing of food systems'. The declaration stresses that, 'How food is grown, processed, distributed, sold, prepared, cooked and consumed is crucial to its quality and nature, and to its effect on well-being and health, society and the environment'.

The philosophy of public health nutrition is not static; it continues to evolve, mature and innovate. In this way, as with science-at-large, it can underpin public health policy, and public policy in general (see chapter 18, on public health nutri-tion policy and politics, for more details).

There is some controversy about whether the name 'public nutrition' may be a more valuable term than 'public health nutrition'. As long as 'health' is collective for 'personal, population and planetary health', this controversy is largely redundant and the descriptors are interchangeable.

Some public health nutrition advocates have a number of concerns, includ-ing the question of public 'ownership' of the nutrition agenda when a top-down approach is used. This is usually part of a human rights approach to nutrition (Eide 2002). Another, somewhat different concern is the lack of professional interest in the problems and opportunities of 'public food' or 'street food'; that is, the food we are bound or encouraged to eat with little choice, which is prepared for us by others, for example at school or in workplace environments, at sporting events, or while commuting (Wahlqvist et al. 2000).

Philosophy is bound with ethics, and the fostering of the public's health through nutrition means would be seen as highly ethical. Problems arise, however, in relation to:

- how we do this
- how we deploy resources
- what extent personal autonomy is respected
- what the risks of our interventions are
- how supported they are with evidence.

The ethics of promoting an unsustainable food supply, even for putative health reasons (for example, encouraging consumption of fish to help reduce coronary mortality) are also relevant. Moreover, as we become more risk- and cost-benefit sensitive in our work as public health nutritionists, there may be greater temp-tations that may influence the ethical status of our judgments and actions (Solomons 2002; Solomons 1993).

Evidence-based public health nutrition

As introduced in chapter 1, public health nutrition needs a solid evidential base in order to inform policy and programme activities. Scientists and healthcare professionals expect evidence to be peer-reviewed, and governments, budget-holders and funders increasingly also require this. The idea has gained much currency as evidence-based medicine and now as evidence-based nutrition (Mann 2002; Wahlqvist et al. 2001; Trichopoulos et al. 2000).

Evidence-based medicine uses hierarchies of evidence, with randomised double-blind clinical trial as the preferred kind of evidence. However, this will not always be feasible or appropriate with evidence-based public health nutrition. In the case of evidence-based nutrition, portfolios of evidence are more relevant and helpful as espoused by the joint IUNS–World Cancer Research Fund–Food and Agriculture Organization (FAO) Task Force on Evidence-Based Nutrition (World Cancer Research Fund International 2003; Brunner et al. 2001; Heggie 2003). For example, the clinical nutrition trial or the feeding trial can rarely or never be double-blind, nor can they test anything other than formulated food without the intervention being recognisably different to the reference or control group (Wahlqvist et al. 1999). What may matter from a public health point of view may be the relationships the cuisine, the culinary aspects, and the food patterns and habits have with the health outcomes of the population.

An even more fundamental issue is that of causality. A randomised control trial tests the efficacy of an intervention, which may or may not have an aetiological, or even a pathogenic role. The study population may not be the one for which application is sought, and yet extrapolation is common and probably often more harmful than we know.

A longitudinal cohort study, in accordance with the pre-observational hypothesis, tests the proposition that certain antecedents are required for certain outcomes. It can accord the relative importance to these antecedents, allowing for other factors. It can adduce complex models, or systems, or frameworks that are conducive to health outcomes, as well as adverse consequences. However, longitudinal cohort studies may not operate for long enough to know the full risks and benefits, especially in unevaluated populations, in which the linkage is nevertheless of interest. And, of course, what is observed is what is measurable; and there may be a causal factor or cluster of factors that are not measured or measurable at present.

This brings us to the much neglected need these days of cross-checking any viewpoint against all kinds of evidence: historical, local and traditional knowledge and various biomedical (mechanistic) and epidemiological (for example, case-control, cohort, cross-sectional, within and between communities, migration, disease registries) studies, and applying the rules of logic and deduction (Popper 1992).

In order to achieve the discipline and policy strengthening role of evidence-based public health nutrition, the culture of public health nutrition science needs to be more and more integrated, as has been pointed out earlier in this chapter, in the section on philosophy.

It should also be possible for public health nutrition to be represented within international nutrition science organisations (see Figure 2.1). The affiliation of the World Public Health Nutrition Association and the New Nutrition Science project with the IUNS are exciting developments illustrating this representation. The international scope is essential if the evidence is to be cogent. This is because:

- nutritionally-related disorders are extensive and present in many countries
- there are no borders for public health nutrition problems or solutions
- commonalities and differences exist from region to region and from country to country
- a community focus is still relevant and possible in international organisations through, for example, inter-community development.

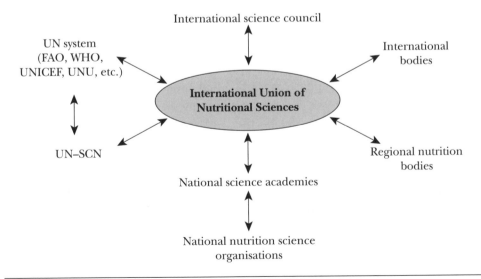

Figure 2.1 Organisational structure of nutritional science internationally

Research design in public health nutrition

This section highlights some important elements that need to be considered when designing public health nutrition research.

The first element of successful research design is to ask the right important questions. In international public health nutrition, there are two broad priorities:

1. *human development*: These include the physical, mental and social growth and development of individuals, and societal health — the development of health promoting processes and policies within societies, such as the provision of mass education, water and sewerage resources and good governance
2. *planetary health*: The promotion of ecologically sustainable bio-systems and food supplies for present and future generations. In practice, this often means the defence of natural and sustainable systems from attacks by short-sighted vested interests.

The second element is to work as a broad biomedical–social–environmental–science partnership. While one's work may be focused, it must also be multi-dimensional for the ultimate findings to be robust and relevant. Such an approach also acknowledges the need for expertise beyond one's own background and training.

The third element is to welcome incongruity as an opportunity to make a paradigm shift (Kuhn 1996). This means that we need to be able to question current practice and be open to new ways of thinking about problems — what Kuhn called 'paradigms'. If current frameworks do not promote public health, then we need to move to frameworks that enable us to work more effectively (paradigm shift). For example, in health promotion there is a shift currently occurring from a dominant emphasis on individual processes to more upstream or environmental processes (see the conceptual framework presented in chapter 1).

The fourth element is to decide the preferred kind of study required, for example:

* *trend analysis and scenario planning*: These allow for the development of long-term, sustainable policies, and often greater appreciation of the effectiveness of health policies; for example, Thompson et al. (2003) claim that the American public health nutrition policies of the past 40 years have brought about considerable benefits for the population (despite the obesity epidemic!)
* *predictive models over various periods of time*: These are more active approaches than analyses of historical trends and are built into the design of programmes.

Essentially, public health nutrition programmes need to have a longer-term life than many do at present. It is important to find ways to make programmes sustainable over periods of years or decades rather than weeks and months, and appropriate long-term evaluation designs and procedures are required.

- *iterative community interventions*: These are based on systematic and targeted data gathering (Scrimshaw and Hurtado 1987; Wahlqvist 2000). While clearly designed experimental interventions are most instructive, at the end of the day, public health nutrition has to promote the health of populations and communities and these may not be amenable to experimental investigation. Instead, sound theoretical thinking is needed to allow public health nutritionists and community leaders to attempt to alter likely key influences on the community's nutrition and health status. The success or failure of such strategies has to be evaluated through systematic monitoring of changes in influences and the health states that they were expected to affect (see Grier and Bryant, 2005).

- *primary, secondary or tertiary prevention studies*: These provide more explanation of the aetiology of disease states (and of health). In public health nutrition, following Rose's thinking (1985), there is likely to be more emphasis on primary and secondary prevention than on tertiary prevention, simply because the pay-off for the population is likely to be greater than from a case-treatment strategy. That being said, there are some considerable advantages to tertiary prevention strategies when the prevalence of frank disease states, such as heart disease, is high.

- *policy analysis, development and reform*: These are essential as we need to know whether current policies are working, and also whether new policies might be more effective. Because public health nutrition is embedded in at least two systems (the food and health systems), policy research in this arena can be extensive; for example, ranging from analysis of the effects of supermarket ownership on food production across countries (see chapter 11) to the effectiveness of kindergarten food policies.

The fifth element is to assemble the relevant, particular and detailed methodologies, set time-lines, cost the resource requirements, and estimate the 'human factor' (yours and your team's strengths and weaknesses). Strength, weakness, opportunities, threats (SWOT) analyses are particularly useful, as are the subsequent development of likely scenarios, contingency plans and exit strategies.

The sixth element is the progressive reporting of findings in the form of plans, reviews, reports of findings and experiences, and discussion of the likely implications of projects and programmes for the community (see chapter 16).

From beginning to end, it is important to undertake public health nutrition research in a constructively critical and supportive environment. Such conditions are not easy to obtain, but with care and tact they can be developed. Part of this process is to be generous with ideas and share success. Ideas and success shared are ideas and success grown – and the reverse is true, although more common. Figure 2.2 illustrates how various public health nutrition research agendas may be formatted and developed – in this example, in the area of eating, activity, cars and the road.

One should try to, but may not, change the world for the better. However, one thing is able to be accomplished by all of us engaged in public health nutrition, and that is to build capacity among those around us and in our successors, which is the ultimate joy of research, beyond the moment of discovery.

Emerging developments in public health nutrition research

Research into public health nutrition continues to evolve. There is currently a reconceptualisation of pathways linking food and health taking place in the following areas (Wahlqvist 2006):

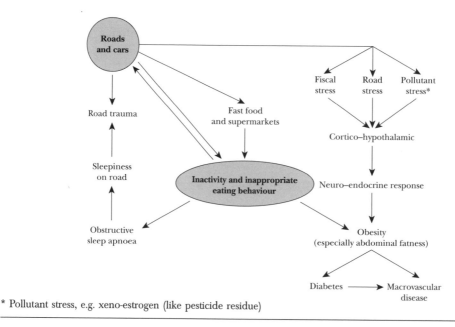

* Pollutant stress, e.g. xeno-estrogen (like pesticide residue)

Figure 2.2 Fundamental and intermediate causes of ecologically and nutritionally related disease (END)

- *planetary health*: Foci such as on the defence and maintenance of bio-diversity and food variety are becoming increasingly important health considerations. The concept of planetary health and eco-nutrition is now well-advanced (Wahlqvist and Specht 1998; Wahlqvist 2002a; Wahlqvist 2002b). The state of food insecurity world wide (FAO 2001) requires us to address not only food production (Tudge 2003), but also governance (Ogun-rinade and Oniang'o 1999; Wahlqvist et al. 1999) and conflict resolution (Wahlqvist 2006).

- *epigenetics and genomic expression*: The ways in which prenatal (and pre-conceptional) environmental influences interact with the human genome are becoming more recognised as important influences on health. The 'Foetal Origins Hypothesis' has helped to show the importance of the peri-natal nutritional environment (see chapter 4). Present work in epigenetics and genetic expression suggests that the surveillance and integrative role of non-mRNA producing DNA may account for integrative responses to the socio-environmental milieu in which we live. This has profound impor-tance for public health nutrition (Wahlqvist 2006); for example, the ways in which nutrients function in the body in later life, putting individuals at greater or lesser risk of diseases such as cardiovascular disease and type two diabetes.

- *socio-environmental injury and the nutritional modulation of inflammatory processes*: Societal, political and economic changes in many countries over the past 30 years have led to maladaptive food consumption patterns and the epidemic of metabolic diseases. At the same time, the importance of nutri-tional factors in the control of inflammatory processes that partly underlie these diseases is also becoming more recognised. There is increasing recog-nition of how widespread inflammatory processes are in disease processes, including so-called chronic diseases like obesity, diabetes and cardiovascular disease; musculo-skeletal disease; neuro-degenerative disease; renal disease; inflammatory bowel disease; upper gastrointestinal disease; certain cancers, and asthma. This encourages the measurement and analysis of the anti-inflammatory potential of foods and food patterns. It is already known that there are foods with inflammatory modulatory properties, including:

  - fruits and vegetables containing polyphenolic compounds
  - foods with high omega-3 to omega-6 fatty acid ratios, such as fish and some seed oils
  - arginine-rich protein sources such as nuts
  - fruits containing salicylates.

[35]

More of the global burden of disease caused by food and food patterns may be accounted for once these linkages are more recognised (Murray & Lopez 1996; Murray & Lopez 1997).

- *sensory nutrition*: Nutrition science is beginning to take account of the important roles the senses play in the modulation of food selection and appetite control. For example, macronutrients, such as certain types of dietary fibre and amino acids, have marked effects on satiety and daily energy intakes. Sensory nutrition represents an important interface between ourselves and the environment. In addition, sensory receptors, as myriad as they are for taste, smell, sight, sound and touch, will have representation beyond the relevant epithelial surface or sense organ itself, as, for example, food sensations are stored in long-term memory (Nishijo & Ono 1992).
- *host-parasite dysbiosis*: Parasitic and infectious diseases such as worm infestations and malaria remain major sources of malnutrition. Nutrition and parasitosis is much neglected, although the nutrition–infection equation is acknowledged for bacteria and viruses (but only recently for HIV). Yet intestinal helminthiasis (disease characterised by the presence of intestinal worms) accounts for much of the global burden of disease, although not nominated as such by the enumerators of this burden.
- *nutrition and wellness*: While focusing on the control of mortality and the extension of longevity is highly important, quality of life and wellbeing are becoming increasingly important to nutrition sciences. The epidemic prevalence of depression, dementia and other forms of cognitive impairment observed in some countries has spurred research into the roles of nutritional factors in their aetiology and prevention. The links between nutrition and wellness are likely to range between the situational to the physiological and molecular (Prilleltensky 2005).

Conclusion

Public health nutrition is poised for an exciting future, but one that could falter if it does not follow a scientifically robust, yet broader evidential road of knowledge, with extensive partnerships and a high level of accountability.

REFERENCES

Brunner, E., Rayner, M., Thorogood, M., Margetts, B., Hooper, L., Summerbell, C., Dowler, E., Hewitt, G., Robertson, A. and Wiseman, M. 2001, 'Making Public health nutrition relevant to evidence-based action' in *Public Health Nutrition*, vol. 4, no. 6, pp. 1297–99.

Cannon, G. and Leitzmann, C. 2006, 'Nutrition science for the new millennium' in *Asia Pacific Journal of Clinical Nutrition*, vol. 15, no. 1, pp. 2–3.

Eide, W.B. 2002, 'Nutrition and human rights' in *Nutrition: A foundation for development*, ACC/SCN, Geneva.

Food and Agriculture Organization (FAO) 2001, 'The state of food insecurity in the world', FAO, Rome, Italy, cited at <http://www.fao.org/documents/show_cdr.asp?url_file=/docrep/003/y1500e/y1500e00.htm> on 10 December 2006.

Giessen Declaration, The, 2005, printed in *Public Health Nutrition*, vol. 8, no. 6A, pp, 783–86.

Grier, S. and Bryant, C.A. 2005, 'Social marketing in public health' in *Annual Review of Public Health*, vol. 26, pp. 319–39.

Heggie, S.J., Wise, M.J., Cannon, G.J., Miles, L.M., Thompson, R.L., Stone, E.M., Butrum, R.R. and Kroke, A. 2003, 'Defining the state of knowledge with respect to food, nutrition, physical activity, and the prevention of cancer' in *Journal of Nutrition*, vol. 133, pp. S3837–42.

Kuhn, T. 1996, *The Structure of Scientific Revolution*, University of Chicago Press, Chicago.

Leitzmann, C. and Cannon, G. (eds) 2005, 'The New Nutrition Science project' in *Public Health Nutrition*, vol. 8, no. 6A, pp. 667–804.

Mann, J.I. 2000, 'Discrepancies in nutritional recommendations: The need for evidence-based nutrition' in *Asia Pacific Journal of Clinical Nutrition*, vol. 11, pp. S10–15.

Murray, C.J. and Lopez, A.D. 1996, *Global Health Statistics: A compendium of incidence, prevalence and mortality estimates for over 200 conditions*, Harvard School of Public Health, Geneva.

—— 1997, 'Global mortality, disability, and the contribution of risk factors: Global burden of disease study' in *Lancet*, vol. 349, no. 9063, pp. 1436–42.

Nishijo, H. and Ono, T. 1992, 'Food memory: Neuronal involvement in food recognition' in *Asia Pacific Journal Clinical Nutrition*, vol. 1, pp. 3–12.

Ogunrinade, A., Oniang'o, R. and May, J. (eds) 1999, *Not by Bread Alone*, Food Security and Governance in Africa, Toda Institute for Global Peace and Policy Research, Witwatersrand University Press, South Africa.

Popper, K.R. 1992, *The Logic of Scientific Discovery*, Routledge, London.

Prilleltensky, I. 2005, 'Promoting well-being: Time for a paradigm shift in health and human services' in *Scandinavian Journal of Public Health*, vol. 66, pp. S53–60.

Rose, G. 1985, 'Sick individuals and sick population' in *International Journal of Epidemiology*, vol. 14, no. 1, pp. 32–38.

Scrimshaw, S.C.M. and Hurtado, E. 1987, *Rapid Assessment Procedures for Nutrition and Primary Health Care: Anthropological approaches to improving programme effectiveness*, United Nations University, Tokyo.

Solomons, N.W. 1993, 'The ethics of prevention' in Wahlqvist, M.L. and Vobecky, J. (eds) 1993, *Medical Practice of Preventive Nutrition*, Smith-Gordon, London, pp. 295–306.

—— 2002, 'Ethical consequences for professionals from the globalization of food, nutrition and health' in *Asia Pacific Journal of Clinical Nutrition*, vol. 11, pp. S653–65.

—— 2006, 'McCollum International Lecturer, Professor Mark L. Wahlqvist, points us "Towards a new generation of international nutrition science and nutrition scientist" from the podium in Durban, South Africa' in *Journal of Nutrition*, vol. 136, pp. 1050–52.

Thompson, B., Coronado, G., Snipes, S.A. and Puschel, K. 2003, 'Methodologic advances and ongoing challenges in designing community-based health promotion programs' in *Annual Review of Public Health*, vol. 24, pp, 315–49.

Trichopoulos, D., Lagiou, P. and Trichopoulou, A. 2000, 'Evidence-based nutrition' in *Asia Pacific Journal of Clinical Nutrition*, vol. 9, pp. S4–9.

Tudge, C. 2003, 'So Shall We Reap: How everyone who is liable to be born in the next ten thousand years could eat very well indeed, and why, in practice, our immediate descendants are likely to be in serious trouble', Allen Lane (Penguin).

Wahlqvist, M.L. 2000, 'Objective orientated project planning (ZOPP)' in *South African Journal of Clinical Nutrition*, vol. 13, no. 1, p. S39.

—— 2002a, 'Chronic disease prevention: A life-cycle approach which takes account of the environmental impact and opportunities of food, nutrition and public health policies – the rationale for an eco-nutritional disease nomenclature' in *Asia Pacific Journal of Clinical Nutrition*, vol. 11, S759–62.

—— 2002b, 'Eco-nutritional disease or nutrition and chronic disease' in *Asia Pacific Journal of Clinical Nutrition*, vol. 11, pp. S753–54.

—— 2006, 'Towards a new generation of international nutrition science and scientist: The importance of Africa and its capacity' in *Journal of Nutrition*, vol. 136, pp, 1048–49.

Wahlqvist, M.L. and Specht, R.L. 1998, 'Food variety and biodiversity: Econutrition' in *Asia Pacific Journal of Clinical Nutrition*, vol. 7, no. 3/4, pp. 314–19.

Wahlqvist, M.L., Hsu-Hage, BH-H. and Lukito, W. 1999, 'Clinical trials in nutrition' in *Asia Pacific Journal of Clinical Nutrition*, vol. 8, no. 3, pp. 231–41.

Wahlqvist, M.L., Kouris-Blazos, A. and Savige, G.S. 1999, 'Food security and the Aged' in Ogunrinade, A., Oniang'o, R. and May, J. (eds) 1999, *Not by Bread Alone*, Food Security and Governance in Africa, Toda Institute for Global Peace and Policy Research, Witwatersrand University Press, South Africa, pp. 206–21.

Wahlqvist, M.L., Worsley, A. and Flight, I. 2000, 'Public (street) foods in Australia' in Karger, B. 2000, *World Review of Nutrition and Dietetics*, vol. 86, pp. 45–52.

Wahlqvist, M.L., Worsley, A. and Lukito, W. 2001, 'Evidence-based nutrition and cardiovascular disease in the Asia-Pacific region' in *Asia Pacific Journal of Clinical Nutrition*, vol. 10, no. 2, pp. 72–5.

World Cancer Research Fund International 2003, *Evaluation of the Evidence on Nutrition and Cancer*, World Cancer Research Fund International, London.

3

Reference standards and guidelines

MARK LAWRENCE
AILEEN ROBERTSON

As nutrition science has evolved, the emerging evidence base has been used to inform policies and programmes designed to help promote and maintain the nutritional health of populations. The cornerstones of these policies and programmes are public health nutrition reference standards and guidelines. These reference standards and guidelines serve as evidence-based benchmarks for assessing the dietary adequacy of individuals and groups of individuals, as well as planning, implementing, monitoring and evaluating public health nutrition policies and programmes directed at influencing the food supply and/or dietary behaviour. There are three especially commonly used and inter-related public health nutrition reference standards and guidelines, namely: reference values for nutrient intakes, dietary goals, and dietary guidelines accompanied with food selection guides.

In this chapter, our emphasis is on analysing these reference standards and guidelines from a public health nutrition perspective. In particular, we draw upon recent reviews of public health nutrition reference standards and guidelines for countries in Australasia, Europe and North America. It is beyond the scope of this chapter to present a detailed examination of the scientific derivation of these reference standards and guidelines. Instead, we provide a broad analysis of their purpose, underlying principles and scientific basis. Our aim is to equip public health nutrition practitioners with a basic understanding for interpreting data analyses based on the reference standards and guidelines, as well as an appreciation of their application to policy and programme practice.

Reference values for nutrient intakes

Background and rationale

The quantification of human requirements for most nutrients followed the identification and elucidation of the vitamins in the first half of the twentieth century. The first national reference values for nutrient intakes were compiled in the late 1930s and early 1940s in Canada and the United States respectively (IOM 2000a). They were set against the aftermath of an economic depression in which food supplies were limited and the poor nutritional status of many recruits for military service in the Second World War. Expressed as population recommendations, they were the amount of nutrients required on an average daily basis for adequate physiological function and prevention of nutrient deficiency diseases. In subsequent decades, reference values for nutrient intakes were regularly published by United Nations (UN) agencies — the Food and Agriculture Organization (FAO) and World Health Organization (WHO) — and many national governments. These reference values were designed with the similar purpose of providing population-based recommendations for nutrient intakes, albeit with variations in the nomenclature used; for example, recommended dietary allowance (US), recommended dietary intake (Australia), and recommended daily amount (United Kingdom).

During the 1990s and 2000s, the conceptual basis of national reference values for nutrient intakes began to be expanded by expert committees, first in the United Kingdom (COMA 1991, 1994, 1998) and the European Union (Scientific Committee on Food 1993), and then North America (IOM 1997, 2000a, 2000b, 2001, 2002, 2004), and more recently in Australasia (NHMRC 2006). There were several reasons for this. There was more understanding of the relationship between nutrients and health, especially in relation to the prevention of diet-related chronic diseases. In addition, there was concern among authorities that users did not always understand how the reference standards were derived and how they were intended to be used. In particular, there appeared to be confusion among certain users that the reference values could be used to assess the adequacy of individuals' diets. The new concepts that were introduced by national authorities extended the conventional population recommendations to include values that could address consideration of:

- dietary guidance at both the individual and population levels
- reduction in the risk of diet-related chronic disease
- reference values for non-traditional nutrients; for example, phytochemicals, for which there is evidence of a health benefit
- upper intake levels to avoid excess consumption.

These additional concepts could not be represented within one type of reference values. Instead, a generic term to refer to at least three types of reference values representing specific concepts was adopted by countries in Australasia (Nutrient Reference Values), North America (Dietary Reference Intakes), Nordic countries (Nordic Nutrition Recommendations) and the UK (Dietary Reference Values).

Underlying principles

Typically, reference values for nutrient intakes are established by expert panels. These expert panels prepare the reference values from reviews of the scientific literature and analyses of the findings of a diversity of epidemiological studies, national surveys and animal and human experimentation that inform the nutrition science knowledge base at a given time. A fundamental challenge when establishing reference values for nutrient intakes is that the physiological requirement for nutrients varies from individual to individual within a population. Hence, reference values for nutrient intakes describe the distribution of required dietary intakes within life stage and gender-specific subgroups of the population. Nutrient requirements for a group are established in relation to a frequency distribution of individual requirements. Recommendations for infants are the exception, as they are based on the nutrient content of breast milk.

Internationally, there is general agreement towards the conceptual basis for the establishment of reference standards for nutrient intakes. Here we provide an overview of the underlying principles to the various reference values to assist public health nutritionists to be more critically aware of their correct use in professional practice. Without this knowledge, it is possible to conduct analyses that ignore the reference values' assumptions and yield incorrect estimates of the prevalence of inadequate intakes in individuals and groups of people and/or lead to their inappropriate application to policies and programmes. The definitions of the different reference values are similar among countries, and we have adopted the specific definitions used in Australasia.

Estimated Average Requirement

The estimated average requirement (EAR) for a nutrient, or average requirement, is 'A daily nutrient level estimated to meet the requirements of half the healthy individuals in a particular life stage and gender group' (NHMRC 2006). When establishing the EAR for a nutrient for a specific life stage and gender group, it is generally assumed that the nutrient requirement is normally distributed around the mean (except for iron, which has a positively skewed distribution). If a group's nutrient requirement pattern is normally distributed, we can apply basic statistical concepts to determine that a range of +/– two standard deviations (2SD) around the mean will include 95 per cent of the group's nutrient requirement values. As outlined in Figure 3.1, this concept provides the basis whereby the EAR for each nutrient is also used to establish the reference nutrient intake (RNI), or equivalent value.

Reference level set at two standard deviations above the EAR

The recommended dietary intake (RDI) in Australasia, population reference intake (PRI) in the European Union, recommended dietary allowance (RDA) in North America, recommended intake in Nordic countries, and the RNI in the United Kingdom, are equivalent concepts that are broadly defined as, 'the average daily dietary intake level that is sufficient to meet the nutrient requirements of nearly all (97 to 98 per cent) healthy individuals in a particular life stage and gender group' (NHMRC 2006). The RDI, or its equivalent, is calculated from knowledge of the EAR. If the requirement for the nutrient is normally distributed and the standard deviation of the EAR is available, then the RDI, or its equivalent, is set two notional standard deviations above the EAR. If data about variability are insufficient to calculate a standard deviation, a coefficient of variation of 10 per cent is generally assumed, and twice that amount added to the EAR is defined as equal to the RDI, or its equivalent.

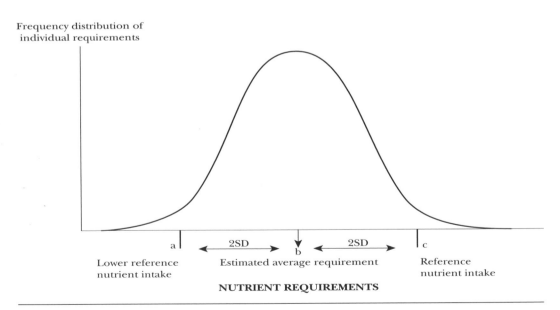

Figure 3.1 The EAR and RNI or equivalent value

Source: adapted from Figure 1.1, COMA 1991

As illustrated in Figure 3.1, an RNI (and also an RDI, PRI and RDA) exceeds the actual nutrient requirements of practically all healthy persons, and is therefore not synonymous with requirements. Indeed, a level of nutrient intake 2SD above the mean estimated average requirement is greater than the individual requirements of 97 to 98 per cent of the population.

Estimated Energy Requirements

Because of concerns about overconsumption and obesity, the dietary energy requirements for a population group are generally set at a level equivalent to the estimated average requirement. The estimated energy requirement (EER), or equivalent, is defined as:

> The average dietary energy intake that is predicted to maintain energy balance in a healthy adult of defined age, gender, weight, height and level of physical activity, consistent with good health. In children and pregnant and lactating women, the EER is taken to include the needs associated with the deposition of tissues or the secretion of milk at rates consistent with good health (NHMRC 2006).

Reference value for nutrients for which an EAR cannot be defined

An adequate intake (AI) in Australasia and North America, safe intake in the United Kingdom, and acceptable ranges in the European Union are equivalent concepts that are established for a nutrient when there is not enough scientific evidence to establish an EAR (and therefore an RDI). The AI, is broadly defined as:

> The average daily nutrient intake level based on observed or experimentally-determined approximations or estimates of nutrient intake by a group (or groups) of apparently healthy people that are assumed to be adequate (NHMRC 2006).

It is set at the median intake of a population that has no apparent health problem with respect to the nutrient. Like the RDI, an AI can be used as a goal for individual intake, but there is less degree of certainty surrounding the AI. If an individual or a population consumes at or above the AI value, there is a low probability of inadequacy. The AI is intended to be a guide for intake that meets or exceeds the needs of a healthy population. It is intended that, as the science base grows and an EAR (and RDI) can be determined, then the AI can be replaced. Because the AI is set when the EAR (and hence the RDI) cannot be defined, no nutrient has all three values.

Upper level of intake

For many minerals and some vitamins such as vitamin A, high levels of intake may pose a health risk, and upper levels of safe intake are recommended. In recognition of the increased use of fortified foods, specially formulated foods and dietary supplements among consumers, there has been growing interest among national authorities to develop a model to help determine the levels of intake that may pose risk, and to provide guidance to avoid excessively high nutrient intakes. In Australasia and North America, an upper level of intake (UL) and tolerable upper intake level, respectively, has been established for each nutrient. The UL is defined as:

> The highest average daily nutrient intake level likely to pose no adverse health effects to almost all individuals in the general population. As intake increases above the UL, the potential risk of adverse effects increases (NHMRC 2006).

From a population perspective, it can be used to estimate the percentage of a group at potential risk of adverse effects from excessive intake. In 2003, the Expert Group on Vitamins and Minerals in the United Kingdom set new recommendations for safe upper levels for vitamin B6, betacarotene, vitamin E, boron, copper, nickel, selenium, zinc and silicon (EVM 2003). The determination of the

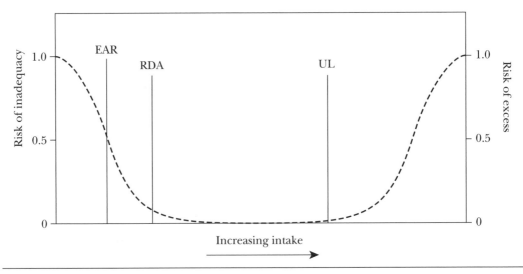

Figure 3.2 Determination of reference values for nutrient intakes from the mean-observed requirement

Source: adapted from Figure 1.1, IOM 2000a

EAR, RDI and UL reference values from the mean-observed requirement are represented in Figure 3.2.

In addition to the four concepts above, in the European Union and the United Kingdom, the lowest threshold intake and a lower RNI level, respectively, have been defined as reference values below which habitual intakes are likely to be inadequate for most individuals. These reference values are set 2SD below the EAR. As illustrated in Figure 3.1, a level of nutrient intake 2SD below the mean-estimated average requirement is less than the individual requirements of 97.5 per cent of the population. The reference values for nutrient intakes published by United Nations' agencies and individual national governments broadly concur. Where differences between tables of reference values might be observed, usually this can be explained by the adoption of different criteria of adequacy and/or different interpretations of the available scientific evidence. In the future, it will be important to explore whether nomenclature and scientific approaches towards establishing reference values might be harmonised among countries. It is not possible here to reproduce the reference values for each national authority. More information on the scientific derivation and tables of reference values for nutrient intakes can be accessed at the following websites:

Australasia: <http://www.nhmrc.gov.au/publications/_files/n35.pdf> and
     <http:// www.moh.govt.nz/publications>
Europe: <http://www.euro.who.int/document/E82161.pdf (p. 341)> and
     <http:// data.euro.who.int/Nutrition/Default.aspx?TabID=77686>
North America: <http://lab.nap.edu/nap-cgi/discover.cgi?term=dietary%
     20reference%20intakes&restric=NAP&ref=NAP>.

Recommendations for prevention of chronic disease

In Europe and North America, consideration for chronic disease prevention is incorporated into the establishment of the EAR and RDIs (or equivalent). In Australasia, the traditional concepts of adequate physiological or metabolic function and/or avoidance of deficiency states are retained as the reference point for establishing the EARs and RDIs, and chronic disease prevention is not included in these values. Instead, in Australasia there are 'suggested dietary targets' addressing specific nutrients, such as dietary fibre, long chain omega-3 fats and sodium, for which there is evidence for setting targets consistent with chronic disease prevention.

Recommendations for macronutrient intakes consistent with chronic disease prevention have been established in the United Kingdom, the WHO in terms of population nutrient intake goals, and Australasia and North America in the form of the Acceptable Macronutrient Distribution Range (AMDR). The AMDR addresses the balance of protein, fat and carbohydrate in the diet in terms of their relative contribution to dietary energy. Whereas the Australasian, United Kingdom, Nordic and WHO recommendations for macronutrients are intended as population average intakes, those in North America are intended for use by individuals. The recommended ranges of macronutrients for the prevention of diet-related chronic disease are listed in Table 3.1.

Practical application of reference values for nutrient intakes

The purpose of the reference values and the principles underpinning their development are sometimes misunderstood, leading to incorrect applications. In this section we examine practical considerations for using reference values for nutrient intakes in public health nutrition practice.

Reference values for nutrient intakes have two broad applications in public health nutrition. First, they can be used for evaluating dietary survey data to assess the likelihood of inadequate or excessive nutrient intake by individuals or groups of people, and thereby identifying high-risk individuals and groups. Second, they can be used as benchmarks for planning, monitoring and evaluating policies and programmes directed at influencing the food supply and/or dietary behaviour.

Assessing diet adequacy evaluations based on the reference values

Here we consider the use of the different reference values to assess dietary adequacy for individuals and groups of people. When assessing dietary adequacy, it is important to remember that all reference values are designed primarily for groups of healthy individuals, and are valid for usual intake over an *extended* period of time. Therefore, although the reference values are expressed as daily amounts, they are not designed to be applied to separate day's intake by an individual or group of people.

Assessing evaluations of the diet adequacy of individuals using reference values

EAR: An EAR value is not intended as a goal for an individual's nutrient intake, as there is a 50 per cent chance that by consuming amounts equivalent to the EAR an individual is not meeting their nutrient requirement. However,

Table 3.1 Ranges of population nutrient intake goals as a proportion of total energy in Australasia, North America, Nordic countries, United Kingdom and WHO

Dietary factor	Australasia AMDRs (NHMRC 2006)	North American AMDRs for adults (IOM 2002)	UK DRVs (COMA 1991, 1994, 1998)	Nordic Recommendations (NCM 2004)	EURODIET* (2001)	WHO Goals (WHO 2003)
Protein	15–25%	10–35%	15%	10–20%	10–15%	10–15%
Total fat	20–35%	UL not set	≤33%	25–35%	< 30%	15–30%
Saturated fat	≤10% (including *trans* fats)	UL not set	≤10%	10%	< 10%	< 10%
PUFAs**	N/A	NA	6%	5–10%		6–10%
Linoleic acid	4–10%			3% of PUFA	< 4–8%	
-linolenic acid	0.4–1%	0.6–1.2%	NA	0.5% of PUFA	2g linolenic + 200mg very long chain	NA
***Trans* fatty acids**	Included within saturated fat range	UL not set	≤2%	Included within saturated fat range	< 2%	< 1%
MUFAs***	N/A	UL not set	12%	10–15%		By difference
Total carbohydrate	45–65%	45–65%	47%	50–60%	> 55%	55–75%
Sugars	Advises carbohydrate be sourced 'predominantly from low-energy density and/or low-glycaemic index foods'	≤25% from added sugars	10%	< 10%	< 10%	< 10%

*   EURODIET also includes population goals for physical activity (PAL > 1.75) and BMI (21–22), both relevant to energy intake. In addition, EURODIET sets population goals for intake of fibre, fruit and vegetables, folate from food, salt and iodine intake, and exclusive breastfeeding.

**   PUFAs = Polyunsaturated fatty acids

***   MUFAs = Monounsaturated fatty acids

comparing an individuals' usual intake to the EAR can be used to examine the probability that their usual intake is inadequate. Although the establishment of an EAR is based on scientific evidence, an individual's true requirement for a nutrient can only be approximated. Moreover, methods for estimating an individual's usual dietary intake are notoriously imprecise. Certainly reference values are not able to be used to diagnose nutrient deficiencies in individuals. If an individual's habitual intake of a nutrient is very low, then nutritional status may be at risk, and further investigation, including biological measures, may be indicated.

RDI and AI: Both the RDI and AI can be used as a goal for individual intake (although the AI provides less certainty). The RDI or AI can be used to indicate the intake at which, or above which, there is low probability of inadequacy. If an individual's usual intake of a nutrient is at a level equivalent to the RDI, then there is a low probability of an inadequate intake (2 to 3 per cent).

UL: As an individual's usual intake increases above this level, their risk of adverse effects from excessive nutrient intake increases.

Assessing evaluations of the diet adequacy of groups using reference values

EAR: At the EAR value, one-half of a specified group would have its nutrient needs met and one-half would not. The EAR is used to estimate the prevalence of inadequate intakes within a group.

RDI: It is not appropriate to use the RDI value for assessing the prevalence of inadequate intakes in a group because it is set at an intake level that exceeds the requirements of 97 to 98 per cent of individuals. By definition, there would be a very low risk of inadequate intakes if the group mean met the RDI, and comparison to the RDI would significantly overestimate the proportion of a group at risk. Assuming that dietary intake data are sufficiently robust, it may be possible to report information on percentiles of intake of the group; for example, X per cent of the group had intakes above or below the RDI.

AI: The correct use of an AI is to determine whether or not the median intake of a group is above or below the AI. A mean usual intake at or above the AI implies a low prevalence of inadequate intakes.

UL: The UL is used to estimate the percentage of the population that may be at risk of adverse effects from excessive nutrient intake.

Application to policies and programmes

Reference standards for nutrient intakes have practical applications to a diversity of policies and programmes, including assessing the adequacy of both food supply reserves and meal provision, informing food regulation policies, educating consumers, marketing of food, and prescribing diets. These applications are discussed below.

Food provision

The reference standards can serve as an assessment tool for monitoring the adequacy of both the food supply for a nation, as well as meal planning for food assistance programmes and institutions with large-scale catering, such as the military, prisons, hospitals and nursing homes. Here, the aim is for the diets and/or food supplies to contain nutrients at the RDI level, the rationale being that, if eaten, the risk of deficiency would be very small in any individual. Indeed, almost all individuals receiving the diet/food supply (if equally distributed) would consume in excess of their requirements.

Food regulation

The development of food standards related to food labelling, food fortification and modified food products is informed by reference standards, and can complement the objectives of national food and nutrition policies (Lewis and Jeffreson 2000).

Food labelling: The food regulations of many countries now incorporate reference standards as the basis of their food labelling provisions, in relation to conveying nutrient information and nutrient content claims to consumers; for example, an average RDI for the purpose of food labelling is set for each nutrient to reflect the requirements of men and women. These RDIs can be used to provide a convenient denominator to convert potentially complex data, such as the amount of a nutrient in a reference quantity of a food product, into a percentage of the labelling RDI value. This is taken a step further with some regulations whereby descriptors such as 'source' or 'good source' of a nutrient are displayed on the food label based on a proportion of the RDI of a nutrient provided in a reference quantity of that food product. The international food standards authority, the Codex Alimentarius Commission (Codex) has specified that a source and good source claim can be made when 15 and 30 per cent, respectively, of the nutrient RDI is present in a serving of the food (Codex 1997). In addition, mandatory information regarding the amount of fat, saturated fatty acids, cholesterol, carbohydrate, fibre, sodium, potassium and/or protein in a reference quantity of a food product in relation to reference standards is prescribed in the food-labelling provisions of many countries.

Food fortification: The reference standards can be used as a benchmark for determining the level of fortification, and when determining a suitable food vehicle(s) for mandatory or voluntary food fortification interventions. Dietary modelling is a scientific procedure that uses information about food consumption patterns among the population to estimate different scenarios of nutrient exposure based on varying the level of fortification and the range of foods fortified with a nutrient. The reference standards provide the reference point against which the findings of dietary modelling activities can be assessed.

Developing modified food products: The reference standards provide a reference point for determining the nutrient composition of modified food products, particularly where such food products are the sole source of nutrition; for example, certain meal replacements.

Education

The reference standards are used to educate individuals and groups of people about selecting types and amounts of foods to meet their nutritional requirements. Also, they provide the foundation for developing and revising dietary guidelines and food selection guides that provide advice on types and amounts of foods consistent with a healthy eating pattern to satisfy nutritional requirements.

Food marketing

Food marketers increasingly defer to the reference standards to inform consumers about the nutrient composition of their products.

Prescribing diets

The reference standards are important benchmarks in planning and prescribing therapeutic diets, such as in clinical dietetic practice. The reference standards can be used as a benchmark for modifying the diets of individual patients requiring therapeutic diets, including where it is important that the diet contains nutrients at the RDI level so that the risk of deficiency would be very small in any individual.

Dietary goals and guidelines

Since the late 1950s, there has been emerging epidemiological evidence of the relationship between dietary patterns and dietary components and nutritional health and the development of risk factors for certain diet-related chronic diseases. There is general agreement among most national and international nutrition agencies about dietary profiles that are consistent with wellbeing and prevention of disease. These nutrition agencies have sought to provide advice to the general population so that their usual diet contributes to a healthy lifestyle consistent with minimal risk for the development of diet-related diseases. These dietary profiles can be quantified to provide dietary goals towards which the population's diet should strive. Also, advice in the form of a list of dietary guidelines can be provided to assist the population's dietary profile shift towards achieving dietary goals. In the next two sections, we consider dietary goals and then dietary guidelines.

Dietary goals

Dietary goals are a general statement of intent and aspiration that are used for planning policies and programmes at the national level. For example, the primary nutrition goal of the Australian food and nutrition policy is to increase the proportion of the population who consume a diet consistent with the dietary guidelines (Commonwealth Department of Health, Housing and Community Services 1992). Dietary targets state the amount of dietary change that could reasonably be expected for a given population within a given time. Therefore, dietary goals generally are quantified as national targets for selected macronutrients and micronutrients aimed at preventing diet-related chronic diseases. Ranges of population macronutrient intake goals in Australasia, EU, Nordic countries, North America, United Kingdom and WHO were listed previously in Table 3.1.

After establishing national recommended nutrient intakes, ministries of health often establish dietary goals for their population. The European Population Goals, as defined by the EURODIET EU-funded initiative, are included in Table 3.1, and are in line with those recommended by WHO and FAO (WHO 2003). These goals are important in establishing specific targets against which dietary intake can be assessed and monitored, and display the extent of change necessary to achieve good health in the EU population. The goals also provide a basis for health-promotion interventions, and a focus for policy development and required resources. The relevant sectors can be identified more easily, and responsibilities allocated to the appropriate stakeholder. The WHO, European Union and national goals aim to help the respective authorities allocate resources to priority areas.

Dietary guidelines

Dietary guidelines are public health recommendations by expert panels based on the analysis of data from published original research. In most countries, the guidelines are intended to provide advice for the general population and healthy individuals so that their usual diet contributes to a healthy lifestyle consistent with minimal risk for the development of diet-related diseases.

Dietary guidelines are expressed in qualitative terms, and are less technical than population goals and reference standards for nutrient intakes. The corollary is that they are less precise and open to interpretation; for example, what is meant by 'eat less fat' or 'eat moderate amounts of sugar'? They are developed as a coherent set of guidelines, and are not designed to be implemented as individual guidelines in isolation from the complete set. Dietary guidelines apply to the total diet and are not intended to be used to assess the 'healthiness' of individual foods. Within some countries, there may be various versions of dietary guidelines and food selection guides available, reflecting the interest of certain non-government organisations in promulgating a particular emphasis. The availability of different guidelines within a country can be confusing; here we focus on official national versions.

Examples from Australasia, Europe and North America

The first dietary guidelines were developed in Scandinavia in the late 1960s. Since that time, dietary guidelines have been published by UN agencies and individual national governments. Examples of dietary guidelines from Australasia, Europe and North America are as follows.

Australia

The Australian government has prepared separate dietary guidelines for adults (NHMRC 2003), children and adolescents, incorporating infant feeding guidelines (NHMRC 2003), and for older Australians (NHMRC 1999). The dietary guidelines for Australian adults (see <http://www.nhmrc.gov.au/publications/_files/n33.pdf>) are listed:

- enjoy a wide variety of nutritious foods
  - eat plenty of vegetables, legumes and fruits
  - eat plenty of cereals (including breads, rice, pasta and noodles), preferably wholegrain
  - include lean meat, fish, poultry and/or alternatives
  - include milks, yoghurts, cheeses and/or alternatives — reduced-fat varieties should be chosen, where possible

    – drink plenty of water.

- and take care to:
  - limit saturated fat and moderate total fat intake
  - choose foods low in salt
  - limit your alcohol intake if you choose to drink
  - consume only moderate amounts of sugars and foods containing added sugars
  - prevent weight gain — be physically active and eat according to your energy needs
  - care for your food — prepare and store it safely
  - encourage and support breastfeeding.

Canada

Canada's Guidelines for Healthy Eating (see <http://www.hc-sc.gc.ca/fn-an/nutrition/diet-guide-nutri/fg-ga-guide_e.html>) were developed as five key messages to be communicated to healthy Canadians over two years of age. They are:

1. Enjoy a variety of foods.
2. Emphasise cereals, breads, other grain products, vegetables and fruit.
3. Choose lower-fat dairy products, leaner meats and food prepared with little or no fat.
4. Achieve and maintain a healthy body weight by enjoying regular physical activity and healthy eating.
5. Limit salt, alcohol and caffeine.

Europe

The WHO food-based dietary guidelines for the European Region (see <http://www.euro.who.int/Document/E7982.pdf>) aim to provide food-based dietary guidelines that can be used as a consistent communication tool and as a springboard to planning, implementing, and evaluating public health nutrition strategies (Stockley 2001). The twelve WHO European dietary guidelines (CINDI 2000) are:

1. Eat a nutritious diet based on a variety of foods originating mainly from plants, rather than animals.
2. Eat bread, grains, pasta, rice or potatoes several times a day.
3. Eat a variety of vegetables and fruits, preferably fresh and local, several times per day (greater than 400 grams per day).

4. Maintain a body weight between the recommended limits (a BMI of 18.5 to 25) by taking moderate levels of physical activity, preferably daily.
5. Control fat intake (not more than 30 per cent of daily energy), and replace most saturated fats with unsaturated vegetable oils or soft margarines.
6. Replace fatty meat and meat products with beans, legumes, lentils, fish, poultry or lean meat.
7. Use milk and dairy products (sour milk, yoghurt and cheese) that are low in both fat and salt.
8. Select foods that are low in sugar, and eat refined sugar sparingly, limiting the frequency of sugary drinks and sweets (less than 10 per cent energy).
9. Choose a low-salt diet. Total salt intake should not be more than one teaspoon (5 grams) per day, including the salt in bread and processed, cured and preserved foods. (Salt iodization should be universal where iodine deficiency is endemic.)
10. If alcohol is consumed, limit intake to no more than two drinks (each containing no more than 10 grams of alcohol) per day.
11. Prepare food in a safe and hygienic way. Steam, bake, boil or microwave to help reduce the amount of added fat.
12. Promote exclusive breastfeeding up to six months and the introduction of safe and adequate complementary foods from the age of six months while continuing breastfeeding during the first years of life.

New Zealand

The New Zealand Food and Nutrition Guideline statements (see <http://www.moh.govt.nz/moh.nsf/0/07BC60BE764FDABBCC250DB006B9ABA/$File/foodandnutritionguidelines-adults.pdf>) list six points:

1. Maintain a healthy body weight by eating well and by daily physical activity. At least 30 minutes of moderate-intensity physical activity on most, if not all, days of the week and, if possible, add some vigorous exercise for extra health and fitness.
2. Eat well by including a variety of nutritious foods from each of the four major food groups each day:
   • plenty of vegetables and fruits
   • plenty of breads and cereals, preferably wholegrain
   • milk and milk products in your diet, preferably reduced or low-fat options
   • lean meat, poultry, seafood, eggs or alternatives.
3. Prepare foods or choose pre-prepared foods, drinks and snacks:
   • with minimal added fat, especially saturated fat

- that are low in salt; if using salt, choose iodised salt
- with little added sugar; limit your intake of high-sugar foods.

4. Drink plenty of liquids each day, especially water.
5. If choosing to drink alcohol, limit your intake.
6. Purchase, prepare, cook and store food to ensure food safety.

United Kingdom

The UK Food Standards Agency's publication, 'Eat well: Your guide to healthy eating' (see <http://www.food.gov.uk/multimedia/pdfs/eatwell.pdf>) provides the following eight practical tips for eating well:

1. Base your meals on starchy foods
2. Eat lots of fruit and vegetables
3. Eat more fish — including a portion of oily fish each week
4. Cut down on saturated fat and sugar
5. Try to eat less salt — no more than six grams a day for adults
6. Get active and try to be a healthy weight
7. Drink plenty of water
8. Don't skip breakfast.

United States

The Dietary Guidelines for Americans 2005 (see <http://www.health.gov/dietaryguidelines/dga2005/toolkit/background.pdf>) identify 41 key recommendations, of which 23 are for the general public and 18 for special populations. These guidelines are intended primarily for use by policymakers, healthcare providers, nutritionists and nutrition educators. They are grouped into nine general topics:

1. Adequate nutrients within calorie needs
2. Weight management
3. Physical activity
4. Food groups to encourage
5. Fats
6. Carbohydrates
7. Sodium and potassium
8. Alcoholic beverages
9. Food Safety.

The different dietary guideline lists indicate that there is general agreement in recommendations for dietary guidance among the selected countries. Most of the differences between the various lists of dietary guidelines can be attributed to the adoption of different criteria of priority and variations of opinion in the interpretation of sometimes relatively sparse experimental evidence. Some countries' guidelines include advice on individual nutrients, and some refer to the eating environment and enjoying food. Other countries' guidelines refer to food security and sustainable production, and some list guidelines in order of priority.

Development of food-based dietary guidelines

In 1995, the Food and Agriculture Organization (FAO) and the WHO held a joint consultation to begin preparing food-based dietary guidelines. These guidelines were developed in recognition of the need to translate population nutrient goals into food-based dietary guidelines, to express dietary advice in the consumer-friendly terms of foods or dietary patterns and to 'avoid, as far as possible, the technical terms of nutritional sciences' (WHO 1998). They take into account the ecological setting, socioeconomic status and cultural factors, as well as the biological and physical environment in which the population lives. The WHO has outlined principles; because they can be technical, it is recommended that they be implemented with local experts. Also, they should be critically appraised and evaluated.

In order to be understood, nutrient population goals need to be translated into food-based dietary guidelines at the national level, to take account of national and regional dietary patterns. Recommendations in different countries in Europe vary depending on the variety of foods available; for example, consumption of rye bread is promoted in some parts of northern Europe but, since rye is not grown all over Europe, it would be unrealistic to expect all Europeans to eat rye bread regularly. There exist at least 27 examples of national dietary guidelines within Europe. Many of these are based on the WHO Dietary Guide and 'Twelve steps to healthy eating' (CINDI 2000).

Food-based dietary guidelines should be adapted to a country's specific needs; ensure that the nutrient needs of the population are covered; and contribute to reducing the risk of diet-related diseases. In addition, guidelines should be in accord with policies that promote food safety, a healthy sustainable environment and a robust local food economy. Ministries of health are encouraged to review their premature mortality rates, morbidity data and the available data on diet and nutritional status before developing national dietary guidelines. This ensures that the recommendations are tailored to national conditions.

Around half (26) of the European countries had developed food-based dietary guidelines by 2001 (see <http://www.euro.who.int/Document/E79832. pdf>). In 2006, a database became available from the WHO Nutrition and Food Security Programme, where information about Nutrition References Standards, Dietary Guidelines and Food Selection Guides in Europe can be found (see

<http://data.euro.who.int/Nutrition/ Default.aspx?TabID=77686>). At this site, it is possible to view the national dietary guidelines for fourteen European countries. Guidelines are culturally inclusive and incorporate foods that are generally available and accessible at a reasonable price within each country. Most European guidelines include the promotion of physical activity. Few countries in Europe have developed dietary guidelines specifically for children and adolescents, but both WHO and the European Food Safety Agency are working on this.

Food selection guides

Food selection guides are nutrition education tools that translate scientific knowledge of food composition, reference intakes and dietary guidelines into practical food selection advice.

The development of food guides can be traced through several stages in parallel with the evolution of reference standards and guidelines (see chapter 1). The first food guides emerged during the period when the vitamins were being discovered, enunciated and quantified. The emphasis of these first food guides was on reflecting reference intakes in recommending the minimum number of daily food serves for so-called 'protective foods' (Santich 2005) for achieving adequate dietary intakes. With the development of dietary guidelines, food guides became increasingly sophisticated in the concepts they portrayed. Generally, food guides aim to illustrate the types and proportion of foods which make up a healthy balanced diet.

In food selection guides, foods are grouped according to their characteristic nutrient profiles and in reference quantities so that they can be interchanged with other foods in the group to which they have been allocated; for example, within the dairy food group a cup of milk (250 millilitres) has approximately an equivalent nutrient profile as two slices of cheese and a small carton (200 grams) of yoghurt. Food selection guides observe the principle that the best strategy for meeting nutrient needs (established and yet to be defined) is to select from a wide variety of foods and not to rely on nutrient supplements or fortified foods (Lichtenstein & Russell 2005). The recommendations about the number of daily serves from the various food groups are based on achieving a diet consistent with reference standards for nutrient intakes and dietary guidelines. Food guides capture the fundamental food selection concepts of variety, balance and moderation in the following ways:

- variety in food selection (across and within groups) is promoted to obtain sufficient amounts and types of nutrients in the diet, and thereby achieve the reference standards

- balance in food selection is promoted to avoid over-consumption of the macronutrients associated with chronic diseases
- moderation in food selection relates to avoiding excessive energy intake and subsequent problems with overweight and obesity. Some food guides, such as the US MyPyramid and WHO CINDI guidelines, incorporate physical activity concepts within their design, to further illustrate the concept of energy balance.

In contemporary times in high-income countries, food guides have assumed increasing importance as individuals have become progressively removed from the food supply and are faced with the daunting task of making informed selections from the estimated hundreds of thousands of food products in the marketplace. With this substantial choice of food products and an overwhelming amount of dietary information people need simple, clear guidance about amounts and types of foods to select a healthy diet.

There is also a diversity of visual representations among the food guides of different countries (Painter et al, 2002). Examples of food guides from Australia, China, Europe and North America, which illustrate a diversity of images (plates, compass, rainbow, pagoda, circle, pyramids) are shown in figures 3.3 to 3.10. In the space available it is not possible to provide a comprehensive review of the food guides of all countries.

Australia
Australia's most recent food guide is the 'Australian Guide to Healthy Eating' that illustrates five food groups as segments on a plate (see Figure 3.3).

Canada
Canada's 'Food guide to Healthy Eating' depicts four food groups as components of a rainbow segment (see Figure 3.4). It is anticipated that Health Canada will release a revised version of its food guide during 2007. The revised guide and supporting materials will be available at <http://www.hc-sc.gc.ca/>.

China
The Chinese food guide illustrates five food groups, each is portrayed as a separate level in a pagoda (see Figure 3.5).

Denmark
The Danish food guide illustrates eight food and physical activity messages that are portrayed as points on a compass (see Figure 3.6).

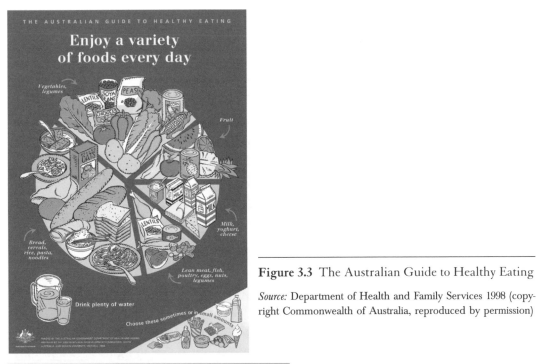

Figure 3.3 The Australian Guide to Healthy Eating

Source: Department of Health and Family Services 1998 (copyright Commonwealth of Australia, reproduced by permission)

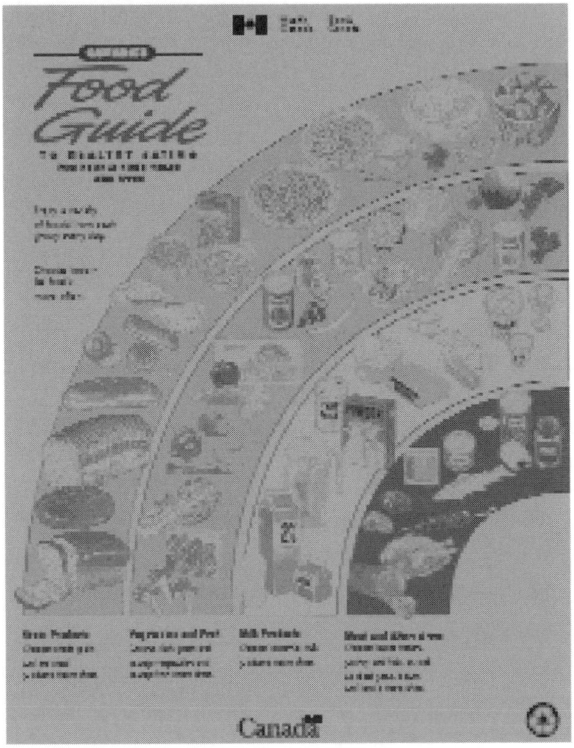

Figure 3.4 Canada's Food Guide to Healthy Eating

Source: Health Canada 2006 (reproduced with the permission of the Minister of Public Works and Government Services Canada)

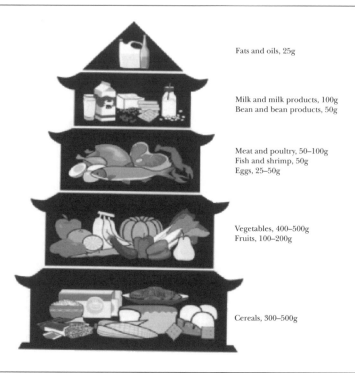

Fats and oils, 25g

Milk and milk products, 100g
Bean and bean products, 50g

Meat and poultry, 50–100g
Fish and shrimp, 50g
Eggs, 25–50g

Vegetables, 400–500g
Fruits, 100–200g

Cereals, 300–500g

Figure 3.5 Chinese food guide pagoda

Source: Chinese Nutrition Society (reproduced with permission)

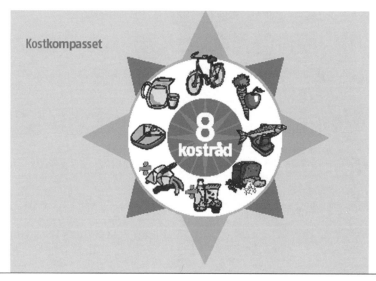

Figure 3.6 Danish food compass model

Source: Danish Veterinary and Food Administration (reproduced with permission)

Portugal

The Portuguese food guide illustrates each of seven food groups as segments of a circle (see Figure 3.7).

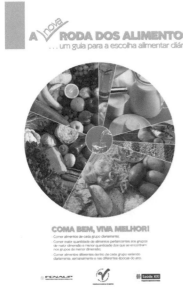

Figure 3.7 The Portuguese food guide

Source: Faculty of Nutrition and Food Sciences from University of Porto and Portuguese Consumer's Institute 2003 (reproduced with permission)

Spain

The Spanish food guide illustrates food groupings in the shape of a pyramid (see Figure 3.8).

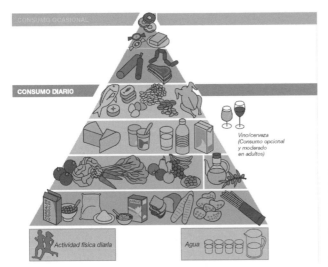

Figure 3.8 Spanish food guide for healthy eating

Source: Sociedad Espanola Nutricion Comunitaria 2004 (reproduced with permission)

United Kingdom

The UK food guide is entitled, 'The Balance of Good Heath' (see Figure 3.9). The guide is portrayed as a plate. It is anticipated that the UK food guide will be revised during 2007. The updated plate model will be published, together with guidelines, on <http://www.eatwell.gov.uk> when available.

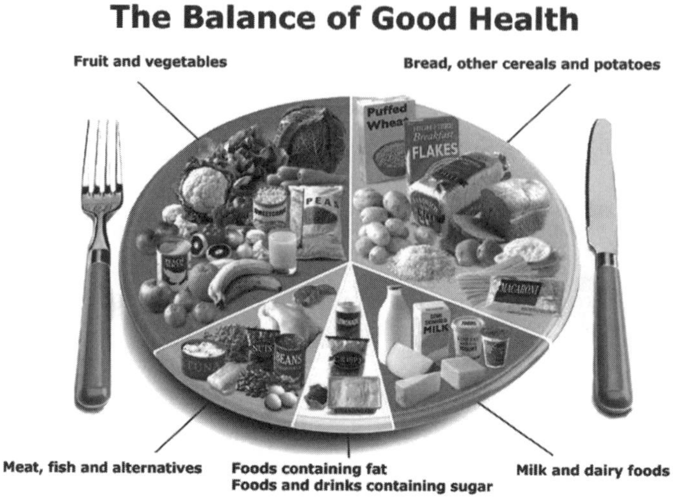

The Balance of Good Health

Figure 3.9 The UK Balance of Good Health food guide

Source: Food Standards Agency (reproduced with permission)

United States

The US food guide, 'MyPyramid', has been developed as an integral component of a comprehensive health education programme which aims to promote a personalised approach to healthy eating and physical activity (see Figure 3.10). As the guide's name indicates it is portrayed as a pyramid.

The images provided in figures 3.3 to 3.10 illustrate that the food selection guides of most countries generally are consistent in their concepts and recommendations. In particular, the guides portray a diversity of foods that are grouped in accordance with common nutrient composition profiles. The aim of the guides is to encourage the consumption of a variety of foods from each of the main food groups every day, with an emphasis on illustrating the types and proportion of foods which make up a well-balanced and healthy diet.

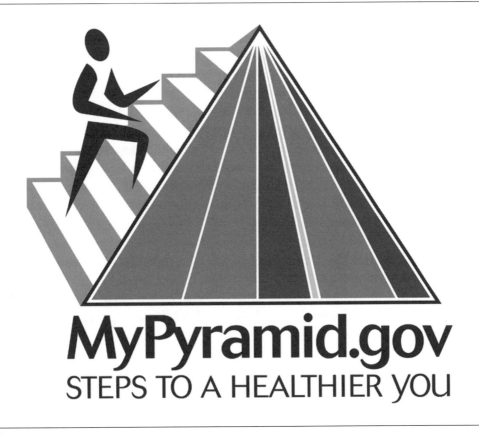

Figure 3.10 The US MyPyramid food guide

Source: United States Department of Agriculture (reproduced with permission)

Nevertheless, there are visual and technical differences among the food selection guides of countries. The foods that are included in food guides reflect the food supply and culture of a particular country. The number of food groupings varies, for example, the guides for some countries combine fruits and vegetables into the one food group and the guides for other countries represent these foods in two distinct groups. Some guides provide advice about the number of serves of various types of food needed to reflect 'foundation' diets, that is they portray core (or nutritious) foods only, and in amounts needed to satisfy minimal nutrient reference intakes. Other guides relate to the total diet, that is they portray both core and non-core (or extra) foods (foods that provide energy but contain insufficient amounts of nutrients to qualify for inclusion in a core food group).

Future priorities in relation to public health nutrition practice

The development of public health nutrient reference standards and guidelines is informed by a combination of the nutrition science evidence base, food technology innovations and policy priorities. The process is dynamic and, as science evolves, the relevance and validity of reference standards and guidelines for public health nutrition practice depends on continual review and development. In turn, as the reference standards and guidelines develop, there will be consequent implications for the diversity of policies and programmes for which they have practical application; for example, food selection guides, food labelling and food fortification programmes would all require consequent review and development.

In this section, we discuss three future priorities for the reference standards and guidelines in relation to public health nutrition practice. We begin by reviewing the need for research to inform and update reference standards, then we consider the possible development of new dietary guidance concepts in accordance with emerging nutrition science knowledge, and finally we consider the challenge to prepare food guides that portray the dynamic nature of the food supply.

Research to inform and update reference standards

Currently, the evidence base that informs reference standards is drawn from a relatively small number of studies, generally with limited numbers of individuals. Inevitably, there are limitations and judgements with the calculation of reference standards; for example, the precise variation in requirement for most nutrients is not known. In the future, the validity of the reference standards for assessing the dietary adequacy of individuals and groups of people will improve as research provides greater knowledge of functional criteria for determining adequacy and physiological processes.

In addition, there will be benefits from increasing our understanding of the bioavailability and safety of traditional nutrients, as well as new dietary components for which recommendations might be established. Also, it will be important to develop more sophisticated research methods, analysis and interpretation procedures to account for possible interactions between nutrients and/or other dietary components in the holistic context of the foods, meals and diets that individuals and groups of people consume; for example, Dupont and Mathias (1994) comment that:

> Reductive strategies for determining nutrient requirements and functions have been
> productive but have led us to think in terms of the paths of a single nutrient, ignoring

its native matrix in food and its complex physical and molecular properties in metabolism. Furthermore, the creation of extremes, such as depletion to severe deficiency and enrichment to excess, leads to massive disruption of physiological processes. Precise causes and effects may be masked by adaptations for survival.

Development of new dietary guidance concepts

The development of dietary guidance has been, and will continue to be, founded in evidence-based practice (Schneeman 2003). Conventional dietary guidance has provided advice for the population based predominantly on epidemiological studies that have identified dietary and physical activity patterns consistent with reduced risk of chronic diseases. However, as the nutrition science evidence base continues to grow, we might anticipate that there may be a need to develop new dietary guideline concepts (Baghurst & Binns 2003). In chapter 1 of this book, an analysis of nutrition science presented the view that the discipline's knowledge base is evolving in the two contrasting directions of molecular nutrition and New Nutrition Science. Proponents of each of these contrasting directions have predicted the need to develop additional types of dietary guidance consistent with their view of public health nutrition.

Advocates of nutrigenomics stress that humans differ in response to diet because of considerable interindividual variations in genetic, epigenetic, and metabolic phenotype status (and the effect on chronic disease risk within the population). They argue that, with tools and knowledge to investigate the molecular basis to genetic variation, researchers will gain understanding of nutrient-specific responses, including genotype expression, which determines the metabolic phenotype that then leads to predispositions to diet-related diseases. This will enable the tailoring of nutritional advice based on a person's specific metabolic profile, that is their personalised dietary recommendations and guidance (Go et al. 2005).

In contrast, proponents of the New Nutrition Science advocate new ways of thinking about food and health relationships, with a need for dietary guidance that is inclusive of social and environmental contexts; for example, Cannon (2003) argues that:

> ... estimations of requirements for protein, and indeed for all nutrients, should derive not just from experiments on animals and humans, but from knowledge of life in the world outside the laboratory, study of long-evolved food systems that produce adequate and varied food supplies, awareness of human evolution, and commitment to sustain not only the human race but also the living and natural world.

It is likely that in future increasing attention will be directed towards evaluating dietary guidelines in terms not only of their nutrient content, but also of the environmental and ethical costs (for example human and animal rights considerations) of implementing the recommended action; for instance, from an environmental perspective, criteria to consider include the cost of food production, processing, packaging, transport, storage and marketing (Gussow & Clancy 1986). The aim should be to support food systems that require less energy for transport and preserve sustainable food production methods. Sweden and their SMART (S: more fruit and vegetables; M: less empty calories; A: more organic food; R: environmentally friendly food products; T: less transport) dietary guidelines and campaign is a good example (see <http://www.folkhalsoguiden.se/Informationsmaterial.aspx?id=1068>). The closer food is grown to where it is consumed, the shorter is its storage and transport time, thus resulting in less loss of nutrients, especially in vegetables and fruit. Improving people's diet in Europe, and elsewhere, requires the promotion of dietary guidelines via information campaigns to be complemented with increased availability, affordability and access to healthy food through political will (Robertson et al. 2006).

Maintaining the relevance of representations in food guides

In the future, more research should be undertaken to find out what types of food guides (and dietary guidelines) are most effective in different circumstances and for specific target groups. As the food supply continues to develop, new challenges will be presented to the principles and concepts underpinning conventional approaches to food guides and how they represent food selection advice. With an increasing diversity of fortified food products and/or novel foods available in the marketplace, does the concept of using characteristic nutrient profiles (and core and non-core foods) as the basis for categorising foods into different food groups become redundant? For example, Beaton questions critically whether it would be appropriate to reconfigure the traditional milk product group to include products such as calcium-fortified citrus drinks (Beaton 2003).

Conclusion

In this chapter, we have compared some of the different reference standards and guidelines that are the cornerstones of public health nutrition policies and programmes. Reference standards for nutrient intakes, dietary goals and guidelines, and food selection guides share a common foundation in that their development is informed by evidence derived from nutrition science. Their establishment is a dynamic process reflecting the assessment and interpretation by experts of the available evidence at a given time. Therefore, the validity of the reference standards and guidelines is dependent on the currency, quality and quantity of the nutrition science evidence base that is available for their ongoing review and development.

Beyond the scientific rigour of their establishment, the utility of the reference standards and guidelines depends upon sufficient professional expertise, resources and mechanisms to enable them to be appropriately interpreted and used in public health nutrition practice. In particular, their application is dependent upon ongoing education of practitioners and the public in what they mean for healthy eating. This education requirement needs to be complemented with regular monitoring of dietary intake and nutrient status, and food composition, to support the reference standards' and guidelines' roles in benchmarking policies and programmes.

REFERENCES

Baghust, K.I. and Binns, C. 2003, 'The role of dietary guidelines: Is it changing?' in *FoodChain*, Strategic Inter-Governmental Nutrition Alliance, vol. 12.

Beaton, G.H. 2003, 'Dietary guidelines: Some issues to consider before initiating revisions' in *Journal of American Dietetic Association*, vol. 103, pp. S56–59.

Canada's Food Guide to Healthy Eating, Health Canada, cited at <http://www.hc-sc.gc.ca/fn-an/food-guide-aliment/index_e.html> on 10 December 2006.

Cannon, G. 2003, 'Fate of Nations', The Caroline Walker Lecture, The Caroline Walker Trust, London.

Chinese Nutrition Society, Food guide pagoda, cited at <http://www.cnsoc.org/asp-bin/EN/?page=8&class= 93&id=145> on 10 December 2006.

CINDI 2000, 'Dietary Guide', World Health Organization Regional Office for Europe, Copenhagen, cited at <http://www.euro.who.int/Document/E7982.pdf> on 10 December 2006.

Codex Alimentarius Commission (Codex) 1997, 'Codex guidelines for the use of nutrition claims CAC/GL 23–1997', adopted at 22nd Session (amended 2001 at 24th Session), FAO/WHO, Rome.

Committee on Medical Aspects of Food Policy (COMA) 1991, 'Dietary reference values for food energy and nutrients for the United Kingdom: Report of the panel on Dietary Reference Values' in *Report on Health and Social Subjects No. 41*, Her Majesty's Stationery Office, London.

— 1994, 'Nutritional Aspects of Cardiovascular Disease' in *Report on Health and Social Subjects No. 48*, Her Majesty's Stationery Office, London.

— 1998, 'Nutritional Aspects of the Development of Cancer' in *Report on Health and Social Subjects No. 48*, Her Majesty's Stationery Office, London.

Commonwealth Department of Health, Housing and Community Services 1992, *Food and Nutrition Policy*, Australian Government Printing Service, Canberra.

Danish Veterinary and Food Administration <http://www.foedevarestyrelsen.dk/FDir/Publications/2005216/Rapport.pdf>, accessed 10 December 2006.

Department of Health and Family Services 1998, *The Australian Guide to Healthy Eating: Background information for nutrition educators*, Canberra, cited at <http://www.health.gov.au/pubhlth/strateg/food/guide/whatis.htm>.

Dupont, J. and Mathias, M.M. 1994, 'Future directions for nutrient requirements: Lipids' in *Journal of Nutrition*, vol. 124, pp. S1743–46.

EURODIET Core Report 2001, 'Nutrition and diet for healthy lifestyles in Europe: Science and policy implications' in *Public Health Nutrition*, vol. 4, pp. 265–74.

Expert Group on Vitamins and Minerals (EVM) 2003, *Safe Upper Levels for Vitamins and Minerals*, Food Standards Agency, Her Majesty's Stationery Office, London.

Faculty of Nutrition and Food Sciences from University of Porto and Portuguese Consumer's Institute. 2003, *Os Alimentos na Roda. Lisboa: Instituto do Consumidor*.

Food Standards Agency (UK), cited at <http://www.food.gov.uk/multimedia/pdfs/eatwell.pdf> on 10 December 2006.

Go, V.L.W., Nguyen, C.T.H., Harris, D.M. and Lee, W-N.P. 2005, 'Nutrient–Gene interaction: Metabolic genotype–phenotype relationship' in *Journal of Nutrition*, vol. 135, pp. S3016–20.

Gussow, J.D. and Clancy, K.L. 1986, 'Dietary guidelines for sustainability' in *Journal of Nutrition Education*, vol. 18, pp. 1–5.

Institute of Medicine (IOM) 1997, *Dietary Reference Intakes for calcium, phosphorus, magnesium, vitamin D, and fluoride*, Food and Nutrition Board, National Academy Press, Washington D.C.

— 1998, *Dietary Reference Intakes for thiamin, riboflavin, niacin, vitamin B6, folate, vitamin B12, pantothenic acid, biotin, and choline*, Food and Nutrition Board, National Academy Press, Washington D.C.

— 2000a, *Dietary Reference Intakes: Applications in dietary assessment*, Food and Nutrition Board, National Academy Press, Washington D.C.

— 2000b, *Dietary Reference Intakes for vitamin C, vitamin E, selenium, and carotenoids*, Food and Nutrition Board, National Academy Press, Washington D.C.

— 2001, *Dietary Reference Intakes for vitamin A, vitamin K, arsenic, boron, chromium, copper, iodine, iron, manganese, molybdenum, nickel, silicon, vanadium, and zinc*, Food and Nutrition Board, National Academy Press, Washington D.C.

— 2002, *Dietary Reference Intakes for energy, carbohydrate, fiber, fat, fatty acids, cholesterol, protein, and amino acids (macronutrients)*, Food and Nutrition Board, National Academy Press, Washington D.C.

— 2004, *Dietary Reference Intakes for water, potassium, sodium, chloride, and sulfate*, Food and Nutrition Board, Food and Nutrition Board, National Academy Press, Washington, D.C.

Lewis, J. and Jeffreson, S. 2000, 'The use of dietary guidelines and recommended dietary intakes in the development of food regulation' in *Australian Journal of Nutrition and Dietetics*, vol. 57, no. 3, pp. 136–38.

Lichtenstein, A.H. and Russell, R.M. 2005, 'Essential nutrients: Food or supplements? Where should the emphasis be?' in *Journal of American Medical Association*, vol. 294, no. 3, pp. 351–58.

National Health and Medical Research Council (NHMRC) 1999, *Dietary Guidelines for Older Australians*, Commonwealth of Australia, Canberra.

— 2003, *Dietary Guidelines for Australian Adults*, Commonwealth of Australia, Canberra.

— 2003, *Dietary Guidelines for Children and Adolescents in Australia: A guide to healthy eating*, Commonwealth of Australia, Canberra.

— 2006, *Nutrient Reference Values for Australia and New Zealand, including Recommended Dietary Intakes*, Commonwealth of Australia, Canberra, cited at <http://www.nhmrc.gov.au/publications/_files/n35.pdf>.

Nordic Council of Ministers (NCM) 2004, *Nordic Nutrition Recommendations* (Fourth edition), vol. 13, Copenhagen.

Painter, J., Rah, J-H. and Lee, Y-K. 2002, 'Comparison of international food guide pictorial representations' in *Journal of American Dietetic Association*, vol. 102, no. 4, pp. 483–90.

Robertson, A., Brunner, E. and Sheiham, A. 2004, *Food and Health in Europe: A new basis for action*, World Health Organization (WHO), Copenhagen, pp. 341–85, cited at <http://www.euro.who.int/eprise/main/who/InformationSources/Publications/Catalogue/ 20040130_8>.

— 2006, 'Food is a political issue' in Marmot, M. and Wilkinson (eds) 2006, *The Social Determinants of Health: Second Edition*, Oxford University Press, Oxford.

Santich, B. 2005, 'Paradigm shifts in the history of dietary advice in Australia' in *Nutrition and Dietetics*, vol. 62, pp. 152–57.

Schneeman, B.O. 2003, 'Evolution of dietary guidelines' in *Journal of American Dietetic Association*, vol. 103, pp. S5–9.

Scientific Committee on Food 1993, *Nutrient and Energy Intakes for the European Community: Report Series no. 31*, Commission of the European Communities, Brussels.

Sociedad Espanola Nutricion Comunitaria. 2004, *Guia de la alimentacion saludable*, Barcelona

Stockley, L. 2001, 'Toward public health nutrition strategies in the European Union to implement food-based dietary guidelines and to enhance healthier lifestyles' in *Public Health Nutrition*, vol. 4, no. 2A, pp. 307–24.

Uauy, R. 2005, 'Defining and addressing the nutritional needs of populations' in *Public Health Nutrition*, vol. 8, pp. 773–80.

United States Department of Agriculture <http://www.mypyramid.gov>, accessed 10 December 2006.

World Health Organization 1998, *Preparation of Food-based Dietary Guidelines: Report of a joint FAO/WHO consultation*, Technical Report Series 880, WHO, Geneva.

—— 2003, *Diet, Nutrition and the Prevention of Chronic Diseases*, Technical Report Series 916, WHO, Geneva, cited at <www.who.int>.

SECTION 2: POPULATIONS

Overview

SIMONE FRENCH

The following section addresses nutrition issues among specific populations defined by the life cycle. Specific biological, social, behavioural and psychological issues are of prominence during older age, adolescence and childhood, and infancy. Scott, Campbell and Davies examine nutritional issues in mothers during pregnancy, and in infants; Brug and Klepp review eating patterns among youth, and interventions that aim to promote healthy eating in children and adolescents; and Hunter, Raats and Lumbers address nutritional issues associated with ageing and health.

Together, these chapters illustrate the important role that food choices and nutrition play at each phase of the life cycle in terms of contribution to biological health and disease prevention. To develop effective promotion interventions, food choices are described in terms of the multiple levels of influence and how these vary across the phases of human development. Certain physiological, social and individual variables may come to the foreground at different phases of the life course.

Among pregnant women, behavioural aspects of nutrition, such as breast-feeding behaviours, have significant influence on infant health. Social norms, behavioural skills, and public and worksite policies represent some of the levels of influence on the adoption and maintenance of breastfeeding behaviours among women with infants. Interventions that can promote and support breast-feeding behaviours among mothers include those that help develop skills around this behaviour, such as hospital-based programmes for mothers and infants. Policies and practices at the worksite and other community settings can support the maintenance of breastfeeding behaviours by providing private spaces for breastfeeding mothers, and by enhancing social normative support through media promotion campaigns.

Among children and adolescents, environmental, behavioural and individual-level variables are prominent influences on food choices, and play an important role in interventions to promote healthy eating patterns. Brug and Klepp highlight the important role of learning and exposure in the development of food preferences, including biological and social-cognitive mechanisms. Behavioural skills and self-efficacy are important socio-cognitive variables that play a role in children's food choices. Individual-level, educational or behavioural interventions may be more effective when implemented in the context of a supportive social and physical environment. Brug and Klepp describe the ANGELO framework, which is used to conceptualise health behaviour environments, and to identify intervention settings and strategies. Environments are scaled on two axes: micro/macro environments; and physical/social/economic environments. The role of neighbourhood, home, school and community environments in shaping children's food choices is described. The Pro Children Study was designed to develop and test intervention strategies to promote fruit and vegetable intake among school children in nine European countries and provides an instructive example of a multi-level intervention that adopts multiple strategies across several settings.

Among older populations, Hunter, Raats and Lumbers convey clearly the importance of multiple levels of influence in dietary quality and food choices. Biological changes that accompany the ageing process uniquely affect nutrition needs. These include a decrease in lean body mass, nutrient absorption, and sense of taste and smell. The decline in taste and smell sensitivity, as well as changes in social and economic living circumstances, may contribute to less healthy food choices and eating patterns. The availability of social networks can foster a greater motivation for healthy eating by more frequent shared-eating settings, rather than eating alone. Social networks can also contribute instrumentally to enhancing access to food. Friends and family may provide transportation to supermarkets and assistance with the food shopping for older people. Changes in food retailing practices, such as the creation of superstores, warehouses and club stores, might uniquely affect older populations by making shopping more difficult in terms of greater distance for transportation to the store, and ability to shop inside the store with taller shelf spaces, larger store square footage, and larger food and beverage package sizes. Food programmes, such as home delivery of meals and prepared frozen convenience meals, are examples of intervention programmes that can support healthy dietary intake among older populations. Data from Food in Later Life, a multinational study of older populations' dietary patterns, provides insights into the environmental, social and interpersonal variables that are most influential on food purchases and consumption in older populations.

4

Mothers and infants

JANE SCOTT
DORIS CAMPBELL
MICHAEL DAVIES

Mothers and infants are among the most nutritionally vulnerable population groups, and nutrition is consistently identified as a major contributor to the health and wellbeing of the mother and the infant, and indeed for later life. Therefore, mothers and infants are priority population groups for public health nutrition policies and programmes. In this chapter, we will concentrate on the importance of adequate nutrition and strategies to improve nutrition during pregnancy and in infancy.

Mothers

Over the years, pregnant women have received advice ranging from needing to eat for two to decreasing food intake to restrict weight gain. Traditionally, the nutritional needs of pregnancy have been computed as no more than the components of the products of conception and their maintenance. This means that the extra requirement for pregnancy should rise as pregnancy progresses *pari passu* with foetal growth. This doesn't take into account however the large number of changes occurring in the maternal body. Pregnancy itself involves a complex interaction of maternal and foetal physiological systems, which presumably ensures that both mother and baby have the best chance of survival, even under conditions of hardship and deprivation. Impaired reproductive performance, as reflected by a high perinatal mortality, has been reported in many deprived populations, both in the developing world and in the slums of better-off countries. This has often been seen as an effect of poor nutrition, but it is remarkable how efficiently the foetus is protected when the mother is malnourished. It is not as simple as the statement 'poor nutrition leads to poor foetal growth' implies. Women with inadequate nutrition during pregnancy have probably always eaten badly, are poorly grown, and in general suffer much disadvantage from poor education, poor housing, general ill-health, an excess of cigarette smoking and the need to do hard physical work, the latter particularly in developing countries.

Nutritional requirements in pregnancy

Normal healthy, pregnant women eating to appetite gain on average 12.5 kilograms over the course of their pregnancy. The components of this increase are shown in Table 4.1. By the end of pregnancy, there remains approximately 3.5 kilograms of weight, which has been shown to be maternal fat stores. This fat serves as an 'energy bank' accumulated during the first two-thirds of pregnancy when foetal growth is relatively slow, to be used as a reserve to support foetal growth in the third trimester of pregnancy, when foetal growth is greatest, and lactation after birth.

Current nutritional recommendations for pregnancy are based on estimates of the cost of supporting the increased maternal tissue mass associated with pregnancy and the delivery of an infant with weight of approximately 3.3 kilogram.

Table 4.1 Components of weight gain during pregnancy for women without generalised oedema

	Increase in weight (grams) up to			
	10 weeks	20 weeks	30 weeks	40 weeks
Foetus	5	300	1500	3400
Placenta	20	170	430	650
Ammotic fluid	30	350	750	800
Uterus	140	320	600	970
Mammary gland	45	180	360	405
Blood	100	600	1300	1250
Extracellular/extravascular fluid	0	30	80	1680
Total weight gained	**650**	**4000**	**8500**	**12 500**
Weight not accounted for	310	2050	3480	3345

Source: Hytten and Leitch 1971

The extra nutritional demands can often be met by maternal adaptation or increased efficiency of utilisation, or from existing nutrient stores. For instance, it is estimated that the total additional energy requirement for the whole of pregnancy is approximately 293 megajoules (MJ) (70 000 kcals). Most studies of pregnant women have, however, failed to demonstrate substantial alterations in energy intake, apparently without adverse effect on outcome, and studies of energy balance in pregnancy have suggested that the specific requirement of pregnancy is less than this calculation (Durnin 1987). The total energy required for pregnancy can be met from two sources – increased dietary intake and diminished energy expenditure. It is likely that both occur in human pregnancy, with each contributing approximately half the specific energy requirement of pregnancy. Reduced energy expenditure is achieved by voluntary reduction in exercise and the taking of more rest, by a general reduction in muscle tone, and a slight general fall in maternal tissue metabolism due to the raised level of thyroid hormones characteristic of pregnancy.

The most recent recommendation for energy intake for the United Kingdom suggests an additional 0.8 MJ (200 kcals) per day over the non-pregnant allowance is reasonable. Such an increase in energy intake would lead to small increases in protein and other specific nutrients, and would most readily be met by the increased food intake that occurs. In women eating to appetite, no study has demonstrated a direct association between energy intake and foetal growth assessed either by crude birthweight or by standardised birthweight, which is adjusted for gestation at delivery, sex and parity, and sometimes for maternal stature.

Nutrition and pregnancy outcome

Birthweight
Infant birthweight is frequently used as an indicator of a successful pregnancy, and a low birthweight (LBW) infant (less than 2500 grams) is considered a poor pregnancy outcome. On assessing the impact of nutrition on foetal growth, it is important not just to consider birthweight, but also to examine the effect of gestation at delivery. Babies born early, that is preterm, are smaller than their counterparts born at term, and low birthweight due to preterm delivery should be considered separately from low birthweight due to intrauterine growth retardation (IUGR). In the developed world, relatively few live births (approximately 6 per cent) are LBW, and the majority of these are due to preterm delivery. In contrast, in developing countries LBW is relatively common, affecting about one-fifth of all newborns, and is a particular problem in the Indian

subcontinent. It is associated with early mortality and morbidity, adverse long-term outcomes, and perpetuates the intergenerational cycle of poverty, under-nutrition and disease (Figure 4.1).

There is evidence that a mother's own birthweight influences infant birth size, independent of her current weight, or other factors known to influence birthweight. In addition to gestational age, parity and sex of the baby, maternal anthropometry (short stature, low body mass index (BMI) and low weight gain during pregnancy, are major determinants of IUGR (WHO 1995). Small, short women tend to have small but appropriately grown babies, whereas low weight gain in pregnancy has been associated with IUGR. Because the most favourable outcome of pregnancy with respect to the development of preeclampsia, IUGR and perinatal deaths is associated with a weight gain of approximately 450 grams per week, health professionals have aimed to keep

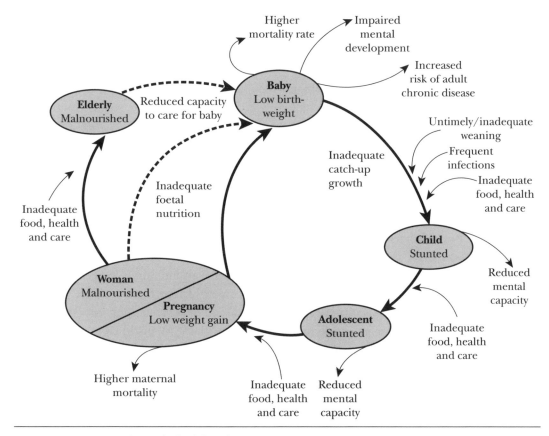

Figure 4.1 Nutrition through the lifecycle

Source: Commission on the Nutrition Challenges of the Twenty-first Century 2000

weight as close to that average as possible by manipulating the diet with nutritional advice. This is clearly illogical. Low weight gain and poor foetal growth are both part of a poor general response to pregnancy. Poor weight gain, particularly in the second trimester may be used as a predictor of poor foetal growth in antenatal care.

In addition to an association with birthweight, maternal anthropometry has been associated with a number of other adverse pregnancy outcomes. Low pre-pregnancy BMI has been associated with an increased risk of having a preterm delivery (Kramer et al. 2000). Conversely, pre-pregnancy obesity has also been associated with a significantly higher frequency of preterm births (Hellerstedt et al. 1997), a higher Caesarean section rate (Brost et al. 1997), as well as an increased risk for neural tube defects (Shaw et al. 2000).

Factors contributing to poor foetal growth and low birthweight are numerous, including socioeconomic and health-related issues that are beyond the scope of this discussion, but it is unlikely that nutrition during pregnancy itself is a major contribution.

Preeclampsia

Preeclampsia, a disease with major mortality and morbidity for the mother and IUGR for the infant, is associated with an above-average weight increase in pregnancy and a relatively high-energy intake. Excess weight gain may be a useful antenatal indicator of developing the disease. In the past, therefore, dietary restriction was advocated in the belief that limiting the amount of weight gain in pregnancy by decreasing energy intake would be beneficial. There is no substantive evidence that dietary restriction aimed at producing very low weight gain during pregnancy has any beneficial effect on the incidence of preeclampsia. Such advice in fact may be detrimental, as evidence from Aberdeen (Campbell & MacGillvray 1975) and Motherwell (Campbell-Brown 1983), Scotland, shows that iatrogenic dietary and energy limitation leads to a depression in foetal growth, as measured by birth weight for gestational age.

Theoretically, calcium supplementation could prevent high blood pressure through a number of mechanisms. To date, there is insufficient evidence to support routine calcium supplementation for all pregnant women, but it may be beneficial for women at high risk of developing gestational preeclampsia or gestational hypertension, or in communities with very low dietary calcium intake prior to pregnancy (Atallah et al. 2002).

A current theory of the aetiology of preeclampsia suggests that oxidative stress is a component of this life-threatening condition and that antioxidants could be used in its prevention. Although pilot studies of supplementation with vitamins C and E have been promising, no direct association has been shown between the amount of antioxidants (mainly vitamins C and E) in the diet and subsequent preeclampsia. Recently one of the large trials of supplementations with vitamins C and E reported no benefit but possible harm was found (Briley et al. 2006).

Anaemia of pregnancy

Physiological changes of pregnancy result in profound changes in the maternal haematological system (Letsky 1998). Plasma volume increases progressively, reaching a peak by the third trimester, which is about 45 per cent above non-pregnant values. The total red cell mass increases proportionately less, by about 18 to 25 per cent. The net result is haemodulation, and hence a decline in haemoglobin concentration, packed cell volume and red cell count. In the absence of iron deficiency the mean cell haemoglobin concentration remains at non-pregnant values, and there is a slight increase in mean cell volume. As a result of these changes, anaemia cannot be diagnosed in pregnancy using the criteria applied to non-pregnant individuals. As haemoglobin values of less than 10.5 grams per decilitre (g/dl) in the second and third trimesters of pregnancy are probably indicative of pathology, WHO recommends that haemoglobin concentration should not fall below the 11 g/dl at any time during pregnancy, and accordingly supplements should be given. Controlled trials of routine oral iron supplementation for all pregnant women do result in fewer women with a low haemoglobin at birth or six weeks post-partum, but demonstrate little benefit on maternal wellbeing or perinatal outcome (Mahomed 2000). There is a lack of data from countries where iron deficiency is common and anaemia is a serious health problem.

Congenital abnormality

It is now policy in many developed countries to recommend that women contemplating pregnancy should take folic acid supplements of 400 micrograms daily to prevent the occurrence of neural tube defects. A recent review has suggested that such supplementation reduced the incidence of neural tube defects, but did not significantly increase spontaneous abortion, ectopic pregnancy or stillbirth, although there was a possible increase in multiple pregnancies (Lumley et al. 2001). This latter incidence is of concern because of the much poorer outcome for neonates resulting from multiple births. There is evidence that this may be linked to a very high intake of folate, particularly among women undergoing infertility treatment where multiple pregnancies are a common consequence of returning multiple embryos to the uterus during treatment (Haggarty et al. 2006). However, once the effect of assisted conceptions is accounted for, the effect of folate on the risk of twinning is small, and has been estimated to produce two additional twin pregnancies per 10 000 gestations per year (Signore et al. 2005). Increases in folate consumption need to be considered in the debate regarding folic acid fortification of the food supply, as dietary intake would then be further increased.

Studies of pregnant women in the United Kingdom (Mathews & Neil 1998) have shown their mean or median folate intake from food sources to be below the recommended nutrient intake (RNI) for non-pregnant women, and well below the RNI of 400 micrograms for pregnant women. Folic acid needs to be taken both pre-conceptionally and during the first twelve weeks of pregnancy for maximum effect. Given that as many as 50 per cent of pregnancies in western countries are unplanned, most women do not begin folic acid supplementation until their pregnancy is confirmed. This, coupled with the low routine intake of folate-rich foods, has led to the call for mandatory fortification of the food supply with folic acid, which is the subject of continued debate, and the ethical dilemma associated with this policy approach is discussed in more detail in chapter 1.

Severe maternal iodine deficiency results in increased pregnancy loss and mental retardation and cretinism in offspring (Ramakrishnan et al. 1999). Iodine remains an important nutrient for pregnant women in those countries where deficiency is still common, as well for women from some developed countries such as Australia, where the re-emergence of iodine deficiency has been reported in certain areas (Guttikonda et al. 2002). It therefore seems prudent for women to use iodised salt during pregnancy in such areas.

An adequate vitamin supply is necessary for normal foetal development, and studies are needed to investigate the associations between nutrition and developmental abnormalities in the periconceptional period, as with folic acid, or very early in pregnancy when organogenesis occurs. Changing dietary practices with consumption of less meat and more refined foodstuffs may mean that sub-optimal trace element and vitamin nutrition is present in western populations, as well as in areas with known low dietary intake. Vitamin D deficiency may occur during pregnancy to the extent that it results in maternal osteomalacia, and may upset foetal calcium metabolism. This is particularly so in women who spend most of their time indoors with little exposure to sunlight; however, there is no evidence of benefit of supplementation during pregnancy above amounts routinely required to prevent vitamin D deficiency (Specker 2004). Likewise, there is no evidence of either vitamin or trace element deficiency and an adverse effect on pregnancy outcome in most pregnant women in Britain and other western countries. It is therefore unsurprising that supplementation with such vitamins and minerals have no effect in pregnancy.

Nutrition and the foetal origins of adult-health hypothesis

Until this point, our discussion has focused on the relation of nutrition in pregnancy and immediate pregnancy outcomes, but it is now widely accepted that foetal nutrition has enduring influences on health during childhood and adulthood, with possible effects into the next generation. This concept is not new, and the scientific literature both in animals and humans is replete with examples of teratagens (an agent or factor causing malformation of an embryo), micronutrient deficiencies, and the risk of congenital abnormalities and related developmental defects. We need only consider iodine deficiency and cretinism, foetal alcohol syndrome, or gross energy malnutrition. There has, however, been a significant shift in our understanding of the relationship between foetal–maternal nutrition and the health of the offspring, particularly with regard to the range of potential outcomes, the latency between pregnancy and health effects, and the type of exposure that may be of importance. Outcomes of interest now include cardiovascular disease and type 2 diabetes. Work in this area was stimulated greatly by the hypotheses of David Barker and colleagues, which placed maternal nutrition in pregnancy in a central role for the aetiology of diabetes and cardiovascular disease (Barker 1998).

Early work demonstrated the geographical pattern of death rates for babies born in Britain during the early 1900s was similar to the geographical pattern of death rates for coronary heart disease in the 1980s (Barker & Osmond 1986). Subsequent studies sought more direct evidence from other cohorts internationally, from living cohorts in addition to the deceased, from survivors of natural experiments such as the Dutch Hunger Winter (the forced starvation of the Dutch population during the seven-month German blockade over the severe winter of 1944–45), and from large cohorts for which data were collected for unrelated reasons, such as the Nurse's Health Study (Rich-Edwards et al. 1999). These epidemiological studies consistently show that individuals who were small at birth have an increased risk of type 2 diabetes and cardiovascular disease in adulthood (Grivetti et al. 1998; Newsome et al. 2003). Results implicate small size for gestational age, rather than preterm delivery.

More recently, the relevance of the environmental context and experiences that span the time from maternal peri-conception through infancy has been recognised. This has given rise to the broader concept of developmental plasticity (Barker 2004; Bateson et al. 2004) and an appreciation of the interaction of pre- and postnatal exposures (Rich-Edwards et al. 2005). Hence, it now suggested that uterine environmental factors, in particular, poor nutrition, might not only influence the relationship between placental weight and birthweight, but also would continue to exert influence into adult life, making individuals more susceptible to the development of cardiovascular disease (Barker 2003). While the experimental evidence in animal models has become compelling (Ozanne 2001; Ozanne et al. 2004; McMillan & Robinson 2005), evidence within free-living human populations is generally poorer. In large part, this is due to the difficulty of conceptualising and assessing the critical dietary exposures within an epidemiological context, the overly focused attention on birthweight as a crude proxy for foetal nutrition, the use of risk factors rather than disease outcomes, and the difficulties in conducting studies of sufficient size and precision for the outcomes of interest (Rich-Edwards et al. 2005).

Nevertheless, within the Generation 1 cohort from Adelaide, the diet of 557 women was assessed at 16 and 30 to 34 weeks of pregnancy, using interviews structured around a semi-quantitative food frequency questionnaire (Moore et al. 2004). The proportion of energy derived from protein in early pregnancy was positively associated with birthweight and placental weight. These effects were stronger in a subset of women considered to have reliable dietary data (n = 429), based on criteria including plausibility when considered in relation to estimated energy expenditure. Within this subset, ponderal index of the baby was also related negatively to the proportion of energy from carbohydrate in early and late pregnancy. Associations were independent of pre-pregnancy weight, pregnancy weight gain, and other potential confounders, including maternal age, height and smoking. The potential for effects to become increasingly apparent under conditions of improved methodological rigour indicate the possibility that null effects in other studies may be due in part to limitations in instrumentation related to the assessment of diet in human populations.

Hence, while the early proliferation of papers related to crude birthweight and various disease entities gave rise to concern over the meaning of relationships, such as that of birthweight and blood pressure (Paneth & Susser 1995), more exhaustive follow-up to death in a very large cohort has confirmed the significance of the original hypothesis (Rich-Edwards et al. 2005).

Dietary intervention in pregnancy
There are two contexts in which dietary intervention might be considered during pregnancy. First, the importance of long-term nutrition and reproductive performance, and second, the impact of acute changes during the course of pregnancy.

Dietary restriction in pregnancy

Acute changes in nutrition, such as occur during famine, relate mainly to a massive fall in conception rates due to amenorrhoea in women and azospermia in men. In those women who do become pregnant, the foetuses grow reasonably well, although there is a deficit in foetal weight, due mainly to loss of subcutaneous fat. This was exemplified in the Dutch Hunger Winter during the Second World War (Susser & Stein 1994).

In western developed countries, the major threat posed to pregnant women is the increasing level of obesity among women of childbearing age. As noted earlier, however, restricting dietary intake during pregnancy in well-nourished communities in women with excess weight gain of varying pre-pregnant body statures is not beneficial, and is detrimental to foetal growth (Kramer & Kakuma 2003). Strategies to address this problem are best targeted outside of pregnancy.

Overall, the impact of acute change in nutrition during pregnancy – for example, on perinatal mortality – is slight, and studies with subsequent follow-up of the offspring to adulthood have failed to show any adverse effect on physical or mental development. This is in contrast to findings in communities that are chronically malnourished. Much of the work from the National Institution of Nutrition in Hyderabad, India, suggests that women belonging to a low socioeconomic group have a very poor dietary intake throughout their lives and during pregnancy. In these situations, the outcome of pregnancy is frequently unfavourable, with low birthweights. This has also been reported from other countries, including Thailand and Central America. Clearly, the impact of famine or acute starvation in such populations is likely to have a devastating effect on reproductive performance.

Supplementation in pregnancy

On account of the noted association between poor nutrition and poor foetal growth, many attempts have been made to increase pregnant women's diet with supplementation. A systematic review of trials involving balanced energy–protein supplementation reported modest but statistically significant increases in mean maternal weight gain (~21 grams/week) and in mean birthweight (approximately 38 grams). Such differences are not clinically significant. A substantial reduction is risk of small for gestational age (SGA) birth (relative risk of 0.68, with a 95 per cent confidence interval of 0.56 to 0.84) was however noted. In studies involving women suspected of IUGR, maternal nutrient supplementation did not alter the numbers of SGA infants (Say et al. 2003).

High protein supplementation in pregnancy is also not advocated, as it confers no benefit for pregnancy outcome, but may lead to an increased risk of neonatal death (Kramer & Kakuma 2003). Such small changes in birthweight in these women, supplemented in non-famine conditions, is not likely to be mediated by maternal energy deposition, and the hypothesis that maternal macronutrient status leads to an increased maternal weight and/or weight gain leading to increased foetal growth and improved survival is no longer tenable (Rush 2001).

Effectiveness of nutritional advice in pregnancy

There is evidence that dietary intervention strategies targeted at pregnant women are effective in achieving modest dietary change. A systematic review of controlled trials of dietary advice to increase energy and protein intake indicates that such interventions are successful in achieving these dietary goals, but no consistent benefit was observed on pregnancy outcomes such as maternal weight gain, foetal growth and gestational duration (Kramer & Kakuma 2003).

Dietary guidelines for pregnancy

While the scientific literature fails to show a clear relationship between maternal nutrition and pregnancy outcome, common sense indicates that women entering pregnancy should consume a diet that is nutritionally adequate to meet the theoretical costs of a successful pregnancy and the delivery of a term infant with a weight of approximately 3.5 kilograms. Women, if eating to appetite, should have little difficulty in meeting the increased energy demands of pregnancy, which, as previously discussed, are relatively small. Women (and their partners) should be guided towards the consumption of a variety of foods, as suggested in the food selection guides (see chapter 3). Meat, poultry, seafood, legumes and nuts are important sources of protein, as well as zinc, iron and magnesium. Wholegrain cereals, leafy green and yellow vegetables, and fruit are important sources of vitamins and fibre. Dairy products are an important source of calcium as well as a range of other nutrients, including protein, vitamin B12, riboflavin, phosphorus, magnesium, potassium, zinc, selenium and iodine. Women with a medically diagnosed allergy to cows' milk should take particular care to ensure that their calcium requirements are met (for example, by consuming calcium-fortified foods and drinks). If a pregnant woman increases her dietary intake to meet her increased energy needs and makes good food choices, then vitamin and mineral supplementation is generally not necessary.

Pregnancy and the months after childbirth offer opportunities (or 'teachable moments') for health practitioners to advise women and their families about food and health issues. The American Dietetic Association's position statement

(Kaiser et al. 2002) provides further information on the key components of a health-promoting lifestyle during pregnancy.

Food safety and pregnancy
In addition to ensuring that they eat a nutritionally adequate diet, pregnant women should take steps to avoid contracting listeria infection. While uncommon, the consequences if contracted during pregnancy are especially serious and can lead to miscarriage, still birth and premature birth. The listeria bacteria are found in nature and in some foods (Box 4.1).

Infants

A small number of preventable causes are responsible internationally for more than ten million deaths of children younger than five years (under-five deaths) each year. Infants less than twelve months of age are particularly vulnerable to these conditions, and account for a large proportion of these deaths. Under-

---

BOX 4.1 STEPS TO AVOIDING LISTERIA IN PREGNANCY

- Avoid eating:
    - soft cheeses such as brie, camembert and ricotta (these are safe if cooked and served hot)
    - takeaway cooked, diced chicken (as used in chicken sandwiches)
    - cold meat
    - pate
    - pre-prepared and stored salads (packaged or from salad bars)
    - raw seafood such as oysters and sashimi
    - smoked seafood such as smoked salmon, smoked oysters (canned are safe).

- Cook foods properly. If reheating food in the microwave, make sure it is steaming hot throughout.

- Only eat food that is hot, do not eat food that is lukewarm.

- Do not eat food that has been prepared and then stored in a refrigerator for more than twelve hours.

- Practice good food hygiene.

Source: Australia New Zealand Food Authority, see www.anzfa.gov.au

---

nutrition is an underlying factor in approximately half of these deaths (Caulfield et al. 2004). Feasible prevention and treatment interventions are available for each of these primary causes and, if universally applied, could prevent more than 60 per cent of under-five deaths each year (Table 4.2). As a group, four nutrition interventions, including exclusive breastfeeding, complementary feeding, vitamin A, and zinc supplementation, could save about 2.4 million lives each year (Jones et al. 2003). In this section, we discuss the first two of these interventions: breastfeeding and complementary feeding practices.

Breastfeeding

Breastfeeding is recognised internationally as the optimal way to feed infants, and the WHO advises that infants should be exclusively breastfed for the first six months of life, and that breastfeeding should continue into the second year of life, and beyond (Kramer & Kakuma 2002). The universal adoption of this recommendation could prevent 13 per cent of under-five deaths annually, primarily through the prevention of diarrhoea and pneumonia (Jones et al. 2003). Formula-fed infants are at increased risk of gastrointestinal, respiratory and inner-ear infection in both developed and developing countries (Labbok et al. 2004). While infants in developed countries do not commonly die from these infections, formula-fed infants nevertheless experience a greater incidence and severity of these infections requiring medical intervention, which places an unnecessary economic burden on the healthcare system (Weimer 2001).

HIV and breastfeeding

Every year, about 700 000 children become infected with HIV via transmission from their parents, approximately one-third of these from breastfeeding. However, babies who are breastfed by HIV-positive mothers have only a 10 to 20 per cent chance of becoming infected. On the other hand, babies who are not breastfed are six times more likely to die from diarrhoea and respiratory infections than babies who are breastfed (UNICEF 2005b). Therefore, the risk of HIV transmission needs to be weighed against the risk of an infant dying from undernutrition and infections related to replacement feeding. The Interagency recommendations (UNFPA/UNICEF/WHO/UNAIDS Interagency Team 2001) for feeding infants born to HIV-positive women are presented in Box 4.2.

As noted, most infants of HIV-positive mothers do not become infected if breastfed, and there is evidence that the vertical transmission of HIV through breast milk is dependent on the pattern of breastfeeding and not simply on

Table 4.2 Under-five deaths that could be prevented through universal coverage of individual interventions with sufficient or limited evidence of effect on reducing mortality

	Diarrhoea	Pneumonia	Measles	Malaria	HIV/AIDS	Birth asphyxia	Preterm delivery	Neonatal teanus	Neonatal sensis	Estimated number of under-5 deaths prevented §	
Preventive intervention										Number of deaths (×10³)	Percentage of all deaths
Breastfeeding*	1	1							1	1301	13
Insecticide treated materials				1			1			691	7
Complementary feeding	1	1	1	1						587	6
Zinc	1	1		2						459	5
Clean delivery								1	1	411	4
Hib vaccine#		1								403	4
Water, sanitation, hygiene	1									326	3
Antenatal steroids							1			264	3
Newborn temperature management							2			227	2
Vitamin A	1		2	2						225	2
Tetanus toxoid								1		161	2
Nevirapine and replacement feeding					1					150	2
Antibiotics for premature rupture of membranes							2		2	133	1
Measles vaccine			1							103	1
Antimalarial intermittent preventive treatment in pregnancy							1			22	< 1
Treatment interventions											
Oral rehydration therapy	1									1477	15
Antibiotics for sepsis									1	583	6
Antibiotics for pneumonia		1								577	6
Antimalarials				1						467	5
Zinc	1									394	4
Newborn resuscitation						2				359	4
Antibiotics for dysentery	1									310	3
Vitamin A			1							8	< 1

Notes: 1 = Level 1 (sufficient) evidence; 2 = Level 2 (limited) evidence
§ = Numbers represent effect if both levels 1 and 2 evidence are included
* = Exclusive breastfeeding in the first 6 months of life and continued breastfeeding from 6 to 11 months
# = Hib = *Haemophilus influenzae* type b
Source: based on data from Jones et al. 2003

Box 4.2 Recommendations for feeding of infants born to HIV-infected mothers

- When replacement feeding is acceptable, feasible, affordable, sustainable and safe, avoidance of all breastfeeding by HIV-infected mothers is recommended. Otherwise, exclusive breastfeeding is recommended during the first months of life.

- To minimise HIV transmission risk, breastfeeding should be discontinued as soon as feasible, taking into account local circumstances, the individual woman's situation, and the risks of replacement feeding (including infections other than HIV and malnutrition).

- When HIV-infected mothers choose not to breastfeed from birth or stop breastfeeding later, they should be provided with specific guidance and support for at least the first two years of the child's life to ensure adequate replacement feeding. Programmes should strive to improve conditions that will make replacement feeding safer for HIV-infected mothers and families.

Source: UNFPA/UNICEF/WHO/UNAIDS Interagency Team 2001

---

breastfeeding per se (Coutsoudis & Rollins 2003). Studies have shown that babies who are exclusively breastfed have lower rates of HIV infection than those who are partially breastfed. Similarly, the risk of infection increases with duration of breastfeeding, and infants who are breastfed for six months have about one-third the risk of HIV infection of children who breastfeed for two years. There is also some evidence that transmission of HIV is greatest among women who have breast conditions including mastitis, breast abscess and nipple fissure, or who are in some other way immuno-compromised.

Contraceptive effect of breastfeeding

Breastfeeding through hormonal mechanisms exerts a natural contraceptive effect and for millions of couples worldwide is the only form of contraception available to them. It is estimated that in sub-Saharan Africa, where breastfeeding levels are high, that approximately 50 per cent more births would occur if there were no breastfeeding (Becker et al. 2003). Through its contraceptive effect, exclusive and prolonged breastfeeding increases the interval between births. This has a direct effect on infant mortality, as a short birth interval carries an increased risk of undernutrition and death for subsequent siblings (Rutstein 2005). It should be emphasised, however, that breastfeeding is not a reliable form of contraception.

Long-term health outcomes associated with breastfeeding

Since the early 2000s, research attention has focused on the potential long-term benefits of breastfeeding in childhood and beyond. Numerous systematic reviews have investigated, among other things, the association of breastfeeding and cognitive development (Drane & Logemann 2000), atopy (Gdalevich et al. 2001), obesity (Arenz et al. 2004; Harder et al. 2005), blood pressure (Martin et al. 2005a), cholesterol levels (Owen et al. 2002) and risk of cancers (Martin et al. 2005b). Most of these studies have demonstrated either a small protective or a null effect of breastfeeding on these outcomes in later life. These effects, although small, may have important public health benefits.

Barriers to breastfeeding

The reasons women decide to initiate breastfeeding and subsequently discontinue breastfeeding are complex and multifactorial, and probably differ in developed and developing countries. In general, in industrialised countries breastfeeding rates are lowest in young, less-educated women from socially deprived groups. Conversely, in developing countries, breastfeeding rates are the highest among less-educated women in rural communities and lowest among better-educated women living in urban areas. Even in traditional societies where the initiation of breastfeeding is almost universal and the duration of breastfeeding extends into the third year of life, few infants are exclusively breastfed, as recommended, for the first six months of life. It has been estimated that in more than 70 per cent of non-industrialised populations, infants are typically supplemented with non-breast milk liquids before six months of age, and often within the first few weeks of life. Furthermore, in 50 per cent of these populations, infants are typically introduced to complementary solid foods before six months (Sellen 2001).

Much of the blame for the rapid decline in breastfeeding experienced in western countries during the 1950s and 60s has been attributed to the hospitalisation of childbirth, and routines that favoured artificial feeding. New mothers were cared for usually by male obstetricians and pre-maternal nurses, neither having first-hand knowledge of breast-feeding (Millard 1990), thus limiting the opportunities for mothers to learn in hospital the art of breast-feeding, which was traditionally handed down from mother to daughter or from older sister to younger sister. The loss of these generations of breastfeeding women is still being felt today in western populations where women may lack successful breastfeeding role models. As a result, many women have lost confidence in their ability to feed their infant, and doubt both the adequacy of the quality and quantity of their breast milk.

In developing countries, a decline in breastfeeding has been associated with increasing urbanisation and the perception by some mothers that bottle-feeding is 'modern' — a notion that has been actively promoted by the unscrupulous marketing of breast milk substitutes by international formula manufacturers.

Strategies to promote breastfeeding

WHO International Code of Marketing of Breast Milk Substitutes

In 1981, the WHO adopted the International Code of Marketing of Breast Milk Substitutes (WHO Code) to control the marketing of infant formula to mothers and health professionals. The WHO Code prohibits certain aggressive infant formula marketing strategies, such as:

- promoting infant formula through healthcare facilities
- lobbying healthcare personnel with free gifts
- providing free formula samples to new mothers
- using words or pictures in advertising which idealise bottle-feeding.

Despite the existence of the WHO Code, numerous examples of code violations are reported each year (IBFAN 2004).

Baby Friendly Hospital Initiative

The Baby Friendly Hospital Initiative (BFHI), launched in 1991, is a joint initiative of UNICEF and the WHO to improve breastfeeding rates worldwide. The requirements for achieving baby-friendly status by maternity services are listed in Box 4.3.

Since its initiation, more than 15 000 facilities in 134 countries have been awarded BFHI status. In Cuba and China, which have large numbers of BFHI facilities, more women are initiating breastfeeding, and the rates of exclusive breastfeeding have more than doubled (UNICEF 2005a). In a randomised, controlled trial in the Republic of Belarus, 'BFHI designation was associated with a significantly increased duration and degree (exclusivity) of breastfeeding, and decreased risk of gastrointestinal tract infection and atopic eczema in the first year of life' (Kramer et al. 2001).

Other breastfeeding-promotion strategies

The success of other strategies to promote and support breastfeeding differs between developing and developed countries. There is general consensus that didactic health education interventions providing factual or technical information about breastfeeding are of limited value. In particular, written materials alone do not increase breastfeeding rates, and have only limited impact on

---

BOX 4.3 BABY FRIENDLY INITIATIVE IN MATERNITY SERVICES
TEN STEPS TO SUCCESSFUL BREASTFEEDING

1. Have a written breastfeeding policy that is routinely communicated to all healthcare staff.
2. Train all healthcare staff in the skills necessary to implement the breastfeeding policy.
3. Inform all pregnant women about the benefits and management of breastfeeding.
4. Help mothers initiate breastfeeding soon after birth.
5. Show mothers how to breastfeed and how to maintain lactation, even if they are separated from their babies.
6. Give newborn infants no food or drink other than breast milk, unless medically indicated.
7. Practice rooming-in — allowing mothers and infants to remain together 24 hours a day.
8. Encourage breastfeeding on demand.
9. Give no artificial teats or dummies to breastfeeding infants.
10. Foster the establishment of breastfeeding support groups and refer mothers to them on discharge from hospital or clinic.

Source: http://www.unicef.org/programme/breastfeeding/baby.htm

---

breastfeeding rates when combined with a more formal, non-interactive method of health education. However, small, informal group health education classes delivered in the antenatal period can be effective in increasing initiation rates, and in some cases the duration of breastfeeding, among women from different income or ethnic groups (Fairbank et al. 2000).

In recent years, peer support programmes and interventions that involve a woman's partner have become increasingly popular. The design of the majority of peer support programmes reported in the literature does not allow for critical evaluation. However, there is some evidence from a few well-designed studies, conducted in both developing and developed countries, that peer support programmes can increase both the initiation of breastfeeding and the duration of exclusive breastfeeding. Programmes involving fathers are based on the premise that partners act as important supports or deterrents to breastfeeding. While there have been frequent calls for the increased participation of partners in existing antenatal breastfeeding interventions, and for interventions specially targeted at partners, relatively few trials have been reported or adequately evaluated. Again, there is some promising evidence that programmes of this kind can increase both the initiation and duration of breastfeeding (Scott 2005).

Family friendly workplaces and policies

Women's involvement in the workforce has also been identified as a deterrent to breastfeeding. In particular, return to employment has been negatively associated with breastfeeding duration. Although there is not a simple relationship between a country's breastfeeding rates and labour policy, Galtry (2003) contends that a country's breastfeeding rates are influenced by, and reflected in, its maternity leave programme. More generous maternity leave provisions in the form of statutory paid leave for both permanent and casual employees may enable women to remain at home with their infants for longer periods. In the absence of this, more flexible working conditions, including increased opportunities for part-time work, improved conditions at work for breastfeeding, and breastfeeding breaks at work will help support breastfeeding among women who work outside the home.

Finally, many breastfeeding mothers find that the external environment (outside their homes) is not conducive to breastfeeding. Workplaces, for example, usually do not provide quiet, private rooms for breastfeeding, and some actively oppose it (McIntyre et al. 1999). Similarly, shops, restaurants, bus and rail terminals, and airports often do not provide adequate facilities. This lack of conducive environments often convinces mothers that it is more practical to cease breastfeeding relatively soon after birth. To address this problem, the Australian Department of Health and Aged Care has created an information kit for businesses about ways in which they can provide supportive environments for women to breastfeed. The kit also includes signs, which can identify premises as baby friendly. For such environmental changes to become widespread, advocacy and awareness-raising programmes are required to shift societal norms about the acceptability of breastfeeding in public. In some countries, legislation has been introduced to protect a woman's right to breastfeed in public and to tackle negative societal attitudes to breastfeeding.

Complementary feeding practices

From around six months of age, the nutritional needs of infants can no longer be met solely by breast milk. The WHO recommends that, from six months up to two years, infants should receive complementary food together with breastfeeding. These first two years of life are a critical period for achieving optimum growth and mental development.

The introduction of complementary foods signals the start of an infant's transition from milk feeds to consuming household foods. In poorer populations, growth faltering among infants often occurs shortly after this transition begins, as most households do not have access to the types of foods needed to meet the nutritional needs of young children, for either economic, cultural or educational reasons. Many traditional weaning foods are based on plants, cereals or roots. They are often nutritionally inadequate in energy density, protein and micronutrients such as vitamin A, calcium, iron and zinc, and may contain digestive enzyme inhibitors and other anti-nutritive factors such as phytates and tannins, which inhibit mineral bioavailability (Mensah & Tomkins 2003). Complementary foods are often introduced too early or too late, and may be prepared, stored and fed to children in ways that increase their risk of illness and death (Caulfield et al. 1999). In many groups, the introduction of complementary feeding results in a reduction in breastfeeding, with some children receiving fewer nutrients from complementary feeds than that provided by breast milk feeds, and the need for maintenance of breastfeeding should be emphasised.

Interventions to improve intake of complementary foods
Interventions to improve intake of complementary foods by infants in developing countries have been successful in improving the energy intake and growth of infants (Caulfield et al. 1999). Successful programmes are those that use a comprehensive approach that combines mass media (radio and/or print) and one-on-one counselling (Box 4.4).

BOX 4.4 COMMON FEATURES OF SUCCESSFUL COMPLEMENTARY FEEDING PROGRAMMES

- Programmes are designed with an understanding of the key context conditions and determinants of current behaviours.
- Communities are involved in the design of programmes that are responsive to the context and local values.
- Programme content is built upon current local practices, beliefs and concerns.
- Mothers are provided with simple *action-oriented* information that is *age-appropriate* and that changes as their infant grows.
- Food products or recipes are culturally appropriate, affordable, and quick and easy to prepare.
- Messages reflect the fact that mothers need advice and information not only on what to feed, but also on how to feed their infants.

Source: Caulfield et al. 1999; Pelto et al. 2003

The causes of malnutrition in infants are multifactorial, and include the immediate causes of inadequate dietary intake and disease associated with a variety of underlying causes, including poverty, food security, access to health care, and sanitation and hygiene. Maternal education is a key determinant of good caregiving behaviours, and there is evidence to suggest that better educated women have a greater awareness of the needs of their child, which in turns leads to changes in childcare behaviours. Associated with this is the gender gap, which exist in many South Asian countries, where significantly more female children aged less than five years are likely to be severely malnourished than male children. In these countries, female children are often discriminated against in intra-family food distribution and healthcare. Policies and programmes aimed at improving infant nutrition must not only target directly inappropriate feeding practices but also the underlying causes of low levels of female literacy.

Monitoring the growth of infants and children
In 2006, the WHO released its new Child Growth Standards for infants and children up to the age of five (see www.who.int/childgrowth/en/). The new Standards are the result of the Multicentre Growth Reference Study (MGRS) initiated by the WHO in 1997 and conducted in Brazil, Ghana, India, Norway, Oman and the United States. The 8440 children included in the study, while from diverse cultures, were all raised in environments that promote healthy growth, such as breastfeeding, good diets, and prevention and control of infections. In addition, their mothers followed healthcare practices such as not smoking during and after pregnancy, and ensuring adequate healthcare for the children. The standards are based on the breastfed infant as the normative growth standard, and show how every child in the world should grow. They prove that children born in different regions of the world and given the optimum start in life have the potential to grow and develop to within the same range of height and weight for age, and that differences in children's growth are influenced more by nutrition, feeding practices, environment and healthcare than gender or ethnicity. There are more than 30 Child Growth Standard charts, which include for the first time standardised BMI charts for infants to age five, which will be useful for monitoring the increasing epidemic of childhood obesity.

Conclusions

It is now widely accepted that foetal nutrition has enduring influences on health during childhood and adulthood, with possible effects into the next generation.

While the relationship between foetal nutrition and maternal dietary intake is unclear, women should be encouraged to make good dietary selections in line with current dietary guidelines for adults.

Exclusive breastfeeding to six months of age, followed by the timely introduction of safe and nutritionally adequate complementary foods, would prevent close to two million under-five deaths annually.

Targeted nutrition-intervention programmes alone cannot address the problem of under-nutrition in mothers and infants. Nutrition programmes need to be conducted in concert with policies and programmes that address poverty, household food security, access to improved health care, female literacy, and the position of women in society.

REFERENCES

Arenz, S., Ruckerl, R., Koletzko, B. and von Kries, R. 2004, 'Breast-feeding and childhood obesity: A systematic review' in *International Journal of Obesity*, vol. 28, no. 10, pp. 1247–56.

Atallah, A., Hofmeyr, G. and Duley, L. 2002, 'Calcium supplementation during pregnancy for preventing hypertensive disorders and related problems' in *Cochrane Data Base of Systematic Reviews*, no. 1, p. CD001059.

Barker, D. 1998, '*Mothers, Babies and Health in Later Life*', Churchill Livingston, Edinburgh.

—— 2003, 'The developmental origins of adult disease' in *European Journal of Epidemiology*, vol. 18, no. 8, pp. 733–6.

—— 2004, 'The developmental origins of chronic adult disease' in *Acta Paediatrica Supplement*, vol. 93, no. 446, pp. 26–33.

Barker, D.J. and Osmond, C. 1986, 'Diet and coronary heart disease in England and Wales during and after the second world war' in *Journal of Epidemiology and Community Health*, vol. 40, pp. 37–44.

Bateson, P., Barker, D., Clutton-Brock, T., D'Udine, D., Foley, R., Gluckman, P., Godfrey, K., Kirkwood, T., Lahr, M., McNamara, J., Metcalfe, N., Monaghan, P., Spencer, H. and Sultan, S. 2004, 'Developmental plasticity and human health' in *Nature*, vol. 430, no. 6998, pp. 419–21.

Becker, S., Rutstein, S. and Labbok, M. 2003, 'Estimation of births averted due to breast-feeding and increases in levels of contraception needed to substitute for breast-feeding' in *Journal of Biosocial Science*, vol. 35, pp. 559–74.

Briley, A.L., Poston, L. and Shennan, A.H. 2006, 'Vitamins C and E and the prevention of preeclampsia' in *New England Journal of Medicine*, vol. 355, pp. 1065–66.

Brost, B., Goldenberg, R., Mercer, B., Iairs, J., Meis, P., Mowad, A., Neuman, R., Miodovnik, N., Caritis, S., Thurnam, G., Bottoms, S., Das, A. and McNellis, D. 1997, 'The Preterm Prediction Study: Association of caesarean delivery with increases in maternal weight and body mass index' in *American Journal of Obstetrics and Gynecology*, vol. 177, no. 2, pp. 333–41.

Campbell, D. and MacGillvray, I. 1975, 'The effects of a low-calorie diet or thiazide diuretic on the incidence of pre-eclampsia and on birth weight' in *British Journal of Obstetrics and Gynaecology*, vol. 82, no. 7, pp. 572–77.

Campbell-Brown, M. 1983, 'Protein energy supplementation in primigravid women at risk of low birth weight' in Campbell, D. and Gillmer, M. (eds) 1983, *Nutrition in pregnancy*, Royal College of Obstetrics and Gynaecology, London, pp. 85–98.

Caulfield, L., de Onis, M., Blossner, M. and Black, R. 2004, 'Undernutrition as an underlying cause of child deaths associated with diarrhea, pneumonia, malaria and measles' in *American Journal of Clinical Nutrition*, vol. 80, no. 1, pp. 193–8.

Caulfield, L., Huffman, S. and Piwoz, E. 1999, 'Interventions to improve intake of complementary foods by infants 6 to 12 months of age in developing countries: Impact on growth and on the prevalence of malnutrition and potential contribution to child survival' in *Food and Nutrition Bulletin*, vol. 20, no. 2, pp. 183–200.

Coutsoudis, A. and Rollins, N. 2003, 'Breast-feeding and HIV transmission: The jury is still out' in *Journal of Pediatric Gastroenterology and Nutrition*, vol. 36, no. 4, pp. 434–42.

Drane, D. and Logemann, J. 2000, 'A critical evaluation of the evidence on the association between type of infant feeding and cognitive development' in *Paediatric and Perinatal Epidemiology*, vol. 14, no. 4, pp. 349–56.

Durnin, J. 1987, 'Energy requirements of pregnancy: An integration of the longitudinal data from the Five Centre Study' in *Lancet*, vol. 2, no. 8568, pp. 1131–33.

Fairbank, L., O'Meara, S., Renfrew, M., Woolridge, M., Sowden, A. and Lister-Sharpe, D. 2000, 'A systematic review to evaluate the effectiveness of interventions to promote the initiation of breastfeeding' in *Health Technology Assessment*, vol. 4, no. 25, pp. 1–65.

Galtry, J. 2003, 'The impact on breastfeeding of labour market policy and practice in Ireland, Sweden, and the USA' in *Social Sciences and Medicine*, vol. 57, no. 1, pp. 167–77.

Gdalevich, M., Mimouni, D., David, M. and Mimouni, M. 2001, 'Breast-feeding and the onset of atopic dermatitis in childhood: A systematic review and meta-analysis of prospective studies' in *Journal of the American Academy of Dermatology*, vol. 45, no. 4, pp. 520–27.

Grivetti, L., Leon, D., Rasmussen, K., Shetty, P., Steckel, R. and Villar, J. 1998, 'Report of the IDECG Working Group on variation in foetal growth and adult disease' in *European Journal of Clinical Nutrition*, vol. 52, pp. S102–03.

Guttikonda, K., Burgess, J., Hynes, K., Boyages, S., Byth, K. and Parameswaran, V. 2002, 'Recurrent iodine deficiency in Tasmania, Australia: A salutary lesson in sustainable iodine prophylaxis and its monitoring' in *Journal of Clinical Endocrinology and Metabolism*, vol. 87, no. 6, pp. 2809–15.

Haggarty, P., McCallum, H., McBain, H., Andrews, K., Duthie, S., McNeill, G., Templeton, A., Haites, N., Campbell, D. and Bhattacharya, S. 2006, 'Genetic and nutritional determinants of the success of IVF treatment: The role of B vitamins' in *Lancet*, vol. 367, no. 9521, pp. 1513–19.

Harder, T., Bergmann, R., Kallischnigg, G. and Plagemann, A. 2005, 'Duration of breastfeeding and risk of overweight: A meta-analysis' in *American Journal of Epidemiology*, vol. 162, no. 5, pp. 397–403.

Hellerstedt, W., Himes, J., Story, M., Alton, I. and Edwards, L. 1997, 'The effects of cigarette smoking and gestational weight change on birth outcomes in obese and normal-weight women' in *American Journal of Public Health*, vol. 87, no. 4, pp. 591–96.

Hytten, F. and Leitch, I. 1971, 'Components of weight gain: Changes in the maternal body' in *Physiology of Human Pregnancy*, Blackwell Scientific Publications, Oxford, pp. 332–69.

International Baby Food Action Network (IBFAN) 2004, 'Breaking the rules, stretching the rules 2004: Evidence of violations of the International Code of Marketing of Breastmilk Substitutes and subsequent resolutions', IBFAN, Penang, cited at <http://www. ibfan.org/english/pdfs/btr04.pdf> on 1 November 2006.

Jones, G., Steketee, R., Black, R., Butta, Z.A. and Morris, S. 2003, 'How many child deaths can we prevent this year? The Bellagio Child Survival Study' in *Lancet*, vol. 362, no. 9377, pp. 65–71.

Kaiser, L., Allen, L. and American Dietetic Association 2002, 'Position of the American Dietetic Association: Nutrition and lifestyle for a healthy pregnancy outcome' in *Journal of the American Dietetic Association*, vol. 102, no. 10, pp. 1479–90.

Kramer, M. and Kakuma, R. 2002, 'The optimal duration of exclusive breastfeeding: A systematic review', World Health Organization (WHO), Geneva.

—— 2003, 'Energy and protein intake in pregnancy' in *The Cochrane Data Base of Systematic Reviews*, no. 4, p. CD003133.

Kramer, M., Chalmers, B., Hodnett, E., Sevkovskaya, Z., Dzikovich, I., Shapiro, S., Collet, J., Vanilovich, I., Mezen, I., Ducruet, T., Shishko, G., Zubovich, V., Mknuik, D., Gluchanina, E., Drombrovskiy, V., Ustinovitch, A., Kot, T., Bogdanovich, N., Ovchinikova, L. and Helsing, E. 2001, 'Promotion of Breastfeeding Intervention Trial (PROBIT): A randomized trial in the Republic of Belarus' in *Journal of the American Medical Association*, vol. 285, no. 4, pp. 413–20.

Kramer, M., Seguin, L., Lydon, J. and Goulet, L. 2000, 'Socio-economic disparities in pregnancy outcome: Why do the poor fare so poorly?' in *Paediatric and Perinatal Epidemiology*, vol. 14, no. 3, pp. 194–210.

Labbok, M., Clark, D. and Goldman, A. 2004, 'Breastfeeding: Maintaining an irreplaceable immunological resource' in *Nature Reviews Immunology*, vol. 4, no. 7, pp. 565–72.

Letsky, E. 1998, 'The haematological system' in Chamberlain G. and Pipkin-Broughtom F. 1998, *Clinical Physiology in Obstetrics*, Blackwell Science, Oxford.

Lumley, J., Watson, L., Watson, M. and Bower, C. 2001, 'Periconceptional supplementation with folate and/or multivitamins for preventing neural tube defects' in *Cochrane Database of Systematic Reviews*, vol. 4, p. CD001056.

Mahomed, K. 2000, 'Iron supplementation in pregnany' in *Cochrane Database of Systematic Review*, vol. 2, p. CD000117.

Martin, R., Gunnell, D. and Davey Smith, G. 2005a, 'Breastfeeding in infancy and blood pressure in later life: Systematic review and meta-analysis' in *American Journal of Epidemiology*, vol. 161, no. 1, pp. 15–26.

Martin, R., Middleton, N., Gunnell, D., Owen, C. and Smith, G. 2005b, 'Breast-feeding and cancer: The Boyd Orr cohort and a systematic review with meta-analysis' in *Journal of the National Cancer Institute*, vol. 97, no. 19, pp. 1446–57.

Mathews, F. and Neil, H. 1998, 'Nutrient intakes during pregnancy in a cohort of nulliparous women' in *Journal of Human Nutrition and Dietetics*, vol. 11, pp. 151–61.

McIntyre, E., Turnball, D. and Hiller, J. 1999, 'Breastfeeding in public places' in *Journal of Human Lactation*, vol. 15, no. 2, pp. 131–35.

McMillan, I. and Robinson, J. 2005, 'Developmental origins of the metabolic syndrome: Prediction, plasticity and programming' in *Physiology Review*, vol. 85, no. 2, pp. 571–633.

Mensah, P. and Tomkins, A. 2003, 'Household-level technologies to improve the availability and preparation of adequate and safe complementary foods' in *Food and Nutrition Bulletin*, vol. 24, no. 1, pp. 104–29.

Millard, A.V. 1990, 'The place of the clock in pediatric advice: Rationales, cultural themes and impediments to breastfeeding' in *Social Science and Medicine*, vol. 31, no. 2, pp. 211–21.

Moore, V., Davies, M., Willson, K., Worsley, A. and Robinson, J. 2004, 'Dietary composition of pregnant women is related to size of the baby at birth' in *Journal of Nutrition*, vol. 134, no. 7, pp. 1820–26.

Newsome, C., Shiell, A., Fall, C., Phillips, D., Shier, R. and Law, C. 2003, 'Is birth weight related to later glucose and insulin metabolism? A systematic review' in *Diabetic Medicine*, vol. 20, no. 5, pp. 339–48.

Owen, C., Whincup, P., Odoki, K., Gilg, J. and Cook, D. 2002, 'Infant feeding and blood cholesterol: AZ study in adolescents and a systematic review' in *Pediatrics*, vol. 110, no. 3, pp. 597–608.

Ozanne, S. 2001, 'Metabolic programming in animals' in *British Medical Bulletin*, vol. 60, pp. 143–52.

Ozanne, S., Fernandez-Twinn, D. and Hales, C. 2004, 'Fetal growth and adult diseases' in *Seminars in Perinatology*, vol. 28, no. 1, pp. 81–87.

Paneth, N. and Susser, M. 1995, 'Early origin of coronary heart disease: The "Barker hypothesis"' in *British Medical Journal*, vol. 310, no. 6977, pp. 411–12.

Pelto, G., Levitt, E. and Thairu, L. 2003, 'Improving feeding practices: Current patterns, common constraints, and the design of interventions' in *Food and Nutrition Bulletin*, vol. 24, no. 1, pp. 45–82.

Ramakrishnan, U., Manjrekar, R., Rivera, J., Gonzales-Cossio, T. and Martorell, R. 1999, 'Micronutrients and pregnancy outcome: A review of the literature' in *Nutrition Research*, vol. 19, no. 1, pp. 103–59.

Rich-Edwards, J., Colditz, G., Stampfer, M., Willett, W., Gillman, M., Hennekens, C., Speizer, F. and Manson, J. 1999, 'Birthweight and the risk of type 2 diabetes mellitus in adult women' in *Annals of Internal Medicine*, vol. 130, no. 4 part 1, pp. 278–84.

Rich-Edwards, J., Kleinman, K., Michels, K., Stampfer, M., Manson, J., Rexrode, K., Hibert, E. and Willett, W. 2005, 'Longitudinal study of birth weight and adult body mass index in predicting risk of coronary heart disease and stroke in women' in *British Medical Journal*, vol. 310, no. 7500, pp. 411–12.

Rush, D. 2001, 'Maternal nutrition and perinatal survival' in *Nutrition Reviews*, vol. 59, no. 10, pp. 315–26.

Rutstein, S. 2005, 'Effects of preceding birth intervals on neonatal infant and under-five years mortality and nutritional status in developing countries: Evidence from the demographic and health surveys' in *International Journal of Gynecology and Obstetrics*, vol. 89, pp. S7–24.

Say, L., Gülmezoglu, A. and Hofmeyr, G. 2003, 'Maternal nutrient supplementation for suspected impaired fetal growth' in *The Cochrane Data base of Systematic Reviews*, no. 1, p. CD00148.

Scott, J. 2005, 'What works in breastfeeding promotion?' *Journal of the Royal Society for the Promotion of Health*, vol. 125, no. 5, pp. 203–04.

Sellen, D. 2001, 'Comparison of infant feeding patterns reported for nonindustrial populations with current recommendations' in *Journal of Nutrition*, vol. 131, no. 10, pp. 2707–15.

Shaw, G., Todoroff, K., Schaffer, D. and Selvin, S. 2000, 'Maternal height and prepregnancy body mass index as risk factors for selected congenital anomalies' in *Paediatric and Perinatal Epidemiology*, vol. 14, no. 3, pp. 234–39.

Signore, C., Mills, J., Cox, C. and Trumble, A. 2005, 'Effects of folic acid fortification on twin gestation rates' in *Obstetrics and Gynecology*, vol. 105, no. 4, pp. 757–62.

Specker, B. 2004, 'Vitamin D requirements during pregnancy' in *American Journal of Clinical Nutrition*, vol. 80, no. 6, pp. S1740–45.

Susser, M. and Stein, Z. 1994, 'Timing in prenatal nutrition: A reprise of the Dutch Famine Study' in *Nutrition Reviews*, vol. 52, pp. 84–94.

UNFPA/UNICEF/WHO/UNAIDS Interagency Team 2001, 'New data on the prevention of mother-to-child transmission of HIV and their policy implications: Technical consultation', cited at <http://www. who.int/reproductive-health/publications/new_data_prevention_mtct_hiv/index.html>.

UNICEF 2005a, 'Baby Friendly Hospital Initiative', cited at <http://www.unicef.org/programme/breastfeeding/ baby.htm> on 1 December 2006.

—— 2005b, 'Infant feeding and HIV', cited at <http://www.unicef.org/nutrition/ 23964_infantfeeding.html>.

Weimer, J. 2001, 'The economic benefits of breastfeeding: A review and analysis', Department of Agriculture (US), Washington D.C.

World Health Organization (WHO) 1995, 'Maternal anthropometry and pregnancy outcomes' in *Bulletin of the World Health Organization*, vol. 73, pp. S1–47.

5

Children and adolescents

Johannes Brug
Knut-Inge Klepp

Why do Mexican children eat and like hot chilli peppers that make a Dutch child cry? Why do Portuguese schoolchildren eat far more fruit and vegetables than their Spanish peers? How is it that food habits among children can be so different across countries?

On the other hand, all children, whether from Mexico, the Netherlands, Portugal, Spain, or anywhere else, seem to like sweet and fatty foods. How can it be that these food preferences are so similar? Eating high fat and sugar foods in abundance contributes to the present epidemic of overweight and obesity that is now affecting children and adolescents across the world. Why is this happening now and not thirty years ago? The present chapter will address the above questions.

A chapter on public health nutrition for school-aged children and adolescents is needeed as diet and nutrition clearly play a critical role during childhood and adolescent development. First of all, during childhood and adolescence children grow to be adults. Therefore, children and adolescents need to cover not only their nutrient and energy needs for maintenance metabolism and physical activities, but also for growth. These needs are especially critical in the distinct periods of very rapid growth in infancy (see chapter 4) and the preschool growth spurt, and in the growth spurt during puberty (Koletzko et al. 2004). Growth means special dietary requirements in terms of quantity and quality of foods, and specific recommendations for childhood and adolescent nutrient intake have therefore been established (see chapter 3). The adverse health consequences of under-nutrition — the lack of macro and/or micronutrients — as well as over-nutrition in childhood and adolescence can be severe, and often are not fully reversible (Koletzko et al. 2004). Furthermore, eating habits may be less established in childhood and adolescence, and may therefore be more modifiable (Birch 1999), and food preferences and habits adopted in childhood and adolescence may track into adulthood.

Thus, in this chapter we will argue that promotion of healthy dietary habits is of specific importance during childhood and adolescence. We will introduce a six-step planning framework that helps to approach healthy diet promotion in childhood and adolescence in a systematic way. This model will subsequently be used to further describe and explain the rationale for public health nutrition in youth. Our focus will mostly be on why children eat what they eat and how healthy diet promotion interventions for children and adolescents should be tailored to these behavioural determinants.

The focus in this chapter will be on school-aged children and adolescents (that is, five to eighteen years of age), with special attention on the critical period of ten to fourteen years, when most children have their pubertal growth spurt, become adolescents and gain more food choice autonomy (Story et al. 2002). This focus will be confined to nutrition issues in children and adolescents in countries with established market economies as defined by the World Bank.

A basic model of planned promotion of population health

Careful, systematic, evidence and theory driven planning of health promotion has long been advocated (Green & Kreuter 1999). The Precede–Proceed model and other planning models (see chapter 17) show great similarities and reviews and meta-analyses of the relevant literature show that applying such planning models improves the chances of success (Contento et al. 1995; Bartholomew et al. 2000). Based on a comparison and integration of the available health promotion planning models, we identified six important steps or phases in health promotion planning (Brug et al. 2005b) as shown in Figure 5.1.

The first two steps cover the epidemiological analysis. When applied to public health nutrition in childhood and adolescence, these steps should identify the most important health and quality of life issues in this age group, their nutritional risk factors, and the populations most at risk. These initial steps result in setting priorities for dietary change interventions and identification of behaviour change goals.

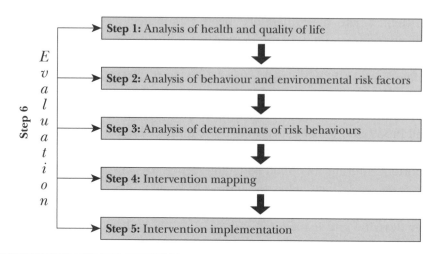

Figure 5.1 A model for planned health education and health promotion

Source: Brug et al. 2005b

What, when and how much children eat is influenced by a complex, interrelated set of so-called behavioural 'mediators' or 'determinants', and successful dietary behaviour change interventions are dependent on the identification of the most *important* and most *changeable* determinants. The third step in planned promotion of healthy eating is therefore the analysis of the determinants of nutrition behaviours. This analysis of behavioural determinants identifies the more proximal, intermediary intervention goals as well as specific target groups for interventions. In the fourth step of the planning process, intervention strategies, methods and materials need to be selected or developed that are tailored to the target populations and the most important and most modifiable determinants of behaviour change. Step 5 constitutes the implementation and dissemination of the intervention, to ensure that the target population is reached and exposed to the nutrition education messages or other healthy diet promotion strategies. Each step should preferably be evidence-based and theory driven, and evaluation (Step 6) is an integral part of the planning process.

In brief, our planning model states that we need to understand the major health problems and related dietary behaviours among children and adolescents, as well as what drives children and adolescent food choices, in order to be able to identify effective healthy diet promotion interventions for these populations. Careful, evidence-based planning of healthy diet promotion interventions increases the likelihood that important health problems are prioritised, and that appropriate behaviour change goals are pursued by focusing on critical determinants, with effective intervention strategies targeting the right audience.

In the remainder of this chapter, we will use this planning model to describe in some detail what the main issues are in childhood and adolescent nutrition, and in more detail what we know about important determinants of nutrition behaviours in children and adolescents. In the final section of the chapter, we will present the Pro Children project as an example of a study in which the planning model was used to develop, implement and evaluate a school-based intervention to promote fruit and vegetable intakes in ten to eleven year-old children in Europe (Klepp et al. 2005).

Childhood and adolescent nutrition and health

Here, a brief overview is given of important nutrition issues in children and adolescents, which are related to health promotion and protection in youth and adulthood. Childhood and adolescence are critical periods characterised by extraordinary rapid growth and change with respect to physical, cognitive and social development. Nutrition plays a key role in this, and children and adolescents are particularly vulnerable if their dietary requirements are not met. Globally, the main issues in childhood and adolescent nutrition are:

- micronutrient deficiencies (iron deficiency and anaemia)
- protein-energy malnutrition and stunting
- nutrition-related chronic diseases, including dental diseases, hypertension, type 2 diabetes, obesity, cardiovascular diseases, osteoporosis, and a number of cancers
- eating patterns and lifestyles
- eating disorders
- nutrition in relation to early pregnancy.

Within established market economies, the main concerns today are related to the development of eating patterns and lifestyles during this age span and how these relate to the development of nutrition-related chronic diseases (Lytle & Kubik 2003). There are at least three ways in which dietary habits during childhood and adolescence affect the risk of chronic disease:

1. the development of risk factors (for example, elevated serum cholesterol levels, blood pressure or overweight) or disease (such as dental caries or cognitive disorders)
2. the tracking of risk factors throughout life (such as tracking of serum cholesterol levels, blood pressure or weight-status)

3. the development of healthy or unhealthy dietary habits that tend to stay throughout life (for example, fruit and vegetable intake or consumption of high-sugar beverages).

While the establishment of risk factors at an early age and their high degree of tracking throughout life has been long established and documented (Wynder et al. 1981; Bao et al. 1995), less is known about the tracking of dietary behaviours from childhood and adolescence throughout life. There are, however, studies indicating that food behaviour and concrete food choices are established early in life and show some long-term stability (Kelder et al. 1994; Lien et al. 2001; Mikkila et al. 2005).

While there appears to be wide consensus regarding the critical role of nutrition during childhood and adolescence, there is less consensus and comparable data regarding the actual nutritional requirements, nutritional intake and nutritional status among these young target groups. This is illustrated by a recent study in 29 European countries, where it was demonstrated that 'considerable disparities in the perceived nutritional requirements of European children and adolescents' are present (Prentice et al. 2004). Furthermore, a parallel study investigating dietary intake and nutritional status pointed to the lack of standardisation and generally poor intake data across Europe, and that insufficient data on nutrition status exist 'to be able to draw any conclusions about the nutritional quality of the diets of European children and adolescents' (Lambert et al. 2004). The situation in Europe is probably not much different from what is seen elsewhere, as indicated by a recent review of nutritional issues for adolescents in the United States, where it was concluded that a top priority for a future research agenda should be improved methods for assessing the diets of youth (Lytle & Kubik 2003).

In spite of this disparity in nutritional guidelines and lack of standardised assessment methods, a number of nutrition-related health concerns have been raised in countries with established market economies. Large proportions of children and adolescents seem to have excess energy intake (in relation to their energy expenditure levels) and too high intake of saturated fat, sugar and salt, while their intake of fibre, vitamin D (particularly in the northern hemisphere), iron and calcium (for girls only) often are too low to meet dietary requirements or recommended intake levels. In terms of dietary habits, this nutritional imbalance is largely caused by low intake of vegetables, fruit, wholegrain cereals and low-fat dairy products, while the consumption of, in particular, sugar-sweetened soft drinks, sweets and high-fat snack foods is too high. Even relatively small but long-lasting changes in the intake of these food groups, along with increased physical activity levels, are likely to have a major effect on public health in the long run, as their link to the most prevalent chronic diseases, including dental diseases, hypertension, type 2 diabetes, obesity, cardiovascular diseases, osteoporosis and a number of cancers, are well established.

The increasing rates of overweight and obesity among children and adolescents are of particular concern, as it is exceedingly difficult to lose weight later in life, and because obesity is such an important risk factor for several other chronic diseases, such as osteoarthritis, type 2 diabetes, cardiovascular disease and certain cancers (see chapter 9 for more information on obesity and public health nutrition). International criteria and cut-off points have been established for assessing overweight and obesity among children and adolescents based on body mass index (BMI) (Cole et al. 2000), and more recently based on body fat (McCarthy et al. 2006). Such cut-off points are important as they help to provide internationally comparable prevalence rates of overweight and obesity in children.

At the same time as overweight and obesity rates are increasing, an alarmingly high proportion of children and adolescents, mostly girls, report they are dissatisfied with their body weight. Results from the 2001–02 survey of the Health Behaviour in School-aged Children Study (WHO 2004), conducted in 35 countries and regions, demonstrate that as many as three in ten eleven-year-old girls and four in ten fifteen-year-olds reported they were dissatisfied with their body (that is, reporting to be 'a bit too fat' or 'much too fat'). For boys, the corresponding figure was about two in ten for both eleven- and fifteen-year-olds. In the same study, a total of about 15 per cent of the fifteen-year-old girls and 9 per cent of the same aged boys were classified as overweight or obese. While these data are based on self-reported height and weight information with large variations between countries, the results do indicate that a significant proportion of normal-weight adolescents do perceive themselves as being too fat.

Weight-related disorders include anorexia nervosa, bulimia nervosa, binge-eating disorders, anorexic/bulimic behaviours, and dieting behaviours. Anorexia and bulimia nervosa are, even though their observed prevalence rates have increased over the past decades, relatively rare, but they are serious conditions suggesting mental illness requiring specialised, individual treatment (Lytle & Kubik 2003). As most individuals who develop eating disorders are adolescent girls or young women, who typically begin experiencing food-related and self-image problems, it is of great concern that so many normal-weight young girls appear to experience body dissatisfaction and engage in dieting and weight-control behaviours (WHO 2004). However, the public health consequences of obesity are much higher than those of eating disorders, and the sometimes suggested associations between obesity prevention efforts on the one hand, and the likelihood of developing eating disorders on the other, is not based on any strong evidence. Eating disorders such as anorexia and bulimia nervosa are recognised as psychiatric disorders, and will not be further dealt with in this chapter. Nevertheless, it remains a public health challenge to combat the increasing overweight and obesity rates, and at the same time reduce the vulnerability of young girls with respect to body dissatisfaction and food-related problems.

Determinants of child and adolescent nutrition: Why do we eat what we eat?

In affluent countries, most people can generally choose what, when and how much they eat. To induce dietary change, one needs to change people's food choices. To be able to do that, insight is necessary on why people choose to eat what they eat. Studies on personal determinants of food choice have primarily made use of psychology-oriented theories to explain food choice and nutrition behaviours (Conner & Armitage 2002). It has, however, been argued that, since children may have less autonomy in making food choices, environmental rather than personal factors may be more important determinants of their nutrition behaviours. More recently, social-ecological models of health behaviour (Sallis & Owen 2003) have drawn more attention to such environmental factors that may influence nutrition behaviours.

A framework proposed by Rothschild (1999) provides a simple, integrative framework to categorise the large and diverse number of potential personal and environmental determinants from various more specific behaviour theories. Rothschild identifies three distinct categories of determinants: motivation, ability and opportunity, with motivation and ability as important categories of personal determinants and opportunity as a category of environmental determinants. These categories of determinants are interrelated and mutually interacting. For example, in environments with few opportunities for healthy eating, higher motivation and more abilities are needed to maintain a healthy diet.

Motivation: Why would children and adolescents want to eat a healthy diet?

In nutrition education and other health education research, determinants of behaviour have been studied mostly from a social psychology perspective. Within social psychology, different theories and models have been proposed to study nutrition behaviours. These theories and models include the Health Belief Model, Protection Motivation Theory, Social Learning Theory and the Theory of Planned Behaviour. A shared common feature in these is that they recognise behavioural decision, motivation or intention as a primary determinant of behaviour (van Trijp et al. 2005). Each theory proposes different but similar determinants of intentions. Based on an integration of insights from the aforementioned theories, at least three groups of determinants that predict intention are recognised: attitudes, perceived social influences, and self-efficacy.

Attitudes

Attitudes are based on a subjective weighting of expected positive and negative consequences or outcomes of the behaviour. Closely related constructs are decisional balance, outcome expectations, and perceived threat. But which expected outcomes are important for most children and adolescents in making food-choice decisions? In general, expectations about short-term outcomes are more important than longer-term outcomes. Taste, satiety and pleasure are short-term consequences of major importance. People, and young people maybe more so, will eat what they like, and disliked foods will not be chosen (Birch 1999). Certain taste preferences are innate, such as a liking for sweet and salt, and a dislike for bitter and sour. However, taste preferences can be learned and unlearned.

'Hunger' or appetite are strong motivators to eat. In Maslow's (1970) hierarchy of human needs, the need to cover physiological energy requirements, that is, overcoming hunger, is among the highest human priorities, and the urge to eat and drink when hungry is an inborn trait.

Since eating is primarily a way to cover the basic physiological nutrient requirements and calorie requirements, satiety — the feeling that energy require - ments have successfully been met — is a strong reinforcer for eating specific foods, and we therefore quickly learn to like and appreciate energy dense foods (Birch 1999). Children are therefore 'programmed' to like, or to learn to like, the taste of high-energy, sweet and fatty foods. Nevertheless, many people acquire a taste for coffee, tea or beer during childhood or adolescence, and this illustrates that we can even unlearn our innate dislike of bitter tastes. Learning to like and dislike certain tastes follow the principles of basic classical and operant conditioning.

Some specific types of learning strategies that have been identified relate to food and eating. The aforementioned example of learning to like high-energy foods is referred to as 'taste-nutrient learning'. Taste-nutrient learning is an example of operant or instrumental conditioning: a stimulus (eating energy-dense, sweet and fatty food) is positively reinforced ('rewarded') by the pleasant feeling of satiety. Evolutionary psychologists claim satiety is a strong reinforcer of behaviour because learning to like such energy dense foods improved chances for survival during the long history of evolution, when periods of energy shortage were much more likely than periods of abundance. The present-day obesity epidemic has, however, been attributed to this innate tendency to learn to prefer energy dense foods in combination with an 'obesogenic' environment (Swinburn et al. 1999) — see below. In recent decades, when palatable foods have become readily available and accessible for most children in western countries, children and adults alike still tend to like and thus choose foods as if we anticipate the next famine. Since most fruits and especially vegetables have low-energy densities, and since many vegetables have a somewhat bitter taste, preferences for these foods are not so easily learned. Fat and sugar-rich foods are indeed among the most preferred foods among children and adolescents (Cooke & Wardle 2005).

Two other food-preference learning strategies are examples of classical conditioning, and are referred to as 'taste–taste learning' and 'taste–environment learning'. If a new, unfamiliar, taste is combined with a taste for which a preference already exists, children will more easily learn to like the new taste. For example, children will more easily learn to like the somewhat bitter taste of tea or the sour taste of yoghurt or grapefruit, if these are first served with sugar. Similarly, tastes that people are exposed to in pleasant physical and/or social environments are also more easily learned to be liked. Foods first encountered as a child in a friendly, pleasant family environment may become favourite foods for a lifetime. A fourth important learning strategy is 'observational learning' or 'modelling', which will be described later.

Health-related outcome expectations or beliefs are also important in food choice; in adults, health usually comes second (or third) after taste (and cost), if people are asked about what they find important in their diet and food choice, especially in women (Lennernas et al. 1997). Nevertheless, 40 per cent of Americans and 57 per cent of Europeans indicated rarely or never to compromise on taste to improve the healthiness of their diets (Health-Focus 2005). This is likely to be even more the case in children (Story et al. 2002). Furthermore, in everyday life, health expectations may only significantly influence food choices for most people when the health consequences are expected to be soon, severe and easy to recognise. We may therefore very quickly develop negative attitudes toward foods to which we are allergic or intolerant, such as foods that literally make you sick (Capaldi 1996). But most energy dense foods are sweet and/or salty, and provide that comfortable feeling of satiety. The potential negative consequences, like obesity, type 2 diabetes and heart disease, will be present only to some, and most often only decades later, especially in children, although cases of type 2 diabetes and metabolic syndrome are becoming more common now that children are increasingly likely to be overweight (Liu et al. 2004).

In adults, the cost of foods is often mentioned as one of the top-three considerations in making food choices. In adolescence, people often start to buy their own foods, and price becomes relevant, for example in selecting snacks from vending machines (Story et al. 2002).

Perceived social influence

The second category of determinants of intention, perceived social influence, includes subjective norms and descriptive norms. Subjective norms are expectations about what 'important others' want us to do. If, for example, a child thinks that her parents want her to eat vegetables at dinner or her best friends want her to eat snack foods, she will be more likely to do so. Descriptive norms are based on the observed behaviour of important others. If a child's parents eat diets high in fruit and vegetables, she will be more likely to be motivated to do so herself. A third social environmental factor is social support, that is, active and explicit encouragement to eat a healthy diet.

A recent review of the literature on environmental determinants of eating behaviours in children showed that there is convincing evidence that social environmental factors are indeed important and, descriptive norms in particular (Brug & van Lenthe, 2005). These social factors may influence nutrition behaviour via intentions and motivation, as predicted by theories such as the Theory of Planned Behaviour, but social influence may also more directly determine nutrition and eating behaviour in children and adolescents by defining opportunities or lack of opportunities for healthful eating. A more elaborate description of social–environmental influences on nutrition behaviours in children and adolescents is provided below.

Self-efficacy

Sometimes known as perceived behavioural control, self-efficacy is the third predictor of motivation, and it refers to the perception of, or confidence in, one's abilities and skills to engage in certain behaviour. A person who is confident that he or she can cut back on saturated fat intake will be more motivated to do so. Perceived control is behaviour- and context-specific. A person can, for example, be confident to be able to eat less fat, but not to increase vegetable intake; and confidence to cut back on fat may be high for regular meals prepared at home, but not for eating out. Perceived control is strongly related to abilities and skills, which we refer to below. Studies in children and adolescents show that food- and nutrition-related self-efficacy is associated with healthy food choices and dietary behaviour (Heatey & Thombs 1997; Resnicow et al. 1997; Wind et al. submitted).

Motivation and intentions are important determinants of nutrition behaviours, but not all behaviour is intentional, and we do not always act on our intentions. Lack of ability or lack of environmental opportunities may be important barriers to doing what we intend to do. Environmental cues may also trigger automatic behavioural responses.

Ability: What enables children and adolescents to eat a healthy diet?

Previously, we indicated that people with high confidence in their skills and abilities to make healthy dietary choices will be more motivated to do so. If such confidence is based on true personal abilities and skills, people can translate their motivation into action.

Skills and abilities are to some extent dependent on practical knowledge; for example, knowledge of recommended intake levels and healthy alternatives for unhealthy choices help to enable voluntary dietary change. To make conscious dietary changes for better bodyweight maintenance, for example, knowledge is necessary about which dietary changes will be most effective. Some knowledge about which foods are high in calories is helpful to be able to avoid high-calorie foods and for self-monitoring calorie intake. Knowing why to eat healthy, knowing what healthy foods are, and knowing the recommended intake levels is important. But knowledge in itself is unlikely to result in healthy food and nutrition choices, and associations between nutrition knowledge and dietary behaviour have been found to be weak (Story et al. 2002). Nevertheless, some recent studies show that knowledge of recommended intake levels of fruit and vegetables was associated with higher intake in eleven-year-old schoolchildren (Wind et al. submitted).

As outlined before, nutrition behaviours are complex behaviours. To further build on the weight management example: we do not eat calories as such; calorie intake is the result of a series of interrelated specific actions, such as buying, preparing, combining and eating specific foods in different serving sizes. To calculate one's total calorie intake requires extensive knowledge of calorie contents of foods, as well as intensive self-monitoring and advanced arrhythmic skills. This becomes even more difficult if you do not buy and prepare most of your food yourself, as is the case for the vast majority of children and adolescents. If the opportunities for objective self-assessment of dietary intake levels are lacking, people tend to search for other comparison possibilities, and often social comparisons are used: people compare their own perceived intake levels with what they perceive that others do. Such social comparisons are more likely in younger people (Oenema & Brug 2003) and tend to be liable to a so-called optimistic bias. Different studies have shown that people, including adolescents (Kremers et al. 2003), are likely to think that they comply with nutritional recommendations such as for fat, fruit and vegetable intake (see Brug et al. 1994; Lechner et al. 1997), while their actual intake levels are not in line with official dietary guidelines. For example, in studies conducted in the Netherlands we found that only about 10 per cent of the population thought that their diets were too high in fat, while more objective food consumption research showed that about 80 per cent of the population had high fat diets (Brug et al. 1994, Brug & Kok 1995). Similar results were found for fruit and vegetable intake (Lechner et al. 1997). If people think that they already comply with dietary recommendations, they will not be motivated to change (Brug et al. 1994, Lechner et al. 1997), and having the knowledge and skills to gain awareness of personal intake levels is an important first step in improving motivation to change.

Practical skills to prepare healthy foods and meals are also important. This may be less the case among young children, but becomes more important in adolescence when children gain more food choice and food preparation autonomy. Since children and adolescents often depend on others for what they eat, skills to influence the gate keepers' decisions may also be relevant. Success-ful interventions to encourage healthy eating in children have been explicitly aiming to improve such asking skills (Baranowski et al. 2003; Perez Rodrigo et al. 2005). Finally, skills and confidence to be able to resist peer pressure to eat non-healthy foods or diets may be relevant.

Opportunity: Availability and accessibility of healthy choices
In promotion of healthy behaviours in recent decades, most attention has been given to nutrition education as the primary tool to encourage children and adolescents to adopt healthy dietary habits. Nutrition education focuses on conscious behaviour change and on improving individuals' motivations and skills to increase the likelihood of adopting healthy diets. However, children's and adolescents' opportunities to make healthy dietary changes depend strongly on the opportunities in the environments they live in. For example, their social environment, such as their parents and school staff, importantly influence their range of food choices; their physical environment, such as where they live or go to school, importantly influences what foods are available and accessible to them. The ecological health promotion approach, with stronger attention on environmental barriers and opportunities for health behaviours, has resulted

in studies aiming to identify specific relevant environmental determinants of nutrition behaviours in children and adolescents.

Environmental influences on nutrition behaviours are often believed to be mediated or moderated by motivation and abilities. Environments that offer appealing and tasty opportunities for healthy eating may, for example, improve motivation to do so; in an environment that offers easy opportunities for healthy dietary choices, a child may need less motivation and fewer skills to engage in healthy eating; and children or adolescents who have strong motivation and plenty of skills to eat a healthy diet will be more likely to pursue healthy eating, despite environmental barriers. There is, however, ample evidence that environmental factors may also more directly influence eating habits, unmediated or moderated by personal factors. Children and adolescents, for example, eat more when they are offered larger portions, independent of their hunger levels.

Classifying the food environment

Different classifications of environmental determinants of health behaviours have been proposed in ecological models of health behaviour, and these classifications show great overlap and similarities (Sallis & Owen 2003). In early ecological models of health behaviour, five levels of influence were distinguished: intrapersonal factors, interpersonal processes, institutional factors, community factors and public policy. Story and his colleagues (2002) recognise social environmental influences (interpersonal influences), physical environmental influences (influences within community settings), and macrosystems influences (influences at the societal level). Flay and Petraitis (1994) distinguish between the social environment and the cultural environment as important categories of environmental determinants of health behaviour, and within these categories they make a further distinction between ultimate, distal and proximal factors. Based on the distinctions within the environment, combined with the proximity of the factors within these broad categories, a matrix or grid could be designed with six cells that represent different classes of environmental influences.

Such a grid structure is explicitly proposed in the ANGELO (analysis grid for elements linked to obesity) Framework (Swinburn et al. 1999) (see Table 5.1). This framework was specifically developed to conceptualise health behaviour environments, and enables the identification of potential intervention settings and strategies (chapter 9). The ANGELO Framework was primarily developed for investigation and classification of so-called obesogenic environments, that is, environments that promote excess energy intake and lack of

Table 5.1 The ANGELO grid

	Micro-environment	Macro-environment
Physical environment	for example, availability of school fruit at schools	for example, availability of certain fruits in a country
Economic environment	for example, the price of snack foods at the local supermarket	for example, food price policies
Political environment	for example, bans on soft drink machines in schools; family food rules	for example, national school food policies
Socio-cultural environment	for example, parental norms regarding snack foods at home	for example, what is culturally regarded as appropriate foods

Source: adapted from Swinburn et al. 1999

physical activity, but the categorisation of environmental factors seems also applicable for other nutrition behaviours and was recently used for systematic reviews of environmental correlates and interventions for specific nutrition behaviours among children and adolescents (Brug & van Lenthe 2005).

The ANGELO Framework is a grid with two axes. On the first axis, two 'sizes' of environment (micro and macro) are distinguished. Micro-environments are defined as environmental settings in which groups of people meet and gather. Such settings are often geographically distinct, and offer room for direct mutual influence between individuals and the environment. Examples of micro-environments are homes, schools, workplaces, supermarkets, recreational facilities and neighbourhoods. Macro-environments, on the other hand, include the broader, more anonymous infrastructure that may support or hinder health behaviours. Examples of macro-environments are how food products are marketed, taxed and distributed; the media are sometimes also included in the macro-environment.

On the second axis, four types of environments are distinguished: physical, economic, political and socio-cultural. The physical environment refers to availability of opportunities for healthy and unhealthy choices, such as points-of-purchase for fruit and vegetables, and soft drink vending machines in schools, etc. The economic environment refers to the costs related to healthy and unhealthy behaviours, such as the price of soft drinks, fruit and vegetables or energy dense snacks in school cafeterias. The political environment refers to the rules and regulations that may influence food choice and eating behaviour. Bans on soft drink vending machines in schools, rules on what treats can and cannot be brought to school, as well as family food rules are micro-level political–

environmental factors. National school food policies or national legislation regarding food-marketing efforts aimed at children are part of the macro-level political environment. The socio-cultural environment refers to the social and cultural subjective and descriptive norms and other social influences, such as social support for adoption of healthy behaviour, and social pressure to engage in unhealthy habits.

Evidence for environmental determinants of nutrition behaviours in youth

Child and adolescent dietary behaviour is likely to be strongly influenced by environmental factors, since children may have less autonomy in food choice. From the age of about three years, children's eating behaviour is influenced by their responsiveness to environmental cues, and a variety of family and social factors start to influence children's eating behaviours (Patrick & Nicklas 2005). The role of parents and schools is considered to be of particular importance.

Parent and family influences

Parents directly and importantly determine the child's micro-level social, political, physical and economical nutrition environments.

Eating is a social behaviour, especially for children (Birch 1999), and observing eating behaviours of others, especially parents, influences their own preferences and behaviour. Such modelling of eating behaviours can even result in establishing preferences for foods or substances that are inherently disliked. A recent review of the literature on environmental correlates of nutrition behaviours in youth indicates that children's and adolescents' nutrition behaviours are consistently associated with their parents' behaviours (Brug & van Lenthe 2005). Other important models for nutrition behaviours may be siblings, especially older ones.

Parents further influence their offsprings' nutrition behaviours by actively encouraging, discouraging or controlling certain behaviours. Restricting children's access to foods that are believed to be 'bad', such as high-fat or sugar-rich foods, may encourage rather than discourage preferences for such foods, especially if these same foods are also used to reward children for good behaviour and are served at celebrations and other parties. However, a study conducted in Belgium indicated that clear restrictive family rules about high-fat foods during childhood were associated with healthier food choices in adolescence (De Bourdeaudhuij & Van Oost 1996), and a recent cross-European study showed that parental demand, as well as facilitation to eat fruit and vegetables, were associated with higher intake levels in eleven-year-old children, while parents allowing children to eat as much as they like was not (Wind et al. submitted).

From studies on the association between general parenting styles and children's health behaviours, it appears that authoritative parenting, that is, a parenting style characterised by high parental involvement as well as strictness, is associated with more positive health behaviours including higher fruit and vegetable intakes (Kremers et al. 2003; Patrick et al. 2005), compared to adolescents who reported authoritarian (high strictness, low involvement) or neglectful (low strictness, low involvement) parenting styles.

As a result of these parenting practices and rules, as well as parents' own food preferences and choices, parents influence what foods are available and accessible within the home environment. Availability and accessibility of foods have repeatedly been found to be associated with intake levels in children and adolescents (Cullen et al. 2003).

Finally, family socioeconomic position is important. A recent review of the literature again confirmed that low parental education, as well as low parental income is associated with less healthy diets in children and adolescents (Wardle et al. 2003; Brug & van Lenthe 2005).

School influences

A second very important setting for children and adolescent nutrition is the school environment. Children spend much time in schools, where they consume a large proportion of their daily intake because food is provided or sold there, and because nutrition education is often part of the school curriculum.

Accessibility and availability of foods in schools are important physical environmental factors. In many countries, schools provide lunch. In the United States, for example, the large majority of schools participate in the national school lunch programme and schools are required to offer meals that meet the Dietary Guidelines for Americans. Youth who participate in this programme have better nutrient intake than those who do not (Story et al. 2002). In middle and high schools in the United States, adolescents are exposed to à la carte cafeterias, snack counters, fast food outlets and vending machines, which sell foods that are not required to meet the dietary guidelines. Most of these foods are high in fat, sugar and/or salt.

In Europe, there are great differences between countries. The differences between the Netherlands and Belgian Flanders are illustrative. These two neighbouring countries with the same language and similar school systems differ in their school food policies. In Belgium, school lunches are offered in a majority of primary and secondary schools. Parents need to pay for their children to have a school lunch, children are allowed to bring their own lunch to school, and the school lunches are not required to meet official dietary guidelines. Most secondary schools do have vending machines and small snack food outlets. In the Netherlands, school lunches are not offered. In primary schools, children go home for lunch or children need to bring their lunch to school. In secondary schools, adolescents bring their lunch to school, or they can buy lunch in the school à la carte cafeteria. In Sweden and the United Kingdom, primary and secondary schools do offer free school lunches, but while Swedish schools are required to meet official recommended intake levels, nutrition requirements for school lunches in the United Kingdom only state that meals in primary schools should contain at least one item from four major food groups (starchy foods; fruit and vegetables; dairy products; meat, fish or alternative protein source), and in secondary school lunches, at least two items from each of these groups should be offered. In other European countries, schools offer lunch subscription programmes that are sometimes free for children from deprived families. Preliminary evidence from the European Pro Children study indicates that school lunches can make a difference; Swedish kids eat more vegetables at school, and have a relatively high total daily vegetable intake.

Schools do also provide an important environment for social influences on nutrition behaviours. Peers may influence behaviour in general, among adolescents in particular, and peer influences have also been observed for nutrition behaviours (Brug & van Lenthe 2005); however, peer influences on nutrition behaviours appear to be less important than parental influences (Story et al. 2002; Brug & van Lenthe 2005).

Neighbourhood influences

Neighbourhoods may differ in availability of healthy and less healthy foods. In the United States, the notion of food deserts — neighbourhood environments that offer no accessibility to nutritious foods — has received attention. These areas with little access to healthy foods appear to be especially present in poorer neighbourhoods. Similar research conducted in the United Kingdom indicates that accessibility to healthy foods is much more evenly distributed between neighbourhoods (Cummins & Macintyre 2005). Another issue of importance is fast-food restaurants. The number of these restaurants has risen in most western countries over the past decades, leading to better accessibility of fast-food. Meals eaten at fast-food restaurants are higher in fat, saturated fat and sodium, and lower in fibre, and frequency of eating at fast-food restaurants is associated with higher calorie intake (French et al. 2001). Fast-food outlets may also importantly influence dietary intake levels because of the large portion sizes they offer. As mentioned before, portion size is an independent predictor of amount of intake in youth.

Macro-level environment

Differences in nutrition behaviours in children and adolescents between countries indicate that macro-level environment factors do indeed influence eating habits. Food availability differs between countries, as well as what is culturally appropriate to eat. Nevertheless, the popularity of certain foods and identical fast-food restaurants around the globe is an example of the ongoing globalisation of foods.

An important macro-level factor is how foods are marketed to children and adolescents. Children and adolescents are increasingly seen as an important target group for food marketing (Story & French 2004). Young people in affluent countries have money to spend, they may also influence food-buying behaviours of their parents, and they are the future adult buyers and consumers. Foods that are most intensively marketed by means of advertising and marketing campaigns are high in sugar and fats, and often low in micronutrients. In the United States, fast-food restaurants and soft drink companies spent most on marketing their products. The large portion sizes offered at 'value pricing' (that is, larger portions cost relatively less), especially in the United States, is a marketing strategy that has probably contributed to higher caloric intakes and unnecessary weight gain. Food marketing efforts already start among toddlers. Television is the most important channel for marketing food products, especially for younger children, but food marketing among youth also includes school-based marketing, Internet advertising, sponsoring of events, etc.

Although most countries do regard children as an especially vulnerable group for television advertising, there are striking differences between countries in rules and regulations for food marketing to children. Although only few countries have a complete ban on television advertising for younger children, most countries (85 per cent of 73 countries surveyed by the WHO – see WHO 2004) do have statutory regulations for food television advertising to children; regulations that define, for example, in which ways foods can be promoted at particular broadcasting times. The principle underlying many regulations is that advertising must not be misleading.

School-based marketing is of secondary importance. School-based marketing of foods is most notable in the United States, but these marketing practices are growing almost everywhere. Only 33 per cent of countries surveyed by the WHO had regulations for school-based marketing of foods.

The effects of food marketing to children and adolescents on their food choices is not well researched, but evidence does indicate that children ask their parents to buy foods that have been heavily marketed.

Food environments and habitual nutrition behaviours

Different eating behaviours are repeated often, and may therefore become habitual, that is, children and adolescents may engage in nutrition behaviours without any conscious decision-making process. Habitual behaviour is considered to be automatic, triggered by environmental cues instead of evaluations of possible outcomes, the opinion of other people, and confidence about being able to engage in the behaviour (Verplanken & Orbell 2003). Studies among adults and children alike show that past behaviour is the best predictor of future nutrition behaviour. However, tracking of past behaviour is not the same as habitual behaviour (Verplanken & Aarts 1999). Furthermore, even if past behaviour is a strong determinant of future dietary practices, past behaviour is not changeable, and in planned development of interventions to promote healthy dietary practices in children and adolescents (see Figure 5.1), we are mostly interested in important and changeable determinants. In contrast, habit strength, that is, the extent to which eating behaviours are automatic as well as often repeated, may be changeable; for example by changing the environmental cues that trigger the automatic, habitual response. Comprehensive tools to measure habit strength have successfully been tested and used in previous research (Verplanken & Orbell 2003; Wind et al. submitted). Such measures include assessments of repetition as well as 'automaticity' of eating behaviours. A recent series of studies that used such habit-strength measures, which go beyond past behaviour, show that habit strength is indeed a strong predictor and correlate of a range of dietary behaviours (for example, fat, fruit, soft drink intake) among adolescents as well as children (Brug et al. 2005a) and that habit strength may modify the association between attitudes and intentions, as well as intention–behaviour associations (Kremers 2005).

Implications for healthy diet promotion in youth

The Pro Children project example

In this section, we will provide an example of what the present insights about important determinants of nutrition behaviours in youth may mean for interventions promoting healthy diets in this target population. The European Pro Children study will be briefly described for this purpose as an example of the implementation of the model for Planned Promotion of Population Health in healthy diet promotion in youth.

Based on convincing epidemiological data supporting the beneficial role of increased vegetable and fruit intake (WHO 2003), and data indicating that children across Europe eat far less vegetables and fruits (Figure 5.1, Steps 1 to 2) than recommended, the Pro Children study was designed to:

- provide information on actual consumption levels of vegetables and fruits in European school children and on likely determinants of such consumption patterns
- develop and test effective strategies to promote adequate consumption levels of vegetables and fruits among school children (Klepp et al. 2005).

The overall goal of the study was to produce a 20 per cent increase in reported vegetable and fruit intake.

The project was aimed at eleven- to thirteen-year-old children, since children in this age group do have poor intake levels and gain more food choice autonomy. The project consisted of two phases. In the first phase, relevant information was gathered for planned development and implementation of vegetables- and fruit-promoting interventions (see Figure 5.1, Step 3). In the second phase, planned interventions were developed (Step 4), implemented (Step 5) and evaluated (Step 6). The first phase was conducted in nine participating countries (Austria, Belgium, Denmark, Iceland, the Netherlands, Norway, Portugal, Spain and Sweden), while the second phase was restricted to three countries (the Netherlands, Norway and Spain).

Potent and modifiable determinants were identified through extensive literature searches (Rasmussen et al. 2006), qualitative, explorative work with representatives of the target age group (Wind et al. 2005), and through extensive survey work (De Bourdeaudhuij et al. 2005), which enabled a comprehensive theoretical model for guiding intervention planning to be made (Table 5.1).

The intervention programmes were designed through an Intervention Mapping process, employing strategies and methods identified, based on previous systematic reviews of the relevant intervention literature (Contento et al. 1992, French & Stables 2003). Specifically, the programmes:

- focused on specific eating behaviours related to vegetable and fruit consumption
- employed educational strategies that are directly relevant to vegetable and fruit consumption derived from appropriate theory for behavioural determinants

- devoted adequate time and intensity in order to be effective
- included parental involvement and age-appropriate self-assessment and computer-tailored feedback
- included interventions targeting the school environment and the larger community.

In order to further advance the state of the art within the field of school-based public health nutrition intervention strategies, a theoretically and methodological rigorous approach was combined with the health-promotion paradigm, and an attempt was made to utilise the cultural diversity and richness of Europe in designing the intervention strategies. Specifically, we:

- encouraged local participation in planning and implementation of the intervention to secure culturally relevant interventions and foster local ownership
- included sharing of relevant food habits across intervention sites in order to promote the European heterogeneity in terms of eating habits as a positive, motivational element for participants to explore
- conducted a cross-national test of the effectiveness of a comprehensive (theoretically similar, but culturally adapted) intervention approach.

The intervention programmes were designed to ensure approximately twenty hours of exposure to food-based messages delivered to the children. These were behaviour-specific, and the activities provided opportunities for skills development during an eight-month period of intensive intervention, followed by some booster activities in the second year of intervention. The intervention in each of the three countries consisted of core programme components, as well as additional, optional components that differ between the countries. In order to design the programmes, an adapted Intervention Mapping (Perez Rodrigo et al. 2005) process was applied at all three sites.

The final Pro Children programmes all consisted of three main parts: a school-based programme, a family component, and a community component.

School-based programme
Teachers were trained to implement the classroom curriculum, which consisted of a number of worksheets and activities the pupils were to conduct at school or as homework assignments. Furthermore, the teachers provided information regarding the health benefits of fruit and vegetables and current recommendations. A computer-tailored software programme was designed in order to provide the children with personalised feedback on their own intake, and to provide suggestions for how they might set personal goals and find ways to increase

their regular intake. An Internet forum was also created so that children could communicate with participating children from other countries. A fruit and vegetable recipe contest was conducted, with the winning recipes from all three countries presented on the project homepage, which was also made into a cookbook that was distributed to all participating children.

The school environment was changed in the following ways. Introducing fruit breaks at all intervention schools increased the availability of fruit and vegetables. The fruit and vegetables were either brought from home or provided through various national school fruit programmes tested as part of the Pro Children project. Finally, attempts were made to introduce school food policies favouring fruit and vegetable availability and consumption while deterring the availability of unhealthy snacks at schools.

Family component

Parents received information about the project and its objectives through direct mail (letters and regular newsletters), meetings and special events at school. A number of worksheet activities were designed to be carried out jointly by parents and their children. A computer-tailored programme was also made available for parents (through Internet or CD-ROM) to assist them in increasing their own fruit and vegetable intake.

Community-based component

In order to reinforce the educational messages given at school and at home through the Pro Children programmes, a number of optional community-based activities were provided. These included collaboration with the school health services, with the local media regularly publishing news items related to the intervention programmes and the international aspects of the programme, as well as collaboration with local grocery stores, enhancing their produce departments' ways of introducing and presenting it to the local intervention classes.

Preliminary results from the first follow-up survey (eight months after the programme was initiated) indicate that the pupils attending the intervention schools did indeed increase their reported intake of vegetables and fruit to approximately the target goal of 20 per cent. Process measures furthermore indicate that teachers, pupils and parents were all pleased and enthusiastic about the programme. However, we also observed that the extent to which the programme had been implemented varied between schools and across countries. Overall, the degree of implementation was moderate at best, and points to the need for further assessment of barriers to successful health-promotion intervention programmes with children and adolescents (Wind et al. submitted).

Conclusions

Healthy nutrition behaviours are of specific importance in childhood and adolescence, because of the nutritional needs related to growth, and because healthy nutrition behaviours established in youth may influence health through-out the life course. These behaviours in youth are determined by motivation, abilities and opportunities. Food choice motivation is strongly influenced by taste preferences. Food choice opportunities for children and adolescents are highly dependent on their family and school environments. Interventions to promote healthy eating should be tailored to important motivations, abilities and opportunities for healthy eating because this will improve the chances for effectiveness.

REFERENCES

Bao, W., Threefoot, S.A., Srinivasan, S.R. and Berenson, G.S. 1995, 'Essential hypertension predicted by tracking of elevated blood pressure from childhood to adulthood: The Bogalusa Heart Study in *American Journal of Hypertension*, vol. 8, pp. 657–65.

Baranowski, T., Baranowski, J., Cullen, K.W., Marsh, T., Islam, N., Zakeri, I., Honess-Morreale, L. and deMoor, C. 2003, 'Squire's quest! Dietary outcome evaluation of a multimedia game' in *American Journal of Preventive Medicine*, vol. 24, pp. 52–61.

Bartholomew, K., Parcel, G., Kok, G. and Gottlieb, N. 2000, *Intervention mapping: Developing theory- and evidence-based health education programs,* Mayfield, CA.

Birch, L.L. 1999, 'Development of food preferences' in *Annual Review of Nutrition*, vol. 19, pp. 41–62.

Brug, J. and Kok, G.J. 1995, 'Misconceptie van consumenten over eigen vetconsumptie' ['Miscon-ception of consumers about their own fatconsumption'] in *Voeding*, vol. 56, pp. 11–14.

Brug, J. and van Lenthe, F. 2005, *Environmental determinants and interventions for physical activity, diet and smoking: A review,* Erasmus MC, Rotterdam, The Netherlands.

Brug, J., Kroeze, W., Wind, M., van der Horst, K. and Ferreira, I. 2005a, 'The importance of habit strength in dietary behaviors' (abstract) in Fourth Annual Conference of the International Society of Behavioral Nutrition and Physical Activity (ISBNPA), Amsterdam.

Brug, J., Oenema, A. and Ferreira, I. 2005b, 'Theory, evidence and intervention mapping to improve behavioural nutrition and physical activity interventions' in *International Journal of Behavioural Nutrition and Physical Activity*, vol. 2, p. 2.

Brug, J., van Assema, P., Lenderink, T., Glanz, K. and Kok, G.J. 1994, 'Self-rated dietary fat intake: Association with objective assessment of fat, psychosocial factors and intention to change' in *Journal of Nutrition Education*, vol. 26, pp. 218–23.

Capaldi, E.D.E. (ed.) 1996, *Why we eat what we eat: The psychology of eating,* American Psychological Association, Washington, D.C.

Cole, T.J., Bellizzi, M.C., Flegal, K.M. and Dietz, W.H. 2000, 'Establishing a standard definition for child overweight and obesity worldwide: International survey' *British Medical Journal,* vol. 320, pp. 1240–43.

Conner, M. and Armitage, C.J. 2002, *The Social Psychology of Food,* Open University Press, London.

Contento, I., Balch, G.I., Bronner, Y.L., Lytle, L.A., Maloney, S.K., Olson, C.M. and Swadener, S.S. 1995, 'The effectiveness of nutrition education and implications for nutrition education policy, programs and research: A review of research' in *Journal of Nutrition Education*, vol. 27.

Contento, I.R., Manning, A.D. and Shannon, B. 1992, 'Research perspective on school-based nutrition education' in *Journal of Nutrition Education*, vol. 24, pp. 247–60.

Cooke, L.J. and Wardle, J. 2005, 'Age and gender differences in children's food preferences' in *British Journal of Nutrition*, vol. 93, pp. 741–46.

Cullen, K.W., Baranowski, T., Owens, E., Marsh, T., Rittenberry, L. and de Moor, C. 2003, 'Availability, accessibility, and preferences for fruit: 100% fruit juice, and vegetables influence children's dietary behaviour' in *Health Education and Behaviour,* vol. 30, pp. 615–26.

Cummins, S. and Macintyre, S. 2006, 'Food environments and obesity: Neighbourhood or nation?' in *International Journal of Epidemiology*, vol. 35, pp. 100–04.

De Bourdeaudhuij, I. and Van Oost, P. 1996, 'De relatie tussen op jonge leeftijd aangeleerde voedings-regels en voedingskeuze in de adolescentie' ['The influence of family food rules on (un)healthy eating in adolescents' in *Gedrag Gezond*, vol. 24, pp. 215–23.

De Bourdeaudhuij, I., Klepp, K.-I., Wind, M., Due, P. and Brug, J. 2005, 'Reliability of a question-naire to measure personal, social and environmental correlates of fruit and vegetable intake in 10- to 11-year-old children in 5 European countries' in *Public Health Nutrition*, vol. 8, pp. 189–200.

Flay, B.R. and Petraitis, J. 1994, 'The theory of triadic influence: A new theory of health behaviour with implications for preventive interventions' in *Advances in Medical Sociology*, vol. 4, pp. 4–19.

French, S.A. and Stables, G. 2003, 'Environmental interventions to promote vegetable and fruit consumption among youth in school settings' in *Preventive Medicine,* vol. 37, pp. 593–610.

French, S.A., Story, M., Neumark-Sztainer, D., Fulkerson, J.A. and Hannan, P.J. 2001, 'Fast food restaurant use among adolescents: Associations with nutrient intake, food choices and behav-ioral and psychological variables' in *International Journal of Obesity*, vol. 25, pp. 1823–33.

Green, L.W. and Kreuter, M.W. 1999, *Health promotion planning: An educational and ecological approach,* Mayfield, Mountain View, CA.

Health-Focus 2005, 'HealthFocus Study of Public Attitudes and Actions Toward Shopping and Eating' in *Health Focus International*, St Petersburg.

Heatey, K.R. and Thombs, D.L. 1997, Fruit–vegetable consumption self-efficacy in youth in *American Journal of Health Behavior,* vol. 21, pp. 172–77.

Kelder, S.H., Perry, C.L., Klepp, K.I. and Lytle, L.L. 1994, 'Longitudinal tracking of adolescent smoking, physical activity, and food choice behaviours in *American Journal of Public Health,* vol. 84, pp. 1121–26.

Klepp, K.-I., Perez Rodrigo, C., De Bourdeaudhuij , I., Due, P., Elmadfa, I., Haraldsdottir, J., König, J., Sjöström, M., Thorsdottir, I., Daniel Vaz de Almeida, M., Yngve, A. and Brug, J. 2005, 'Promoting fruit and vegetable consumption among European schoolchildren: Rationale, conceptualization and design of the Pro Children Project' *Annals of Nutrition and Metabolism,* vol. 49, pp. 212–20.

Koletzko, B., de la Gueronniere, V., Toschke, A.M. and von Kries, R. 2004, 'Nutrition in children and adolescents in Europe: What is the scientific basis? Introduction' in *British Journal of Nutrition,* vol. 92, S67–73.

Kremers, S.P.J. 2005, 'Habit Strength of energy balance-related behaviors among children and adolescents' (abstract) in *Fourth Annual Conference of the International Society of Behavioral Nutrition and Physical Activity (ISBNPA),* Amsterdam.

Kremers, S.P.J., Brug, J., Vries de, H. and Engels, R.C.M.E. 2003, 'Parenting style and adolescent fruit consumption' in *Appetite,* vol. 41, pp. 43–50.

Lambert, J., Agostoni, C., Elmadfa, I., Hulshof, K., Krause, E., Livingstone, B., Socha, P., Pannemans, D. and Samartin, S. 2004, 'Dietary intake and nutritional status of children and adolescents in Europe' in *British Journal of Nutrition,* vol. 92, S147–211.

Lechner, L., Brug, J. and de Vries, H. 1997, 'Misconception of fruit and vegetable consumption: Differences between objective and subjective estimation of intake' in *Journal of Nutrition Education,* vol. 29, pp. 313–20.

Lennernas, M., Fjellstrom, C., Becker, W., Giachetti, I., Schmitt, A., Remaut de Winter, A. and Kearney, M. 1997, 'Influences on food choice perceived to be important by nationally representative samples of adults in the European Union' in *European Journal of Clinical Nutrition,* vol. 51, S8–15.

Lien, N., Lytle, L.A. and Klepp, K.-I. 2001, 'Stability in consumption of fruit, vegetables, and sugary foods in a cohort from age 14 to age 21' in *Preventive Medicine,* vol. 33, pp. 217–26.

Liu, L., Hironaka, K. and Pihoker, C. 2004, 'Type 2 diabetes in youth' in *Current Problems in Pediatric Adolescent Health Care,* vol. 34, pp. 254–72.

Lytle, L.A. and Kubik, M.Y. 2003, 'Nutritional issues for adolescents' in *Best Practice and Research: Clinical endocrinology and metabolism,* vol. 17, pp. 177–89.

McCarthy, H.D., Cole, T.J., Fry, T., Jebb, S.A. and Prentice, A.M. 2006, 'Body fat reference curves for children' in *International Journal of Obesity,* vol. 30, pp. 598–602.

Maslow, A.H. 1970, *Motivation and Personality* (second edition), Harper & Row, New York.

Mikkila, V., Rasanen, L., Raitakari, O.T., Pietinen, P. and Viikari, J. 2005, 'Consistent dietary patterns identified from childhood to adulthood: The cardiovascular risk in young Finns study' in *British Journal of Nutrition,* vol. 93, pp. 923–31.

Oenema, A. and Brug, J. 2003, 'Exploring the occurrence and nature of interpersonal comparisons of one's own dietary fat intake to that of self-selected others' in *Appetite,* vol. 41, 259–64.

Patrick, H. and Nicklas, T.A. 2005, 'A review of family and social determinants of children's eating patterns and diet quality' in *Journal of American College Nutrition,* vol. 24, pp. 83–92.

Patrick, H., Nicklas, T.A., Hughes, S.O. and Morales, M. 2005, 'The benefits of authoritative feeding style: Caregiver feeding styles and children's food consumption patterns' in *Appetite*, vol. 44, pp. 243–9.

Perez Rodrigo, C., Wind, M., Hildonen, C., Bjelland, M., Aranceta, J., Klepp, K.-I. and Brug, J. 2005, 'The Pro Children Intervention: Applying the Intervention Mapping Protocol to develop a school-based fruit and vegetable promotion programme' in *Annals of Nutrition and Metabolism*, vol. 49, pp. 267–77.

Prentice, A., Branca, F., Decsi, T., Michaelsen, K.F., Fletcher, R.J., Guesry, P., Manz, F., Vidailhet, M., Pannemans, D. and Samartin, S. 2004, 'Energy and nutrient dietary reference values for children in Europe: Methodological approaches and current nutritional recommendations' in *British Journal of Nutrition*, vol. 92, S83–146.

Rasmussen, M., Krolner, R., Klepp, K.I., Lytle, L., Brug, J., Bere, E. and Due, P. 2006, 'Determinants of fruit and vegetable consumption among children and adolescents: Systematic review of the literature' in *International Journal of Behaviour, Nutrition and Physical Action*, vol. 3, p. 22.

Resnicow, K., Davis-Hearn, M., Smith, M., Baranowski, T., Lin, L.S., Baranowski, J., Doyle, C. and Wang, D.T. 1997, 'Social-cognitive predictors of fruit and vegetable intake in children' in *Health and Psychology*, vol. 16, pp. 272–76.

Rothschild, M.L. 1999, 'Carrots, Sticks, and Promises: A conceptual framework for the management of public health and the social issue behaviours, *Journal of Marketing*, vol. 63, pp. 24–37.

Sallis, J.F. and Owen, N. 2003, 'Ecological Models of Health Behavior' in Glanz, K., Rimer, B.K. and Lewis, F.M. (eds) *Health Behavior and Health Education*, pp. 462–85.

Story, M. and French, S. 2004, 'Food advertising and marketing directed at children and adolescents in the US' in *International Journal of Behavioural Nutrition and Physical Activity*, vol. 1, p. 3.

Story, M., Neumark-Sztainer, D. and French, S. 2002, 'Individual and environmental influences on adolescent eating behaviours' in *Journal of American Dietetic Association*, vol. 102, S40–51.

Swinburn, B., Egger, G. and Raza, F. 1999, 'Dissecting obesogenic environments: The development and application of a framework for identifying and prioritising environmental interventions for obesity' in *Preventive Medicine*, vol. 29, pp. 563–70.

van Trijp, H.C.M., Brug, J. and van der Maas, R. 2005, 'Consumer determinants and intervention strategies for obesity prevention' in Mela, D.J. (ed.), *Food, Diet and Obesity*, Woodhead Publishing in Food Science and Technology, pp. 331–56.

Verplanken, B. and Aarts, H. 1999, 'Habit, attitude, and planned behaviour: Is habit and empty construct or an interesting case of goal-directed automaticity?' in *European Review of Social Psychology*, vol. 10, pp. 101–34.

Verplanken, B. and Orbell, S. 2003, 'Self-reported habit: A self-report index of habit strength' in *Journal of Applied Socoiology and Psychology*, vol. 33, pp. 1313–30.

Wardle, J., Jarvis, M., Steggles, N., Sutton, S., Williamson, S., Farrimond, H., Cartwright, M. and Simon, A.E. 2003, 'Socioeconomic disparities in cancer-risk behaviors in adolescence: Baseline results from the Health and Behaviour in Teenagers Study (HABITS)' in *Preventive Medicine*, vol. 36, pp. 721–30.

Wind, M., Bjelland, M., Perez Rodrigo, C., te Velde, S.J., Hildonen, C., Bere, E., Klepp, K.-I. and

Brug, J. (submitted), 'Appreciation and implementation of a school-based intervention are associated with changes in fruit and vegetable intake in 10-11-year-old school children'.

Wind, M., Bobelijn, K., De Bourdeaudhuij , I., Klepp, K.I. and Brug, J. 2005, 'A qualitative exploration of determinants of fruit and vegetable intake among 10- and 11-year-old school children in the Low countries' in *Annals of Nutrition and Metabolism,* vol. 49, pp. 228-35.

Wind, M., De Bourdeaudhuij, I., Te Velde, S.J., Sandvik, C., Klepp, K.-I., Due, P. and Brug, J., 'Correlates of fruit and vegetable consumption among 11-year-old Belgian–Flemish and Dutch schoolchildren' in *Journal of Nutrition Education and Behavior,* vol. 38, pp. 211–21.

World Health Organization (WHO) 2003, *Technical Report 916: Based on expert consultation in diet, nutrition and the prevention of chronic diseases*, WHO, Geneva.

— 2004, 'Young people's health in context: Health behaviour in school-aged children' in *International Report from the 2001/2002 Survey*, Regional Office for Europe, Copenhagen.

Wynder, E.L., Williams, C.L., Laakso, K. and Levenstein, M. 1981, 'Screening for risk factors for chronic disease in children from fifteen countries' in *Preventative Medicine,* vol. 10, pp. 121–32.

6

Older adults

WENDY HUNTER
MONIQUE RAATS
MARGARET LUMBERS

The proportion of older people in the populations of almost all countries is increasing, and it is predicted that in western countries the current 20 per cent of the population aged 60 years or over will have increased to 32 per cent by 2050 (Population Division of the Department of Economic and Social Affairs of the United Nations Secretariat 2005). Consequently, it is projected that population ageing will result in increases in age-related public spending, including age pension payments and expenditure on health and long-term care (Dang et al. 2001).

The ageing process is one of progressive and irreversible biological changes that results in a growing risk of chronic disease, cognitive and functional impairment, and an increased likelihood of dying (Khaw 1997). Successful ageing is regarded as decreasing the risk of diseases and disease-related disability while maintaining physical and mental functioning; and being actively engaged with life, with 'active' referring not only to being physically or economically active, but also to continued societal participation (Rowe & Kahn 1998). The World Health Organization's (WHO) active ageing policy framework (2002) identified and brought together the key concepts of productive ageing (that is, the ability to contribute directly and indirectly in older age) and healthy ageing (the ability to remain physically and mentally fit). Therefore, healthy ageing, in which disability and morbidity are compressed into a relatively short period before death, preceded by a long period in which people age with their vigour and functional independence intact (Campion 1998), is the ideal situation.

Later life is commonly regarded as a period of dependency. There has, however, been a move away from considering old age to be a problem in itself towards focusing on older people's ability to improve their quality of life. Studies of mealtimes on geriatric wards in Sweden showed that older patients adopted the role of dependent patient because they were not given the opportunity to feed themselves (Sidenvall et al. 2001). This chapter presents a review of the public health nutrition priorities of older adults.

Physiological basis of food requirements in later life

The quality of older people's diets decline on average with increasing age for both men and women, furthermore, the diets of older men are typically reported to be much poorer than those of older women within each age group, although there is a smaller difference above age 80 (see, for example, Ginn et al. 1998). One reason this may occur is due to a lessening of the olfactory function and taste, losses which serve to reduce appetite. There is evidence that as people age these become less effective and may result in inadequate dietary intake. This is thought to be a major cause of malnutrition (Hickson 2006). For many older people, physical activity also diminishes with age, resulting in a decrease in the basic metabolic rate (BMR), leading to lower energy requirements and reductions in lean body tissue and appetite (Rosenberg 2001). Other factors that bring about the loss of lean mass include hormonal changes that influence metabolism and the immune system (Hickson 2006). Cytokines, such as interleukin 1 (ILK1), interleukin 6 (ILK6), tumour necrosis factor a (TFNa), and serotonin have been associated with protein breakdown in muscle and fat breakdown in adipose tissue (Hickson 2006). It is also thought that some cytokines interfere with myogenic differentiation into the development of functional muscle fibres (Langen et al. 2001). The loss of muscle or lean body mass with age is known as sarcopenia. For women, this decrease is usually prevalent after menopause; however, for both sexes, the greatest loss of muscle mass occurs after 80 years of age, and the ultimate implication is decreased strength and mobility, which has been associated with an increase in the risk of falls (Rosenberg 2001).

Osteoporosis is the term given to bone loss and bone brittleness. Although it does occur in older males, it is more prevalent among middle-aged and older women (NIH 2000). The consequences of osteoporosis are an increased risk of falling and subsequent increased risk of fractures (Rosenberg 2001). It has been estimated that approximately 80 per cent of all hip fractures are suffered by women who have experienced a history of falls prior to the fracture (WHO 2006). Inadequate intakes of vitamin D and calcium, and lack of physical activity are thought to play a significant role in the development of bone loss (Rosenberg 2001; Flicker et al. 2005). Other contributing factors to osteoporosis include smoking, low weight and body mass index (BMI), being female, having a family history of osteoporosis, a history of prior fractures, and oestrogen deficiency (NIH 2000). Traditionally, researchers have believed that women tend to lose a considerable amount of bone mass during a ten-year period after the menopause because of hormonal changes (Rosenberg 2001), However, it has also been argued that, while a decrease in bone mineral density does occur after menopause, fractures do not start occurring until women are about 80 years of age; furthermore, as men also develop osteoporosis as they age, it is likely that the other risk factors mentioned have a greater contribution that was originally considered (NIH 2000).

Vitamin D is mainly absorbed through the skin, and in later life there is often a deficiency because of less exposure to the sun. Research has found that supplementation of vitamin D can reduce fall frequency among frail older people, thereby reducing the risk of fractures (Flicker et al. 2005), but recent research in nursing homes has found that dietary intakes of vitamin D among residents were insufficient to overcome the deficiency caused through lack of sun exposure, thereby increasing their risk of fracture (Nowson et al. 2003). Although there is no recommended dietary intake (RDI) in Australia for vitamin D, the accepted adequate intake for people aged between 51 and 70 years is 10 microgram per day, and for those aged over 70 years, this increases to 15 microgram per day. Insufficient vitamin D may also result in osteomalacia in adults, which causes bone pain, deformity and weakness in muscles (Rosenberg 2001).

Calcium is important for preventing and treating osteoporosis. Calcium helps to build bone mass and, in Australia, the RDI for calcium for women aged 51 to 70 years and over has recently been increased to 1300 milligram per day, which is higher than that recommended for men of the same age and for younger women. A daily intake of 1300 milligram of calcium is also recommended for all adults aged 70 years and over (NHMRC 2006).

Protein-energy malnutrition is an increasing problem in the oldest-old (those over 80 years of age), discussed in more detail under 'Malnutrition' below. Other nutrients that are often low with increasing age include vitamin B6, which is needed for amino-acid metabolism and glycogen metabolism, and it is thought that approximately one in three people aged 70 years and over 'have limited secretion of stomach acid, which affects absorption of vitamin B12, folic acid, iron and zinc' (Rosenberg 2001).

Malnutrition

Policymakers and health-promotion campaigns are generally aimed at reducing obesity and improving eating habits. While it has been commonly reported that many older hospital patients may be malnourished on admission, it still goes unrecognised in hospitals, nursing homes and the community. Malnutrition refers to specific nutrient deficiencies and is a multidimensional health problem for older people, particularly protein energy malnutrition (PEM), which has many detrimental health consequences, including increased mortality, prolonged hospitalisation and increased falls, as well as an increase in life-threatening health problems such as stroke, bleeding, respiratory failure, cardiac complications, infections, poor immunity and pressure ulcers (Chen et al. 2001). A recent study of older female patients with hip fractures in the United Kingdom found that many were malnourished, and these patients often had slower recovery times (Lumbers et al. 2001).

Malnutrition is a particular problem for older people, especially those over 80 years of age. Metabolic and physiological changes related to the ageing process make older people more susceptible to nutrient deficiencies. A study of the malnutrition and mortality in two Sydney teaching hospitals found that there was a significantly higher prevalence of malnutrition among subjects aged 65 years and over (43 per cent), compared to 27 per cent for those under 65 years. This increased the patients' length of stay in the hospital, and more malnourished subjects died while in the hospital than those who were well nourished (Middleton et al. 2001).

Furthermore, a number of risk factors, including living circumstances, socio-economic factors, as well as clinical conditions, have been identified (Herne 1995; Visvanathan 2003):

- low intakes of fruit and vegetables, and limited dietary variety
- social class
- knowledge about food
- food insecurity
- lack of food variety
- health issues such as chronic medical conditions, drug-nutrient interaction
- poor dentition, resulting in difficulty in chewing and reduced intakes
- lack of physical activity, due to poor mobility, physical disability or lack of incentive to undertake exercise
- economic circumstances
- social isolation and loneliness.

Insufficient importance or priority is attached to ensuring that adequate diets are maintained by older people living in their own homes, particularly those living alone. With the advent of greater drives to efficiency, older people are often discharged home earlier than in previous times when their nutritional needs for rehabilitation are still high and when access to food may be compromised (Gazzotti et al. 2003). The extent of poor diets and compromised nutritional status of the people living in the community is demonstrated by the high prevalence of malnutrition found among older people on admission to hospital (Gazotti et al. 2003). However, the prevalence of malnutrition in the community reported varies according to different researchers and for different patient groups; it also varies on the range of parameters used to diagnose malnutrition. In geriatric hospitals and nursing homes, the situation is worse. It has been reported that the prevalence in malnutrition in these institutions can range from 30 to 60 per cent of the residents/patients (Gazzotti et al. 2003). In 2003, research into diets in Australian nursing homes found that that energy, protein, and fibre intakes were low compared to hostel diets, particularly for those on soft and pureed diets (Nowson et al. 2003).

Although malnutrition is a serious public health problem, it has not yet appeared on the political agenda of most countries, and awareness of the problem is still low among the general public, clinicians, nurses, healthcare managers and insurers, patients, policymakers and politicians. Malnutrition is not only in itself a problem, it also compromises the health outcomes of individuals, and may delay recovery from acute episodes of illness, increases morbidity and mortality, and is extremely costly for the healthcare system.

Cardiovascular disease, metabolic syndrome and obesity

Increases in life expectancy have seen the leading causes of death shifting dramatically from infectious diseases to non-communicable diseases, and from younger to older individuals. In industrialised countries, about 75 per cent of deaths in people over 65 are from cardiovascular diseases and cancer. Dietary and lifestyle changes can reduce the toll of such diseases. Indeed, in a recent survey of 1500 people over 70 years from eleven European countries, studied over a ten-year period, Knoops and colleagues (2004) showed that the risk of deaths could be cut by 60 per cent through the single and combined effects of a Mediterranean diet, being physically active, moderate alcohol use, and not smoking.

The clustering of closely related risk factors for cardiovascular disease and diabetes is also known as the metabolic syndrome, and is considered to be one of the major public health challenges facing older people. Although there is contention surrounding nature and extent of the syndrome, diagnostic guidelines and treatments have been published. For example, guidelines from the Third Report of the National Cholesterol Education Program (National Heart, Lung and Blood Institute 2001) suggest that identification of the metabolic syndrome should be based on the presence of three or more of the following: abdominal obesity, fasting serum triglycerides, blood pressure, and specific levels of fasting plasma glucose. The risk factors for metabolic syndrome identified in the National Health and Nutrition Examination Survey (NHANES) III study included lifestyle factors such as smoking, physical inactivity, low income, postmenopausal status, high carbohydrate diet, no alcohol (Janssen et al. 2002). However, it should be noted that metabolic syndrome is an incomplete predictor of absolute risk for cardiovascular disease, which should also include factors such as age, sex, total cholesterol, triglyceride, blood pressure, BMI, glucose status, smoking and family history. The safest and most effective way to reduce insulin resistance in overweight and obese people is likely to be weight loss and increased physical activity, and therefore older people would be advised to continue to monitor their weight by keeping a regular record together with waist circumference; however caution is needed with these health messages, as severe weight loss can lead to health problems for older people, such as frailty, leading to an increased risk of falls, as well as increased mortality (Wahlqvist & Savige 2000).

Relatively few studies have investigated overweight and obesity in representative country samples of older populations. Gutierrez-Fisac and colleagues (2004) found the prevalence of overweight and obesity in older Spanish men was 49 and 31.5 per cent respectively (overweight BMI 25 to 29.9; obesity BMI greater than 30). In addition, the loss of real and apparent height occurs after the age of 65, particularly in men, leading to an overestimation of obesity when based on BMI (calculated as weight divided by the square of height) alone. This may be compensated for by the loss of lean body mass with age, meaning that they would have larger relative proportion of body fat than a younger individual with the same BMI. Waist circumference is strongly predictive of cardiovascular risk, and does not suffer the same age-related changes, and therefore may be a useful measurement in clinical practice. Abdominal obesity is linked with resistance to the effects of insulin, leading to type 2 diabetes (Gutierrez-Fisac et al. 2004).

Although it is important to understand the physiological influences on nutrition intake and absorption, and to be aware of the increasing prevalence of sub-optimal nutrition, it should be remembered that these problems still affect the minority of this population, and many people over 65 years live relatively healthy and active lives. It is also too simplistic to argue that the ageing process will inevitably result in poor nutrition and poor health. There are many confounding psychosocial factors that play important roles in the older people's nutritional status, their food choices and general health, such as availability, access, costs, living circumstances, health status and beliefs.

Nutrition intervention in later life: Is it worthwhile?

Studies (Knoops et al. 2004, for example) suggest that healthy lifestyle choices can result in important reductions in morbidity and mortality, and increase the changes of successful ageing. To achieve healthy dietary habits, successful intervention strategies are needed. There is, however, currently limited evidence as to which interventions aimed at older people might be most effective, although a recent review of 25 nutrition interventions targeting adults aged over 55 years (Sahyoun et al. 2004) concluded that the interventions were limited in their ability to induce behaviour change, suggesting that success was more likely if interventions:

- were limited to one or two educational messages
- used reinforced and personalised messages
- provided hands-on activities, incentives, cues, and access to health professionals
- used appropriate behaviour-change theories.

The need for the development and testing of appropriate evaluation instruments, development of appropriate behavioural and educational theoretical frameworks, as well as designs and intervention strategies has been highlighted. Higgins and Clarke Barkley (2004) suggest that the success of nutrition interventions aimed at older people can be limited by the barriers experienced by healthcare professionals, and can include misconceptions and stereotypes about older people and their nutritional concerns, lack of attention to and funding for older adult educational programmes and difficulties recruiting older learners. Furthermore, they found that older people themselves can also experience barriers, including those of an attitudinal, motivational or environmental nature, and those related to low literacy and poverty.

CASE STUDY 6.1
THE FOOD IN LATER LIFE PROJECT

The Food in Later Life Project was set up in 2002 to look at the drivers of food selection and at the whole process of food procurement — from shopping through to the meal preparation, the way food is stored and cooked, the types of meals they have, and the social significance or meaning of the meal for older people, such as whether they are eating alone, with others or in community settings. The project involved nine partners in eight different countries, covering northern, western, eastern and southern Europe, with participants in Denmark, Germany, Spain, Italy, Poland, Portugal Sweden and the United Kingdom. Six studies were conducted in all of the countries:

Study 1: Food selection in later life — functional and convenience
Study 2: Procuring foods and preparing meals in later life
Study 3: Older people's satisfaction with food-related services
Study 4: Formal and informal networks affecting food provisioning and consumption
Study 5: Meals in later life
Study 6: Assessing food-related quality of life.

A variety of data-collection methods were used within the project, as shown below.

All studies	Specific studies
Background questionnaire:	Study 1:
• where they shop	Repertory grid method
• where they eat out	
• reason for choosing foods	Study 2:
• transport available	Observed/accompanied shops
• health (including SF36 or SF8)	
• physical activity	Study 3:
• nutritional screening	Critical incident technique
• social characteristics.	
	Study 4:
In-depth one-on-one interviews	Food diary
	Shopping diary
	Study 5:
	In-depth open interviews
	Study 6:
	Food-related Quality of Life Survey

Each method or instrument was tested for reliability and validity. The survey used in study six was developed from the outcomes of the previous studies. The overriding outcomes of the study were:

- the importance of life transitions on food choice
- the importance of health transitions on food choice
- the importance of trust — of the product, service — of the health professional
- for many aspects, gender more important than age
- shopping experiences and shopping patterns change with age and health (and by country)
- the need to focus marketing of services and products to suit older people's needs, but at the same time not single out older people in a way that can be perceived as negative
- the importance of older people's willingness to embrace new products and services, often influenced by cost, exposure and concern for wastage
- the importance of evaluating products and services
- the conflicting needs and wants of the youngest-old and the oldest-old
- older people's concerns about environmental issues related to food stronger than previously thought
- older people's reluctance to formally complain about food services for fear of losing access to the service
- in many of the countries, participants used supermarkets regularly and enjoyed the convenience of the 'one-stop shop' but where they shopped was influenced by access to public transport or adequate car parking delivery services and easy access to food within the store
- often special offers on food could not be taken up because portion sizes were too large so unlikely to be consumed before the use-by date
- packaging also influenced some older people, with ring-pull lids on cans often considered to be more of a hindrance than a help.

Influences of older people's food choices

The Social Ecological Framework (Welton et al. 1997) offers a framework for understanding the levels through which people's behaviour can be influenced, and the following levels can be distinguished:

- intrapersonal (such as an individual's knowledge, skills, attitudes, values, preferences, emotions, values, behaviour)

- interpersonal (for example, an individual's social networks, social supports, families, peers, and neighbours)
- organisational (like businesses, public agencies, churches, service organisations)
- community (for instance, community resources, neighbourhood organisations, social and health services)
- public policy (such as legislation, policies, taxes, and regulatory agencies, health system, social care system, political/geographic environment).

Intrapersonal level

To some older adults, food is simply fuel for the body, and preparing a meal is a task that has to be undertaken as quickly as possible with as little inconvenience; however, for most people food fulfils more than a biological need, and there are social, cultural and economic associations connected to the procurement, preparation and consumption of food. It has been proposed that:

> cohorts of consumers are groups of people who are born during the same time period and travel through life together. They experience similar external events . . . such as the Great Depression in the USA (Ahmad 2002).

Therefore, it is likely that older people's values, attitudes and food preferences will reflect their life-course experiences.

It is commonly thought that most people develop their food preferences at a young age, and these will be influenced by the food that was available when they were young, the parents' food preferences and cooking skills, along with the food traditions embedded in the culture in which the individual lived (Lilley 1996), and it is thought that the present population of older adults, particularly those people aged 75 years and over, are more likely to continue to eat the types of foods and meals that they were given as children. But Connor (1999) argues that regardless of age, individuals have their own needs, preferences and expectations. Food preferences developed in childhood remain important throughout life, therefore the food choices of older people are likely to be as varied as those of the young. Furthermore, as people age they may be exposed to new food experiences, and these may expand the variety of food they consume.

As older people go along the continuum of health from being independent, healthy and able to care for themselves, to needing a minimal level of care, and finally requiring a high level of care, there will be changes in the types of food chosen. Older people with physical disabilities may modify their food choices by forgoing food that is difficult to prepare and cook; for example, people who have arthritis in their hands have reported difficulty in chopping food, they drop utensils and cooking equipment, and the aftertaste of medication can decrease their enjoyment of food (Wylie et al. 1999).

Older people in the Food in Later Life project (see case study) reported making changes to foods if they could no longer drive and had to carry their shopping home, and instead of heavy packaging such as bottles and cans, they looked for products that would be lighter to carry, such as dehydrated soups. Changes in shopping habits occur for men during transition periods. Generally men in this age group start shopping after they have retired, or if their spouse has become ill or died. Life course transitions, such as widowhood or illness, may also affect women, restricting their access to transport and a range of shops, particularly large out-of-town supermarkets, thereby limiting the amount and types of food they purchase. Furthermore, widows are more likely to be receiving lower incomes and have less money to spend on food.

There is, however, also evidence that people in the face of life course transitions maintain stable food and nutrition-related thoughts, beliefs, and strategies. Edstrom and Devine (2001) used a life course framework in a qualitative study with women aged 44 to 75 years, and found consistent orientations to food and nutrition at interviews ten years apart, even where expected and unexpected changes in health, social environment and roles were experienced fourteen of the seventeen women perceived that their nutrition had been consistent over the ten-year period.

Many of today's older generation are on limited incomes, due to lack of access to private pensions when they were younger or because of interruption to work patterns or careers, such as war for many of the older men and child-bearing for the older women. Where income is considered insufficient to spend on food, the foods the older generations restricted buying were chicken, fish and fruit (Wylie et al. 1999).

Interpersonal level
For many older people, a consequence of ageing is the loss of social networks. It would appear that older people's living arrangements are changing, they are less likely to live with other family members or unrelated individuals, and more likely to live alone with an increased probability of eating alone (Iacovou 2000). There is evidence that older people living alone are more likely to enter an institution than those living with at least one other person. Even where institu-

tionalisation does not take place, older people who live alone are more likely to require inputs of care from the state, in the form of home helps and other social services, than those who live with others (see, Iacovou 2000, for example). The significance for service providers is that living alone is the highest risk factor, after age itself, for admission to hospital or to long-term care.

Many studies (Quandt et al. 2000) suggest that widowhood has the potential for negative impact on food intake. Older men who live alone are also known to be at increased nutritional risk, particularly following bereavement or divorce. Furthermore, in a study comparing men and women's experiences in bereavement, Bennett and colleagues (2003) found that men believed that women are better equipped to deal with widowhood, explaining this in terms of women's domestic abilities and social skills, and men's inability to talk about their emotions. It was also found that women believed men received more support than they did after bereavement. Davidson (2001) found that, for older women, widowhood could lead to a newfound sense of freedom and autonomy, whereas widowers can feel less free because of their need to take on tasks previously carried out by their spouse.

Certain groups of older people, including those living alone, face the risk of social exclusion leading to social isolation. This situation may in part result from poverty and the low incomes experienced by many older people, especially those living alone. Women account for almost two-thirds of the population above 65 years. Yet many older women have been left with insufficient pension cover because of the lack of occupational pension provision and, as such, are the worst-exposed group in terms of financial resources and higher levels of disability (Quandt et. al. 2000). Social exclusion compounded by low income may also affect the uptake of food-related services.

Organisational and Community levels

Food retailing
Retailers appear to often disregard the needs of this growing segment of the community, and problems previously discussed regarding in-store signage, efficiency at checkouts and package sizing are often not been addressed (Hare et al. 2001). Even though package labelling is considered to be a useful source of nutrition information (Satia et al. 2005), frequently labelling on food packages is difficult to read.

The nature of retailing has changed in many western countries over the past twenty years, in particular the growth of large out-of-town hyper- or supermarkets and the closure of the traditional community-based local shops (Borghesani et al.

1997). While the degree to which this development has advanced differs between countries, the direction of the development has been the same. Large multiple food retailers dominate western societies. Recent developments in the retail industry have created barriers to food choice among older people. Decisions made by retailers and food manufactures can play a vital role in the successful procurement of food for this segment of the population, and it has been found that the location of stores was important for older people (Moschis 2003).

Older people have been found to be among those most dependent upon local declining towns and villages, and have reported that they are dissatisfied with the facilities for food shopping, including the higher prices and limited choice of food found in many local shops or convenience stores (Barrett 1997). Easy accessibility to food because of a store's fixtures and layout has been identified as playing a crucial role in the satisfaction of older shoppers (Moschis 2003). If products are placed on shelves too high or too low, some older consumers may ask for assistance, but many will simply not bother purchasing that item. The internal store environment also plays an important role determining where older people do their shopping. Difficulties in manoeuvring supermarket trolleys through narrow or crowded aisles or doorways, lifting heavy shopping bags out of deep trolleys, and poor lighting have also been identified as reasons some older people might have to avoid using particular stores (Hare et al. 2001). However, older people are also influenced by the type of food the store has on sale and the helpfulness and friendliness of the staff (Hare et al. 2001).

A number of recent research projects look at food, nutrition, health and ageing. One of these is highlighted in Case study 6.1 and it illustrates the interrelationship of issues that influence food choices of older people and how these can in turn affect their quality of life and their ability to maintain independence.

Food services

The roles played in the provision of food services to older people by industry, community health organisations, local authorities and government vary between countries. In the past, research on food products has focused on individual foods. Similarly, the industry areas dealing with hospitality, food service and catering have also dealt with individual foods, although most food is eaten as part of a meal. When exploring what older people do eat and the reasons for their food choice, first, it should be remembered that people do not eat nutrients, they eat food, usually in the form of meals or snacks, and it is in these terms that older people relate to food and meals.

The Food in Later Life project found that older people's expectations of food services are low, and they are inclined to demonstrate a sense of gratitude that might inhibit frank feedback. As such, the food service providers may not be aware of the reasons for poor uptake of particular food-related services, or fail to recognise the market opportunity to develop acceptable product ranges for this population group. However, without such support older people may be forced to give up their own homes and independence and move into nursing and residential homes, at significant cost to the community. This point is illustrated by reports in the United Kingdom that only 50 to 60 per cent of patients return to their own home following hospitalisation for hip fractures (Parker et al. 1996). In addition, with the advent of shorter hospital stays, older people are often discharged home when their nutritional needs for rehabilitation are still high and when access to food may be compromised. Early hospital discharge without adequate nutritional support being given to older people can result in readmission at a later stage or entry into nursing home care. This problem is compounded in those living alone. As stated earlier, the proportion of older people living alone is increasing.

Although food service providers may be meeting the Food Safety and Hygiene regulations, food practices, such as preparing meals early in the day and then holding them at the required temperature for four or five hours, have a detrimental effect on the nutritive value of the food. Likewise, untrained staff may be unaware of the needs of older people, providing meals that are unappetising and poorly presented (Connor 1999). Therefore, food service providers need to ensure that training of staff is far more extensive than simply complying with the Food Safety and Hygiene regulations.

In a recent review on food intake and the elderly (Fjellström et al. 2001), it was concluded that flexibility in home help and community service would help older people achieve a better quality of life. There has been a recent growth of commercial schemes that deliver convenience meals to older people living in sheltered housing on a weekly basis. These frozen meals are selected and paid for independently by older people. As yet, these schemes have not been widely extended to older people living in their own homes, and there has been no evaluation of the extent to which such home-delivery schemes might improve the diet of older people. Further, there are differences in the uptake of such services (Finch et al. 1998). Unfortunately, home-delivered meal services do not always overcome problems of social isolation, but the presence of a Meals-on-Wheels delivery volunteer during meals was found to improve service recipients' dietary intakes (Suda et al. 2001).

Public policy level
The WHO developed the Global Strategy on Diet, Physical Activity and Health (2004) in response to the increased prevalence of chronic, non-communicable diseases, the risk factors of which all related to lifestyle, including high blood pressure, tobacco use, high blood cholesterol level, high BMI, low fruit and vegetable intake, physical inactivity and a high alcohol consumption (WHO 2002). It has been recognised that there is a need to maximise the quality of life and not just the number of years that people live. To achieve this, many countries are developing and implementing policies to promote healthy ageing (see, for example, US Department of Health and Human Services 2003).

Preparing for consumption

This section describes the phases prior to the consumption of foods by older people: food marketing, food procurement and food preparation.

Food marketing
The business community has had a tendency to view older consumers as not an important market segment, with the advertising and marketing industry somewhat ignoring the mature market (Long 1998). In the United Kingdom, Long found evidence of marketers viewing older people negatively. According to Moschis (2003) the development of the 'mature market' can be divided into three phases:

1. neglected – prior to 1980s, older consumers were not considered to be a significant segment, and were thus ignored
2. redefined market – during the 1980s, the mature market was defined both in terms of size and buying power
3. two trends – the stage since early 1990s in which there is a dual trend, where some companies have marketing programmes targeted at the mature market, and others are hesitant to develop products or messages aimed at this market.

There is evidence that older people are not homogeneous in their food preferences, and the existence of different market segments within the older community make it difficult to make generalisations (Szmigin & Carrigan 2001). Gerontographics, a segmentation technique based on factors associated with biological, social and experiential ageing (Moschis 2003) has four segments of older persons who are at four different, yet not necessarily sequential, stages in later life:

1. healthy indulgers (that is, their main focus is on enjoying life rather than making it in life)
2. healthy hermits (healthy and relatively more socially withdrawn)
3. ailing outgoers (still active and are likely to maintain a high level of self-esteem despite their adverse life condition)
4. frail recluses (in isolation and are likely to think of themselves as 'old persons').

These types of segmentation methods provide useful insights to help the food sector, service providers and policymakers understand how to best design systems of food delivery and distribution that fit the needs of older people.

There has been an increasing recognition in the food sector that the older population is becoming an important consumer group (Hollingsworth 2003). Food products specifically targeted at older people are appearing on the market, while other companies prefer to target more broadly, and focus on broader age groups with common interests such as health (Hollingsworth 2003).

Food procurement

The social life of many older people is focused on food and eating. Indeed, the procurement of food is an activity of social significance in all societies, but can be of greater importance, yet more difficult to achieve, for the older community. Research with older women found they valued being active with familiar routines that enabled them to live independently (Sidenvall et al. 2001), and that they gained physical exercise and social contacts when they went shopping. The findings of researchers support the view that food shopping is seen as a 'social activity' and an 'opportunity to meet friends' (Hare et al. 2001). They suggest that the inaccessibility of large out-of-town supermarkets and the nature of home-delivery schemes mitigate against maintaining social networks of support in the community associated with the procurement of food for older consumers. Managing of food in everyday life is an important way for an individual to exercise freedom where they might otherwise come to lead a restricted life, depending on others. Older people have been found to be among those more likely to be limited to shopping for groceries at retail locations closer to home, and report dissatisfaction with the food shopping facilities (Bromley & Thomas 1995).

Using the Critical Incident Technique, Hare and colleagues (2001) identified positive and negative aspects of food shopping, with the main factors contributing to the quality of the shopping experience to be merchandise-related, retail practices, and staff issues. The internal store environment, accessibility, external shopping environment and personal factors were also identified, and featured both positive and negative incidents, with social aspects only having positive incidents.

Older people on low incomes and in poor health particularly reported difficulty in either getting to the shops or in shopping (Wylie et al. 1999). Older people can experience food procurement problems as a result of inadequate public transportation. The interaction between mobility and social support is important. Bromley and Thomas's (1995) study of small-town shopping behaviour demonstrates that disadvantaged consumers are more likely to be limited to shopping for groceries at retail locations closer to home, while families with cars and higher incomes shop at supermarkets outside the immediate area. The level of disadvantage experienced by older consumers is reduced when families are able to offer social support by doing the main food purchases for their older relative, but where older people had to rely on neighbours and home helpers for shopping, local shops were used and, consequently, they failed to get best value for money (Piacentini et al. 2001). Poor mobility results in individuals being less able to exercise control over food shopping, thus exacerbating feelings of disadvantage, particularly where social networks are weak. Herne (1995) suggests that, as well as these external barriers, older people also have individual constraints to their food choice, including cultural and biological factors.

Food preparation

Food choices made by older consumers are constrained not only by the availability/access to their preferred foods from retail outlets, but also by their ability to combine these foods into enjoyable and sustaining meals (McKie 1999). The interplay between the availability of foods, cooking skills and the meal as a final outcome is an under-researched area in food and nutrition studies, although many older people report difficulty and/or disinterest in cooking. In addition, dissatisfaction with available merchandise has been reported by older consumers (Hare et al. 2001). It is the combination of meal preparation skills and products available for purchase that, under given economic conditions, sets the limits for both gastronomic enjoyment and nutritional wellbeing. Furthermore, the meaning of cooking as an expression of friendship can be lost when living alone, with people less likely to enjoy meals and running the risk of becoming malnourished (Lyon & Colquhoun 1999).

Food selection and meal preparation among older people can be hindered by perceived effort in food preparation, the presence of physical disabilities, and lack of enjoyment and skills in cooking. People can find it difficult to obtain acceptable food as a result of functional limitations such as physiological decline (for example, sight, hearing, dental health), and other conditions may also result in older people having related mobility problems, thus finding it difficult both to procure and prepare food, and further restricting access to adequate amounts and types of food, and limiting variety and a satisfactory nutrient intake (Keller et al. 2004).

Older men may particularly lack the motivation, knowledge and skills for meal preparation, resulting in less healthy food choices. For example, Hughes and colleagues (2004) found that older men living alone with good cooking skills reported better physical health and higher intake of vegetables. The study revealed that poor cooking skills and low motivation to change eating habits may constitute barriers to improving energy intake, healthy eating and appetite in older men. An evaluation of an intervention in which older men were taught cooking skills reported that participants gained confidence in cooking, increased their cooking activities at home, developed healthier cooking skills, and improved cooking variety as a result of the programme (Keller et al. 2004). Social benefits were also identified by participants, suggesting that community based nutrition and cooking education for older men is a beneficial activity to support. Keller and colleagues (2004) also reported participants wishing to improve cooking skills, both out of interest but also as a preventative measure, in case family roles changed due to their wives becoming ill or dying — a form of behaviour change that Laditka and Pappas-Rogich (2001) termed 'anticipatory caregiving anxiety'.

Conclusion

Population ageing is likely to lead to a growing demand for formal and informal systems of food provision. Easy access to foods acceptable to older people is central to the maintenance of their health, independence and quality of life. Through shopping, choosing and preparing foods, deciding where and what to eat and with whom, older people are engaged in activities that keep them connected with their friends, families and community. Inevitably, as people age they face a number of barriers and constraints in the procurement and preparation of food, and these social networks have a huge impact in helping people to access foods and food services, improving health, independence and quality of life, thereby ensuring successful ageing.

The development of targeted food products and services, health and social support to reduce barriers should help to prevent the risk of sub-optimal nutrition that exists among some older people living at home. The enjoyment of life of older people will ultimately be enhanced if they are not compromised in their choice of food and meals.

REFERENCES

Ahmad, R. 2002, 'The older or ageing consumers in the UK: Are they really that different?' *International Journal of Market Research*, vol. 44, no. 3, pp. 337–60.

Barrett, J. 1997, 'The cost and availability of healthy food choices in southern Derbyshire' in *Journal of Human Nutrition and Dietetics*, vol. 10, pp. 63–9.

Bennett, K.M., Hughes, G.M. and Smith, P.T. 2003, '"I think a woman can take it": Widowed men's views and experiences of gender differences in bereavement' in *Ageing International*, vol. 28, pp. 408–24.

Borghesani, W.H., de la Cruz, P.L. and Berry, D.B. 1997, 'Controlling the chain: Buyer power, distributive control, and new dynamics in retailing' in *Business Horizons*, vol. 40, pp. 17–24.

Bromley, R.D.F. and Thomas, C.J. 1995, 'Small town shopping decline: Dependence and inconvenience for the disadvantaged' in *The International Review of Retail, Distribution and Consumer Research*, vol. 5, pp. 433–56.

Campion, E.W. 1998, 'Aging better' in *New England Journal of Medicine*, vol. 338, pp. 1064–66.

Chen, Schilling and Lyder 2001, 'A concept analysis of malnutrition in the elderly' in *Journal of Advanced Nursing*, vol. 36, no. 1, pp. 131–42.

Connor, R.J.G. 1999, 'Is healthy eating only for the young?' in *Nutrition and Food Science*, vol. 1, January/February, pp. 12–18.

Dang, T., Antolin, P. and Oxley, H. 2001, *Fiscal Implications of Ageing: Projections of age-related spending,* Economics department working papers no. 305, ECO/WKP(2001)31, Organisation for Economic Co-operation and Development, Paris.

Davidson, K. 2001, 'Late life widowhood, selfishness and new partnership choices: A gendered perspective', *Ageing and Society*, vol. 21, pp. 279–317.

Edstrom, K.M. and Devine, C.M. 2001, 'Consistency in women's orientations to food and nutrition in midlife and older age: A 10-year qualitative follow-up' in *Journal of Nutrition Education and Behavior*, vol. 33, pp. 215–23.

Finch, S., Doyle, W., Lowe, C., Bates, C.J., Prentice, A., Smithers, G. and Clarke, P.C. 1998, *National Diet and Nutrition Survey: People aged 65 years and over. Volume 1: Report of the Diet and Nutrition Survey,* Her Majesty's Stationery Office, London.

Fjellström, C., Siddenvall, B. and Nydahl, M. 2001, 'Food intake and the elderly-social aspects' in Frewer, L.J., Risvik, E., Schifferstein, H.N.J. and von Alvensleben R. (eds) 2001, *Food and Society: A European perspective*, , Springer-Verlag London Ltd, London, pp. 197–210.

Flicker, L., Macinnis, R., Stein, M., Scherer, S., Mead, K. and Nowson, C. 2005, 'Vitamin D to prevent falls in older people in residential care'in *Asia Pacific Journal of Clinical Nutrition*, vol. 14, pp. S18.

Gazzotti, C., Arnaud-Battandier, F., Parello, M., Farine, S., Seidel, L., Albert, A. and Petermans, J. 2003, 'Prevention of malnutrition in older people during and after hospitalisation: Results from a randomised controlled clinical trial' in *Age and Ageing*, vol. 32, no. 3, pp. 321–25.

Ginn, J., Arber, S., Cooper, H. 1998, 'Inequalities in older people's health behaviour: Effect of structural factors and social relationships' in *Journal of Contemporary Health*, vol. 7, pp. 77–82.

Gutierrez-Fisac, J.L., Lopez, E., Banegas, J.R., Graciani, A., Rodriguez-Artalejo, F. 2004, 'Prevalence of overweight and obesity in elderly people in Spain' in *Obesity Research*, vol. 12, no. 4, pp. 710–15.

Hare, C., Kirk, D. and Lang, T. 2001, 'The food shopping experience of older consumers in Scotland' in *International Journal of Retail and Distribution Management*, vol. 29, pp. 25–40.

Herne, S. 1995, 'Research on food choice and nutritional status in elderly people: A review' in *British Food Journal*, vol. 97, no. 9, pp. 12–29.

Hickson, M., 2006, 'Malnutrition and ageing' in *Postgraduate Medical Journal*, vol. 82, pp. 2–8

Higgins, M.M. and Clarke Barkley, M. 2004, 'Barriers to nutrition education for older adults, and nutrition and aging training opportunities for educators, healthcare providers, volunteers and caregivers' in *Journal of Nutrition for the Elderly*, vol. 23, no. 4, pp. 99–121.

Hollingsworth, P. 2003, 'Food and the aging consumer' in *Food Technology*, vol. 57, no.?7, pp. 28–40.

Hughes, G., Bennet, K.M. and Hetherington, M.M. 2004, 'Old and alone: Barriers to healthy eating in older men living on their own' in *Appetite*, vol. 43, pp. 269–76.

Iacovou, M. 2000, *Health, Wealth and Progeny: Explaining the living arrangements of older European women*, Essex University, Institute for Social and Economic Research, Colchester.

Janssen, I., Katzmarzyk, P.T. and Ross, R. 2002, 'Body mass index, waist circumference, and health risk: Evidence in support of current National Institutes of Health guidelines' in *Archives of Internal Medicine*, vol. 162, no. 18, pp. 2074–79.

Keller, H.H., Gibbs, A., Wong, S., Vanderkooy, P. and Hedley, M. 2004, 'Men Can Cook! Development, Implementation, and Evaluation of a Senior Men's Cooking Group' in *Journal of Nutrition for the Elderly*, vol. 24, no. 1, pp. 71–87.

Khaw, K.T. 1997, 'Healthy aging' in *British Medical Journal*, vol. 315, pp. 1090–96.

Knoops, K.T., de Groot, L.C., Kromhout D., Perrin, A-E., Moreiras-Varela, O., Menotti, A. and van Staveren, W.A. 2004, 'Mediterranean diet, lifestyle factors, and 10-year mortality in elderly European men and women: The HALE project' in *Journal of American Medical Association*, vol. 292, pp. 1433–39.

Laditka, S.B. and Pappas-Rogich, M., 2001, 'Anticipatory caregiving anxiety among older women and men' in *Journal of Women and Aging*, vol. 13, pp. 3–18.

Langen, R.C., Schols, A.M. and Kelders, M.C. et al. 2001, 'Inflammatory cytokins inhibit myogenic differentiation through activation of nuclear factor-kappab' in *FASEB Journal*, vol. 15, pp 1169–80.

Lilley, J. 1996, 'Food choice in later life' in *Nutrition and Food Science*, vol. 2, March/April, pp. 4–7.

Long, N., 1998, 'Broken down by age and sex: Exploring the ways we approach the elderly consumer' in *Journal of the Market Research Society*, vol. 40, pp. 73–91.

Lumbers, M., New, S.A., et al. 2001, 'Nutritional intake and status in elderly female patients with fractured neck of femur: Comparison with age-matched controls' in *British Journal of Nutrition*, vol. 85, pp. 1–8.

Lyon, P. and Colquhoun, A. 1999, 'Home, hearth and table: A centennial review of the nutritional circumstances of older people living alone' in *Ageing and Society*, vol. 19, pp. 53–67.

McKie, L. 1999, 'Older people and food: Independence, locality and diet' in *British Food Journal*, vol. 101, no. 7, pp. 528–36.

Middleton, M.H., Nazarenko, G., Nivison-Smith, I. and Smerdely, P. 2001, 'Prevalence of malnutrition and 12-month incidence of mortality in two Sydney teaching hospitals' in *Internal Medicine Journal*, vol. 31, pp. 455–61.

Moschis, G.P. 2003, 'Marketing to older adults: An updated overview of present knowledge and practice' in *Journal of Consumer Marketing*, vol. 20, pp. 516–25.

National Health and Medical Research Council (NHMRC) 2006, *Nutrient Reference Values for Australia and New Zealand, including reference dietary intake*, Commonwealth of Australia.

National Heart, Lung, and Blood Institute 2001, *Third report of the National Cholesterol Education Program (NCEP) Expert Panel on Detection, Evaluation, and Treatment of High Blood Cholesterol in Adults (Adult Treatment Panel III)*, US Department of Health and Human Services, Public Health Service, National Institutes of Health, National Heart, Lung and Blood Institute, Bethesda M.D.

Nowson, C., Sherwin, A.J., McPhee, J.G., Wark, J.D. and Flicker, L. 2003, 'Energy, protein, calcium, vitamin D and fibre intakes from meals in residential care establishments in Australia' in *Asia Pacific Journal of Clinical Nutrition*, vol. 12, no. 2, pp. 172–77.

Parker, M.J., Twemlow, T.R. and Pryor, G.A. 1996, 'Environmental hazards and hip fractures' in *Age and Ageing*, vol. 25, pp. 322–25.

Piacentini, M., Hibbert, S. and Al-Dajanie, H. 2001, 'Diversity in deprivation: Exploring the shopping behaviour of disadvantaged consumers' in *International Review of Retail, Distribution and Consumer Research*, vol. 11, pp. 141–58.

Population Division of the Department of Economic and Social Affairs of the United Nations Secretariat 2005, *World Population Prospects: The 2004 Revision Highlights*, United Nations, New York.

Quandt, S.A., McDonald, J., Arcury, T.A., Bell, R.A. and Vitolins, M.Z. 2000, 'Nutritional self-management of elderly widows in rural communities' in *The Gerontologist*, vol. 40, pp. 86–96.

Rosenberg, I.H., 2001, 'Nutrition and ageing' in Garrow, J.S, James, W.P.T. and Ralph, A. (eds) 2001, *Human Nutrition and Dietetics*, Churchill Livingstone, London, pp. 465–9.

Rowe, J.W. and Kahn, R.L. 1998, *Successful Ageing*, Pantheon, New York.

Sahyoun, N.R., Pratt, C.A. and Anderson, A. 2004, 'Evaluation of nutrition education interventions for older adults: A proposed framework' in *Journal of the American Dietetic Association*, vol. 104, pp. 58–69.

Satia J.A., Galanko J.A., Neuhouser M.L. 2005, 'Food nutrition label use is associated with demographic, behavioral, and psychosocial factors and dietary intake among African Americans in North Carolina' in *Journal of the American Dietetic Association*, vol. 105, no. 3, pp. 392–402.

Sidenvall, B., Nydahl, M. and Fjellström, C. 2001, 'Managing food shopping and cooking: The experiences of Swedish women' in *Ageing and Society*, vol. 21, pp. 151–68.

Suda, Y., Marske, C.E., Flaherty, J.H., Zdrodowski, K., Morley, J.E. 2001, 'Examining the effect of intervention to nutritional problems of the elderly living in an inner city area: A pilot project' in *Journal of Nutrition, Health and Aging*, vol. 5, pp. 118–23.

Szmigin, I. and Carrigan M. 2001, 'Learning to love the older consumer' in *Journal of Consumer Behaviour*, vol. 1, pp. 22–34.

Visvanathan, R. 2003, 'Under-nutrition in older people: A serious and growing global problem!' in *Journal of Postgraduate Medicine*, vol. 49, pp. 352–60.

Wahlqvist, M. and Savige, G. 2000, 'Interventions aimed at dietary and lifestyle changes to promote healthy aging' in *European Journal of Clinical Nutrition*, vol. 54, pp. S148–56.

Welton, W.E., Kantner, T.A. and Katz, S.M. 1997, 'Developing tomorrow's integrated community health systems: A leadership challenge for public health and primary care' in *Milbank Quarterly*, vol. 75, pp. 261–88.

World Health Organization (WHO) 2002, *Active Ageing: A Policy Framework,* WHO (document WHO/NMH/NPH/02.8), Geneva.

—— 2004, 'Global Strategy Diet, Physical activity and health', WHO, Geneva.

Wylie, C., Copeman, J., and Kirk S. 1999, 'Health and social factors affecting food choice and nutritional intake of elderly people with restricted mobility' inb *Journal of Human Nutrition and Dietetics*, vol. 12, no. 5, pp. 375–80.

Section 3: Priorities

Overview

Barrie Margetts

The chapters in this section of the book identify priorities for public health nutrition at various levels, from the local and regional within countries to the international between countries. There is also a chapter on the global issues that affect the environment and access to and control over food production and distribution.

Defining public health priorities requires some sense of what may be ideal or optimal in an absolute sense, but more commonly priorities are defined in relative terms – one group or sector in a country compared with another, or one country compared with another, either cross-sectionally or over time. At the crudest level, international comparisons are based on macro-level differences in infant and childhood mortality, maternal mortality, and cause-specific mortality in adults. Internationally, the Millennium Development Goals have set a benchmark for monitoring progress towards reducing variation between countries. Knowledge about the main age-specifc causes of death and disability, and trends over time in these measures, are helpful to monitor progress toward agreed goals, but having goals in and of themselves do not help unless they galvanise action to address the reasons for the high rates of death and disability. Comparison with these goals highlights good progress in some parts of the world, but little or no progress in sub-Saharan Africa. Exploring why there has been differential success is important to understand the key drivers to effective change, but national trends often mask important local and regional variation within countries. The chapter on indigenous communities highlights that, even in supposedly affluent countries, some sectors of society are very much worse off than expected, and worse than should be tolerated.

In many countries, trends over time in dietary supply, and body composition, highlight what is often termed the nutrition transition, where populations move from a relatively low-energy density diet to a higher-energy density diet associated with urbanisation and moving from growing the food that is consumed, to earning money to eat the food produced by others. Even in the low-income countries, there is more than enough food to go around, but access is not even, and there is now the complex situation of over- and under-supply coexisting within the same countries. Rates of obesity are growing rapidly in most countries around the world, while every day nearly 15 000 children die from malnutrition-related illnesses. It is not uncommon to see obese women with micronutrient deficiencies, highlighting the problem of oversupply of relatively cheap energy-dense, nutrient-poor foods. In all countries, the burden and impact of poor nutrition is greatest in the poorest in society. There may be a common underlying pathway to this apparent anomaly. It may be that what happens in utero alters the metabolic competence of the foetus, which makes it more susceptible to certain patterns of dietary exposure after birth. Thin babies that are relatively fat appear to be at particular risk, and if as children they are exposed to more energy than they may be expecting to receive (as signalled by the in utero experience), they are less able to cope metabolically and become even more relatively fat, and have a much higher risk of diabetes and a number of related factors (often grouped as the metabolic syndrome). This adds another important dimension to identifying at-risk groups: knowing a child's birthweight and subsequent growth may predict a much higher-than-expected rate of chronic diseases, particularly in populations that have moved continents, or changed their economic circumstances and access to foods by moving to urban areas where energy-dense foods are relatively cheap.

Many studies describe differences in diet and risk factors in these groups of people, but less often identify the basic and underlying causes as to why they are at particular risk. Being poor or having little or no education may be markers of a deeper basic problem. Chapter 8, on indigenous communities, identifies a set of risk factors that apply to these groups of people, some of which are common to socially deprived groups, and some of which appear to be unique to indigenous peoples, often expressed in terms of clashes of culture or the way the world is viewed. A number of the chapters in this section identify conceptual frameworks or models to help identify those key constraints that need to be changed to affect outcomes. Knowing, for example, that older people from a particular region are more likely to have a problem does not provide the solution: the challenge is to move beyond description to the identification of the basic and underlying causes (see Darnton-Hill and Chopra's chapter 10), or as modifiable and dynamic responsive factors, as described by Swinburn and Bell (chapter 9). The solutions may be a long way removed from the individual: they may reflect a need to alter the wider or even global environment that alters the access to, and control over, the food people eat (or do not eat). The evidence therefore needs to be viewed and disaggregated in a number of different ways to ensure that the key constraint to a family or community's behaviour can be identified.

Without evidence, it is not possible to understand where we are, or whether we are making progress, but evidence alone does not cause change. The information that is collected needs to be used to inform policy, to help identify priorities for action, and to monitor progress. Evidence alone is rarely the main driver of policy, and it is therefore important to understand the complex environment in which governments do or do not (or can or cannot) make decisions that may seem obvious. It is important to understand where the levers of power operate and how these can be influenced to achieve change. Most governments in the low-income countries have little control over the price they receive for the goods they produce, and generally are not allowed to compete in the world economy on a level playing field. The impact of the way food is grown and moved around the world, the resources taken to produce and distribute food, and the control individual governments and their citizens have over this may constrain the effectiveness of programmes aimed at improving health that do not take this wider context into account. For example, while the United States and Europe espouse free markets and demand open access to the goods they produce, they do not allow low-income countries the same fair access to their markets. Without resources, governments cannot spend more on educating children, building local infrastructure, and ensuring household food security for the worst-off in society. Large multinational companies exploit the physical and political environments in low-income countries to produce cheap energy-dense foods for already oversupplied consumers in the rich developed countries. It makes little sense to destroy vulnerable natural habitats to grow feed for cattle, and then use valuable fossil fuels to transport them many miles to supply markets that are already oversupplied.

Priorities need to be viewed in a context that includes ideology about responsibilities and solutions. This raises issues about professional responsibility and whether there are the structures and systems in place in public health nutrition to identify problems and support solutions that really make a difference. What I do know is that the way we currently operate is not good enough, and a part of this is related to a lack of professional competence and accountability among those of us engaged in public health nutrition. If this book is to make any difference, it has to enable public health nutritionists to be better informed, more critical, and less naive about the causes, and therefore solutions, to major international public health problems. We need to move beyond telling people what to do and assuming knowledge is the key constraint to behaviour. We would be wrong to think that our job, and responsibilities as professionals and citizens, stopped with the provision of information. We have to do more than stand on the sidelines and report; we have to engage actively to solve problems. If the profession wants to be taken seriously, it (we, you and I) must act seriously. This means understanding and influencing the wider context to enable individuals and communities to solve their own problems in ways that are appropriate for them.

7

Economically, geographically and socially disadvantaged communities

CATE BURNS
SHARON FRIEL
STEVEN CUMMINS

If we acknowledge health as one of the basic pillars of human dignity, then redressing these health inequities is a matter of social justice. This chapter explores how access to food is influenced by social stratification and isolation. First we explore the underlying societal reasons for the differences in the opportunity to consume nutritious food that is experienced by various population groups. Then we will look at how financial resources, physical location, neighbourhood levels of social disadvantage, and political and social isolation determine food and nutrient intake in specific at-risk populations. Finally we will discuss approaches, both individual and community-based, to improving food access for socially disadvantaged groups, and examine broader approaches to community and national food equity and security.

Overall, the chapter will look at four disadvantaged or marginalised populations, and discuss how social disadvantage or exclusion affects their intake of food and nutrition. Four case studies from the authors' specific research programmes are provided to highlight the nutrition issues for these populations and innovative interventions that have been developed to meet these needs.

The social context of health

Chronic diseases account for a huge proportion of human illness. Cardiovascular diseases, diabetes, cancers and obesity-related conditions now make up 59 per cent of the 56.5 million deaths that occur globally every year (WHO 2002). These diseases are not exclusive to rich nations; 80 per cent of all cardiovascular disease-related deaths now occur in low- and middle-income countries.

Remarkable improvements have been recorded in human health over the past 50 years. Unfortunately, there are very significant discrepancies in the levels of chronic diseases among people from different social and economic circumstances, with those from low socioeconomic backgrounds consistently more likely to experience poor health outcomes (World Bank 2005). To understand why this is the case, we need to explore the social determinants of health.

The social determinants of health

As the limitations of interventions that simply target individuals at risk became clear in the 1970s, a refocus away from individual risk factors to wider population level determinants with respect to the causes of disease took place. The determinants include economic, environmental and social factors, which operate at the individual and population level and are powerful influences on the level of health of individuals and societies. They help to explain not only average population health levels, but also why some people are healthy and others are not (Marmot 2005).

Graham (2004) characterised the framework conceptualising social determinants of health as a web of influence, identifying the structures of society at the most distal level. Marked variations in health have been observed by various measures of social position, including socioeconomic status (SES), which is measured using indicators of occupation, social class and education. Asset-based measures, for example, income, car ownership and home tenure, have increasingly been used as indicators of social stratification in health, showing consistent differentials in morbidity, mortality and health-related risk factors (Davey Smith et al. 1998). It is not only socioeconomic-based factors that pattern the health of society; the social stratification of health is also affected by differences in gender, marital status, residential area and ethnicity (Elstad 2000).

The chance of an individual encountering health risks throughout his/her lifetime is strongly dependent on that 'individual's position in the social hierarchy'. The following example of two children who were born into very different social circumstances and their resulting life chances could be recognised anywhere in the world:

Consider two South African children born on the same day in 2000. Nthabiseng is black, born to a poor family in a rural area in the Eastern Cape province, about 700 kilometres from Cape Town. Her mother had no formal schooling. Pieter is white, born to a wealthy family in Cape Town. His mother completed a college education at the nearby prestigious Stellenbosch University. On the day of their birth, Nthabiseng and Pieter could hardly be held responsible for their family circumstances: their race, their parents' income and education, their urban or rural location, or indeed their sex. Yet statistics suggest that those predetermined background variables will make a major difference for the lives they lead. Nthabiseng has a 7.2 per cent chance of dying in the first year of her life, more than twice Pieter's 3 per cent. Pieter can look forward to 68 years of life, Nthabiseng to 50. Pieter can expect to complete 12 years of formal schooling, Nthabiseng less than 1 year. Nthabiseng is likely to be considerably poorer than Pieter throughout her life. Growing up, she is less likely to have access to clean water and sanitation, or to good schools. So the opportunities these two children face to reach their full human potential are vastly different from the outset, through no fault of their own . . . (World Bank 2005)

A *social determinants approach to food issues*

Disease can be attributable in large part to chronic conditions, and is preventable partly through modifiable behavioural risk factors (WHO 2002). Recent analysis of the burden of disease figures highlights that in developed economies 15 per cent of all disability adjusted life years are food related (Rayner & Scarborough 2005).

Population-based studies worldwide have repeatedly shown that individuals from lower socioeconomic groups are least likely to comply with dietary recommendations, and have significantly lower intake of the foodstuffs regularly advocated by health professionals as promoting better health (WHO 2002). Hence, those who are socioeconomically disadvantaged are at greater risk of developing diet-related diseases. Restricted dietary habits, in relation to both nutritional adequacy and access to nutritious foods, are observed in wealthy societies among particularly disadvantaged members, including those who are unemployed, homeless, elderly, asylum seekers, refugees or from low-income families.

The internationally observed social gradients in dietary behaviour clearly indicate the influence of macroeconomic, structural, psychosocial and personal factors on food choice and resulting health status. It has been suggested that the unequal distribution of these resources in society differentially equips people to make healthy food choices (Shaw et al. 1999), resulting in the observed social inequalities in food and nutrient intake, and often in food poverty, among some population groups.

There are a number of pathways mediating and factors contributing to food and nutrient intake and health status. Figure 7.1 summarises this complex array of factors, interconnecting societal, structural and intermediary determinants of access to healthy food with the food and nutrition system that drive food availability issues. In the figure, the following definitions apply:

- availability indicates the food available for consumption either through self-provision or purchase
- accessibility indicates the food accessible for consumption, either physically by foot or transport, or economically, that is, the individual has sufficient economic resources to purchase food that is affordable
- acceptability is the appropriateness of food to accepted social norms.

Therefore, the socioeconomic status is a strong determinant of an individual's health and nutritional status. This impact plays out in numerous ways from

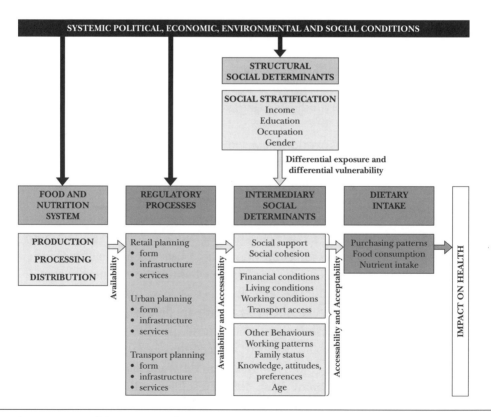

Figure 7.1 Conceptual framework of the social determinants of food, nutrition and health

the financial and social resources to the environment and conditions in which an individual lives and works.

Factors affecting food access

It is useful to consider meeting food and nutrition needs in terms of 'food security'. This term encompasses not only the economic determinants of an adequate diet, but also the need for food habits to meet social and cultural needs. The term can be applied to both individuals and whole communities. Food security has been defined by the Expert Working Group of the American Institute of Nutrition as:

> Access by all people at all times to enough food for an active, healthy life. Food security includes at a minimum the ready availability of nutritionally adequate and safe foods, and an assured ability to acquire acceptable foods in socially acceptable ways, i.e. without resorting to emergency food supplies, scavenging, stealing or other coping strategies (Anderson 1990).

There are a number of factors that impact on an individual or community's food security.

Economic access — Food issues for individuals living in poverty

People are living in poverty if their income and resources (material, cultural and social) are so inadequate as to preclude them from having a standard of living that is regarded as acceptable by society generally. As a result of inadequate income and resources, people may be excluded from participating in activities that are considered the norm for other people in society.

Poverty occurs in all countries. The Social Summit Programme of Action 1995 (United Nations 1995) articulates it as:

> mass poverty in many developing countries, pockets of poverty amid wealth in developed countries, loss of livelihoods as a result of economic recession, sudden poverty as a result of disaster or conflict, the poverty of low-wage workers, and the utter destitution of people who fall outside family-support systems, social institutions and safety nets.

Absolute poverty, as generally experienced in developing countries, is a condition characterised by severe deprivation of basic human needs, including food, safe drinking water, sanitation facilities, health, shelter, education and information. The poverty experienced in the developed world is considered relative. In Australia and other developed countries, people are considered poor if their living standards fall below an overall accepted community standard, and they are unable to participate fully in ordinary activities of society.

Income poverty can be measured in different ways. It can be expressed in relation to a poverty line, a defined income that is updated regularly. A poverty line estimates the amount of money that families of different sizes need to cover essential needs. In Australia, a recent study examining the trends, using a range of poverty lines from 1990 to 2000, indicated that in all but one study poverty rates in Australia did not decrease over the decade, in spite of the nation's economic growth (Commonwealth Government of Australia 2004). Even using a conservative estimate, more than a million-and-a-half Australians (more than one in twenty) were living below the poverty line at the beginning of the twenty-first century.

Another measure of poverty is income relative to a living wage. Again in Australia, wages and salaries were the principal sources of income for households with middle and high income levels, while government pensions and allowances dominated low income households (76 per cent). However, income support payments are often 20 to 30 per cent below the poverty line (ACOSS 2000). It is also possible to have a job and still be living in poverty. It is estimated that one in five poor Australians are in paid work – they may be called the 'working poor' (Harding 2000). Many people in Australia also get trapped in the cycle of insecure low-paid casual jobs, followed by periods spent living on income support. On average, the Australian household weekly food expenditure amounts to 18.2 per cent of income on food and non-alcoholic beverages. Those in the lowest income bracket spend proportionally more, at 20 per cent, than those in the top income bracket, at 17 per cent (ABS 2000).

It is possible for people to live in poverty despite strong economic growth in the country in which they live. For example, using data from the 2005 Luxembourg Income Study, a comparison of relative incomes (poverty line set as 60 per cent of the national median income) across OECD countries, demonstrated that the Republic of Ireland, with one of the highest economic growths in the OECD, exhibited the highest level of poverty (see Figure 7.2).

Veit-Wilson recommends that governments employ an income benchmark, known as a Minimum Income Standard (MIS) (Veit-Wilson 1994). An MIS is a set of criteria for evaluating the adequacy of income levels (based on welfare rates, pensions and minimum wages) required for people to be able to take part in ordinary social life and to stay out of poverty. One of the approaches used in the development of an MIS is to look at budget standards. These are baskets

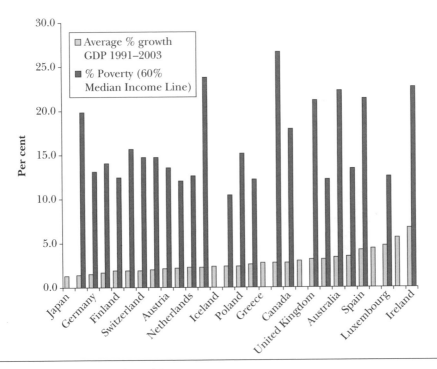

Figure 7.2 Economic Growth and Poverty

Sources: Luxembourg Income Study 2005 <http://www.lisproject.org/>; OECD Factbook 2005 <http://www.oecd.org>

of goods, such as food, household services and leisure goods, which, when priced, can represent the income required by households of different composition to reach predefined living standards (Parker 1998).

In their study of food poverty in Ireland, Friel and Conlon (2004), using a budget standards approach, found that lone parents with one child, two adults with two children, and single older people would have to spend an incredible 80 per cent, 69 per cent and 38 per cent respectively of their weekly household income in order to purchase the food basket based on economy line products (Figure 7.3).

Friel and Conlon commented that, given the flexible priority that food occupies within financially constrained households, it is unlikely that the required allocation of household income to purchase food compliant with national dietary recommendations will be obtainable unless more realistic financial provision is made. Interviews and observed shopping trips have demonstrated that those living in poverty feel excluded from the mainstream food system (Hitchman et al. 2002). Hence, poverty is inextricably linked to social exclusion, a term we will define and discuss later in this chapter.

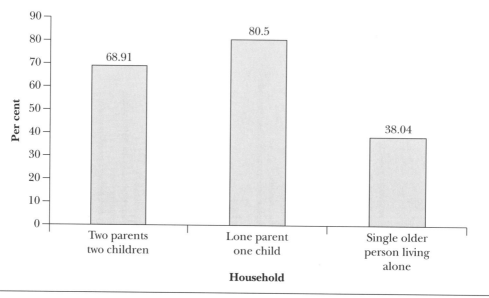

Figure 7.3 Food basket cost as a proportion of weekly social welfare entitlements
Source: Friel & Conlon 2004

Physical and economic access — Food issues for individuals living in socioeconomically disadvantaged neighbourhoods

In recent years, there has been increasing interest in the role that physical access to food has in determining food security and the nutritional status of residents of vulnerable and disadvantaged communities. It has been suggested that the price and availability of food may be one important mediating factor in this relationship, and it has been argued that socially disadvantaged populations have less choice at a higher cost. In the United Kingdom, deprived areas, where 'healthy' food is more expensive and relatively unavailable, have been termed 'food-deserts', a term first attributed to a resident of a public housing scheme in the West of Scotland in the early 1990s. In recent years, such terminology has been used in a variety of UK policy documents from various government departments that have focused on diet and health (Department of Health 1996) and neighbourhood renewal (Social Exclusion Unit 1998).

Studies undertaken in the United States provide the most convincing evidence for the existence of such a relationship, with healthier foods generally more expensive and less readily available in poorer, compared to wealthier, communities (Morland et al. 2002a). Such food access issues appear to be particularly problematic in African–American neighbourhoods (Zenk et al. 2005).

US studies have also found dose–response relationships between local physical access to food and diet and health outcomes (Rose & Richards 2004). For example, in black neighbourhoods a 32 per cent increase in fruit and vegetable intake was found for each additional supermarket situated in a neighbourhood designated by a census district (Morland 2002b).

Though the evidence from the United States appears reasonably consistent, observational work undertaken outside of the United States appears to be much more equivocal. Recent work undertaken in the United Kingdom has found no independent association between food retail provision within neighbourhoods and individual fruit and vegetable intake (White et al. 2004), and little evidence for differences in food price, food availability and access to supermarkets between deprived and affluent areas (Cummins & Macintyre 2002). Similar findings have also been made in Australia (Winkler et al. 2006), in the Netherlands (Giskes et al. 2006) and Northern Ireland (Furey et al. 2002). Therefore, poor neighbourhoods do not necessarily have poor food access. The association between neighbourhood disadvantage and food access may be culture or country specific.

Foods purchased from fast-food outlets, restaurants and other places are becoming an increasingly important part of an individual's diet (Nielsen et al. 2002). Such foods are up to 65 per cent more energy dense than the average diet (Prentice & Jebb 2003), and intake of selected nutrients is lower in the population groups that consume more of them (Burns et al. 2002). Portion sizes of out-of-home meals are also relatively large compared to home-prepared foods (Rolls et al. 2004). It has been hypothesised that the prevalence of outlets that serve such foods might be greater in poorer communities, which might help explain the higher rates of diet-related mortality and morbidity in such communities. Associations between area deprivation and the density of fast-food outlets have been found in Melbourne, Australia, with poorer neighbourhoods having 2.5 times more fast-food outlets than richer neighbourhoods (Reidpath et al. 2002). In the United States, a greater prevalence of fast-food outlets in black census tracts was found in New Orleans (Block et al. 2004), and in Los Angeles, poorer neighbourhoods with higher proportions of African–Americans had fewer healthy options and more advertising and promotional prompts to consume unhealthy alternatives in out-of-home outlets (Lewis et al. 2005). The location of McDonald's restaurants has been associated with area deprivation in England and Scotland (Cummins et al. 2005a). However, conflicting findings have also been reported within each of these countries. Density of fast-food and other outlets was not found to be associated with area deprivation in Glasgow, Scotland (Macintyre et al. 2005), nor was density associated with area-base measures of wealth and racially based residential segregation in areas of the United States (Morland et al. 2002a). In one study undertaken in New Jersey and Pennsylvania, fast-food restaurants were found to charge more for food in black neighbourhoods (Graddy 1997).

Recent studies evaluating the impact on diet of larger supermarkets being opened in deprived neighbourhoods (Figure 7.4) have produced conflicting results. Studies undertaken in Leeds indicated an improvement in fruit and vegetable consumption, especially in the lowest consumption groups at baseline (Wrigley 2003), while a study in Glasgow indicated no improvement (Cummins et al. 2005b). Discrepancies in results may be due, in part, to differing study designs. The Leeds study utilised an uncontrolled 'before and after' approach, while the Glasgow study employed a quasi-experimental design with a control community with which to compare change. However, the lack of evidence makes it difficult to draw any firm conclusions at present, and it is difficult to disentangle whether increased opportunities to consume healthy food are outweighed by similar increased opportunities to consume unhealthy food.

Overall, it appears that the observational evidence for systematic spatial differences in physical access to food varies by country for the grocery-store food environment, and is equivocal and mixed for the fast-food and out-of-home food environment. Such differences may be accounted for by differences in national-level policies and processes associated with the spatial planning of

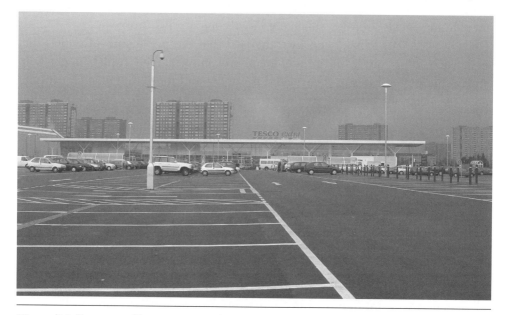

Figure 7.4 Presence of large supermarket in deprived neighbourhood

stores, which can have a direct effect on where shops and services are located. In addition, dynamic changes in the way commercial institutions operate within their respective markets will also govern where stores locate.

One of the lessons learned from the UK experience is that the food retail economy can produce adverse outcomes for some disadvantaged groups through the production of inequities in physical access to food. However, the processes that produce such inequities are dynamic and evolving, and more recent evidence suggests that the 'market' has corrected itself and that physical access to grocery stores and supermarkets is again becoming more equal in the United Kingdom. Despite this, it is still entirely possible that some areas in some cities in the United Kingdom may continue to suffer from 'retail disadvantage', though it remains to be seen whether state intervention to improve physical access to food will be very beneficial.

Neighbourhood level socioeconomic disadvantage may have a direct effect on food cost and availability. It should be noted that there are cultural differences in food retailing and consumption that make lessons learnt in one country not necessarily applicable in another (Cummins & Macintyre 2006).

Physical access — Food issues for individuals living in rural and remote communities and those with poor access to transport

Those who live in rural and remote areas can have their food access and intake compromised by their very geographic location. Nowhere is this more apparent than in outback and rural Australia. It has been shown that there is poor food access in remote areas in Australia (Lee et al. 2002). Case study 7.1, however, was undertaken in a rural community that could not be described as remote. This example demonstrates that even relative physical isolation can compromise food access.

Food issues for socially excluded communities or individuals

Social exclusion has been defined as:

> More than income poverty. Social exclusion happens when people or places suffer from a series of problems such as unemployment, discrimination, poor skills, low incomes, poor housing, high crime, ill health and family breakdown. When such problems combine they can create a vicious cycle. Social exclusion can happen as a result of problems that face one person in their life. But it can also start from birth. Being born into poverty or to parents with low skills still has a major influence on future life chances (Social Exclusion Unit 1998).

CASE STUDY 7.1

FOOD ACCESS IN RURAL SOUTH-WESTERN VICTORIA

This study (Burns et al. 2004) was undertaken to determine availability of access to a healthy food access basket (HFAB) in a 70 000-square-kilometre rural area of south-western Australia in Victoria, with a population of 225 000. The study involved a cross-sectional survey of the costs and availability of a standard selection of HFAB. The availability and cost of certain popular family food purchases, tobacco and takeaway food items were also surveyed. All towns surveyed were classified as highly accessible or accessible, indicating minor or relatively unrestricted access to goods, services and opportunities for social interaction in a regional service centre. All food-related premises in towns with a population in excess of 100 persons were considered eligible. Food outlets were identified through the Yellow Pages®. This list was cross-checked with local government records. The final survey sample was 53 of eligible shops (72 per cent) in 42 towns across the five local government areas.

The HFAB is a standard method used in the assessment of food availability and cost (Lee et al. 2002). Made up of 44 commonly available and eaten foods, the HFAB meets the nutritional requirements of a family of six people for two weeks, and provides 70 per cent of recommended dietary intake (RDI) for all nutrients, excluding energy (Cashel & Jeffreson 1994). Please note that these RDI have since been revised.

On average, only 56 per cent of stores surveyed stocked the complete HFAB (the range of availability across shires was 29 to 78 per cent). The study found that the complete HFAB was significantly more likely to be available in a town with a chain-owned store. The complete HFAB was less likely to be available from an independently owned store in a town with only one grocery shop.

From the table below, it is apparent that these rural residents would be able to access some basic food items locally, but that a range of foods to make up a complete healthy diet would not be available to them. In 15 out of 42 towns surveyed, access to a basket of basic healthy foods was poor. This is a particular problem for those without transport, money for transport and/or the physical ability to go to large service centres to shop.

Most commonly available food items from the HFAB*

HFAB items	Popular items	Takeaway/Tobacco
Carrots	Packet spaghetti	Packet tobacco
Lettuce	Pasta sauce	Can of Coke™
Apples	Family block chocolate	Packet cigarettes
Bananas	Litre of Coke™	Meat pie

Tomatoes
Beef stew (tinned)
Potatoes
Instant noodles
Onions
Weetbix
Dry spaghetti
Tinned beetroot
Canned spaghetti
Margarine
Rice
Eggs
Sugar
Fresh milk fat-reduced
Fresh milk
Wholemeal bread
White bread
Cheese

* Results are given for all items that were available in at least 90 per cent of stores

The average cost of the HFAB across the study region was \$A380.30 ± \$25.10 (mean ± SD). The mean cost of the HFAB in the larger chain stores, \$359.42 ± \$19.74 (mean ± SD) was significantly cheaper than in independent stores. The cost of components of the basic food basket was highly variable. In particular, high variability was found in the cost of fruit and vegetables. Across the study area, there was a range of cost of the order of \$36 for the entire contents of the HFAB. The cost range observed was not as great as that observed in remote and very remote areas, but the average weekly cost of the HFAB in south west Victoria, \$190, is still well in excess of the average weekly household expenditure on food in Australia: \$127 (ABS 2000). Even allowing for differences in household size, this represents a large difference in money required to be spent and currently spent by Australian families.

The limited access to healthy food shown here may explain the high burden of disease suffered in rural Australia (Victorian Department of Human Services 1999). The universal availability of soft drink and some takeaway food may further compound this diet-related ill health.

Poor food access has also been demonstrated for those in urban communities who are without cars or adequate public transport (Social Exclusion Unit 2003; White et al. 2004). Both geographic isolation and a lack of transport can limit access to healthy food in both urban and rural situations.

There are many groups within society that could be considered socially excluded. This social exclusion is often compounded by or proceeding from economic or political exclusion. Socially excluded groups include refugees, the homeless, those coping with drug or alcohol abuse or those living on government allowances. The nutritional impacts of social exclusion can be financial, social and emotional. Nutrition issues for the homeless and users of emergency food relief or food banks and those on government pensions are well known. In Case study 7.2, we discuss Somali asylum seekers in Australia (Burns 2004). The nutritional issues encountered by socially excluded groups include limited money to buy food, limited access to culturally appropriate foods, poor understanding of food supply system in the host community, and a different socialisation around food to that of the host society.

For refugees, establishing and maintaining food security is important for health, and enhances the capacity to deal with the stresses of settlement in a new country. Food serves a role in post-trauma healing processes. Food may facilitate the settlement process as a:

- vehicle for re-establishing cultural and religious traditions and rituals
- focus for bringing families and friends together and fostering relationships between them
- means of commencing the acculturation process by exposing new arrivals to local food and cultural practices.

Some individuals recovering from past trauma have an overwhelming need for psychological counselling and assistance with the immediate tasks of settlement (VFST 2002); however, once the immediate problems of settlement have been met, the health risks for many refugees are essentially those of obesity and the chronic diseases common in their Australian-born compatriots. There is some evidence to suggest that the stresses associated with settlement in a new country may be particularly acute for those migrating from a developing to an industrialised country, since these people face the double challenge of adjusting to both cultural and modernisation gaps (VFST 2002).

CASE STUDY 7.2
FOOD INSECURITY AND NUTRITIONAL ISSUES IN ASYLUM SEEKERS
IN AUSTRALIA

Each year, Australia receives more than 12 000 entrants as refugees from conflict zones around the world through its Humanitarian Program (DIMIA 1997). On average, this number includes 4000 Sub-Saharan Africans. Most of these refugees have been subject to trauma, including prolonged periods of deprivation, the loss of loved ones in violent circumstances, or a perilous escape from their homelands.

This case study describes food security issues as experienced by Somali refugees settling in Melbourne. Data was collected using both focus group discussions (Burns et al. 2000) and a photo-assisted food frequency questionnaire (Burns 2004).

In this study, Somali refugees reported food preparation and shopping practices (for example, bulk buying, shopping at markets, and preparing food from scratch) that are conducive to economising. Nevertheless, many Somali families have arrived in Australia only recently, are on fixed and low incomes, and are, moreover, at a stage in the settlement process where they face the enormous costs of establishing a new household. Many are supporting relatives in refugee camps or similar difficult circumstances overseas. These commitments limit the amount of money that refugees in Australia have to spend on food for their own families. Not surprisingly, a number reported having run out of food. This financial difficulty can be hard to detect because of the shame and cultural sensitivity surrounding the reporting of the fact that the household food supply is compromised. Using standard questions to determine household food security in migrant populations such as these may prove to be unreliable (Burns 2004). In general, these families have preferred to borrow money from friends and relatives rather than to seek assistance from an emergency relief agency.

With respect to food shopping, participants reported that on arrival in Australia they experienced some difficulties in locating cheap supplies of traditional foods. Since most Somali entrants are of the Muslim faith, they follow Islamic dietary law, and require halal food products. The supply of these is limited and often difficult to access. Participants reported that in Somalia they had shopped at local markets at least daily, with perishable foods generally being consumed on the day of purchase. In Australia, most women had adopted the practice of a once-weekly shop in response to the ready availability of refrigeration, less accessible shopping facilities, transport difficulties, and competing demands on their time. Often the Somalis were unfamiliar with much of the fruit and vegetables available on the Australian market, in particular broccoli, mushrooms and stone fruits such as plums and peaches. The fruits with which they were familiar, for example mangoes, were often more expensive.

Some of the women were concerned about the safety of the food supply in Australia. While participants observed that there was a greater variety of foods available, concern was expressed about the safety of the food supply with respect to physical condition and composition of the food available. There was the perception that food was less fresh and there were 'more chemicals used in it'.

From the dietary assessment, foods such as sweetened yoghurt, cheese, potato chips, ready-prepared foods and soft drinks and cordial, which are not traditionally familiar to Somali families, were now included in the diet, particularly for younger children. The dietary changes for these Somali refugees thus reflected their exposure to cheap, readily available and highly promoted energy dense food. As one Somali woman commented, 'In Australia it is easy to get fat'. Whether this is considered by refugees or migrants to be a good or a bad consequence will be explored in future research.

This research highlights the impact on food access and consumption of social exclusion. It indicates also the importance of understanding the cultural context of food security and the need to explore fully and understand every aspect of food security that is in the economic, social and cultural context of any group, but particularly as regards marginalised populations.

How can public health nutrition improve food access?

Public health nutrition interventions directed at socially excluded individuals or communities

Interventions directed at socially excluded individuals or communities can operate on several levels: micro (the individual or household), meso (community or local level) or macro (national or global initiatives). Interventions directed at the individual could include meal access programmes and emergency food relief. These largely relieve individual hunger and meet immediate nutritional needs. Interventions directed at local or community food access have included community gardens, food delivery services, local transport policy, and community education programmes. Macro interventions are directed upstream at leverage points in the food supply and nutrition system (see Figure 7.1) to achieve changes that ideally will make the food system equitable (that is, to make healthy, affordable food equally available to the whole population).

Micro-food security programmes, such as food banks or meal handouts, are at risk of being socially excluding in themselves. Case study 7.3 details a subsidised meal programme that offered food and specifically aimed to encourage social inclusion.

CASE STUDY 7.3

SUBSIDISED CAFE MEAL PROGRAMME

The Yarra Cafe Meals Programme (VicHealth 2005) was developed through partnership between the local (North Yarra) community health service and the local council's Department of Aged Care. It provided increased provision of socially acceptable low-cost meals (75 per cent subsidised from project funds with a minimum payment from client) in several local cafes (Doljanin & Olaris 2004). This project provided the clients with more frequent meals, opportunities for social interaction, and encouraged their attention to food and eating. It provided the referring workers with a tangible response for clients, a means of building trust with clients, and partnerships with other organisations. The cafe proprietors who participated in the programme were able to impact directly on clients' lives. The programme appears to reduce prejudice within the community against marginalised groups who form its client base. It provides 'food with dignity' (VicHealth 2005). This programme fostered social inclusion by using mainstream food outlets that were acceptable to the programme participants and enabled them to have social interactions with proprietors and other patrons, increasing their life skills and confidence to participate in social activities, and, for some, eventually paid employment. Sustainability was assured through new and recurrent funding and subsidisation of meals from the Victorian state government.

A comprehensive literature review of community food security projects (McClone et al. 1999) indicates that weaknesses, barriers and unexpected outcomes are hard to identify in the available project reports, and that these difficulties are compounded by a general lack of evaluation. This report also indicates that local community food projects are unsustainable in the absence of upstream policy or programme changes:

> Local people and organisations can easily identify problems and propose solutions. Very often these solutions cannot be implemented because of the inflexibility of centrally devised programmes and policies (McClone et al. 1999).

Local government has potentially a key role to play in improving community food security by making it more integral to local policymaking and the business of Council (Yeatman 1997). Two major local government initiatives in Sydney, Australia, (Penrith and South Sydney) have been maintained over some ten years (Yeatman 1997). Common features appear to have been commencement in the health sector and their successful transfer to local government, with provision of adequate resources enabling continued strong and consistent involvement of the health sector. Case study 7.4 describes a fruit and vegetables home delivery service auspiced by a local council, which aimed to improve community supply of affordable fruit and vegetables (VicHealth 2005).

CASE STUDY 7.4

BRAYSTONE FRUIT AND VEGETABLE INC.

In Maribyrnong, a municipality of inner Melbourne, a partnership began between the local council, a state government local day-care disability centre (WestNet Disability Inc.), local residents, and a rural fruit growers association, the Braystone Fruit and Vegetable Shop and Delivery Service – WestNet Incorporated (VicHealth 2005). In 2003 WestNet commenced a fruit and vegetable delivery service to local residents, which has subsequently been integrated into other WestNet client programmes to support its sustainability. The neighbourhood had no other local fruit and vegetable supply. The service not only provides produce, but also relief from social isolation and improved integration into the community for the clients of the service, particularly elderly high-rise residents. For the WestNet clients, it helped build work and social skills, and promotes the acceptance of people with an intellectual disability within the community. The WestNet clients unpacked supplies, packed and delivered boxes of fruit and vegetables and stock, and provided customer service for the streetfront fruit and vegetable shop. The clients are very much the public face of the service.

The Braystone Fruit and Vegetable Shop and Delivery Service provides a good working model of an intersectoral partnership operating at community level. This has provided the opportunity to link WestNet and its clients into the community. The project has an impact on community food security, and is sustained not only by the partnership between the groups but also by advocacy on the part of WestNet and the Council to the state government for infrastructure costs. The sustainability of the project and community-wide awareness of food security as an issue has been promoted by the ratification by the Local Council of a Municipal Food Security Policy.

This case study indicates that the needs of socially excluded or vulnerable populations can be addressed by specific food relief programmes that are socially inclusive. For community food insecurity, a multi-pronged approach is necessary, based on intersectoral partnerships within the community and embedded in local government policies (VicHealth 2005).

Food for All — National food security interventions

A more embracing approach to national food security is increasingly been seen as the approach to be encouraged. As Maxwell (quoted in Lang & Heasman 2004) stated:

"A country and people are food secure when their food system operates in such a way as to remove the fear that there will not be enough to eat. In particular, food security will be achieved when the poor and the vulnerable, particularly women and children and those living in marginal areas, have secure access to the food they want. Food security will be achieved when equitable growth ensures that these people have sustainable livelihoods. In the meantime, and in addition, however, food security requires the efficient and equitable operation of the food system". These words were written about food security in Sudan in the late 1980s. They are equally applicable today in many developed countries.

Fundamental changes to make a national or even global food system equitable will require social, economic and agricultural policy change and political advocacy in their favour (Lang & Heasman 2004). As Kumanyika (2006) comments with respect to interventions directed at childhood obesity in minority groups and those on low income in United States:

policymakers aiming to prevent obesity can use many existing policy levers to reach ethnic minorities and those on low income . . . Ultimately, winning the fight against childhood obesity in minority and low-income communities will depend on the nation's will to change the social and physical environments in which these communities exist.

There are international examples that demonstrated the benefits of a national approach to food security. These include equitable food policy and planning that is addressed at a national level by Fome Zero (Zero Hunger), Brazil's Food Security Programme <www.fomezero.gov.br> and The Toronto Food Policy Council, <http://www. toronto.ca/health/tfpc_index.htm>, which partners with business and community groups to develop policies and programmes promoting food security in the city of Toronto. It should be remembered that in 1948 the Universal Declaration of Human Rights asserted the right to food for health for all. This should be the guiding principle underpinning food security interventions at all levels.

Conclusion

Public health nutrition for economically, geographically and socially disadvantaged communities is increasingly important. Economic, geographic and social exclusion have an affect on the food security and nutritional wellbeing of individuals as well as on populations. Specific methodologies are required to identify and fully describe these issues. Public health nutrition interventions for marginalised communities should be multi-strategied, including immediate food relief programmes that encourage social inclusion, but should also involve upstream changes to the food and nutrition supply system to improve the community food security of the neighbourhoods and cities in which these populations live. There are an increasing body of research into and examples in public health practice of interventions directed at individual food security and the broader issue of community food security. Future research and public health endeavour should concentrate on novel methods of engaging socially or economically excluded population groups, and investigating leverage points in the food and nutrition system at which to intervene to improve national and global access to healthy, affordable and acceptable food.

REFERENCES

Anderson, S.A. 1990, 'Core indicators of nutritional state for difficult to sample populations' in *Journal of Nutrition*, vol. 120, no. 11S, pp. 1557–1600.

Australian Bureau of Statistics (ABS) 2000, *Household Expenditure Survey 1998–99*, cat. no. 6530.0, Commonwealth of Australia, Canberra.

Australian Council of Social Services (ACOSS) 2000, *Doling out punishment: The rise and rise of social security penalties*, ACOSS Info 220, Sydney.

Block, J.P., Scribner R.A. and DeSalvo, K.B. 2004, 'Fast food, race/ethnicity, and income: A geographic analysis' in *American Journal of Preventive Medicine* vol. 27, no. 3, pp. 211–17.

Burns, C. 2004, 'Effect of migration on food habits of Somali women living as refugees in Australia' in *Ecology of Food and Nutrition*, vol. 43, no. 3, pp. 213–29.

Burns, C., Webster, K., Crotty, P., Ballinger, M., Vincenzo, R. and Rozman, M. 2000, 'Easing the transition: Food and nutrition issues of new arrivals' in *Health Promotion Journal of Australia*, vol. 10, no. 3, pp. 230–236.

Burns, C.M. and Gibbon, P., Boak, R. Baudinette, S. and Dunbar, J.A. 2004, 'Food cost and availability in a rural setting in Australia' in *Rural and Remote Health*, vol. 4, no. 4, p. 311.

Burns, C.M., Jackson, M., Gibbons, C. and Stoney R.M. 2002, 'Foods prepared outside the home: Association with selected nutrients and body mass index in adult Australians' in *Public Health Nutrition*, vol. 5, no. 3, pp. 441–49.

Cashel, K. and Jeffreson, S. 1994, *The Core Food Groups*, National Health and Medical Research Council (NHMRC), Canberra.

Commonwealth Government of Australia 2004, *A hand up not a hand out: Renewing the fight against poverty; Report on poverty and financial hardship'* Senate Community Affairs Reference Committee, Canberra.

Cummins, S. and Macintyre, S. 2002, 'A systematic study of an urban foodscape: The price and availability of food in Greater Glasgow' in *Urban Studies*, vol. 39, no. 11, pp. 2115–30.

— 2006, 'Food environments and obesity: Neighbourhood or nation?' in *International Journal of Epidemiology*, vol. 35, no. 1, pp. 100–04.

Cummins, S., McKay, L. and Macintyre, S. 2005e, 'McDonald's restaurants and neighbourhood deprivation in Scotland and England' in *American Journal of Preventive Medicine*, vol. 4, pp. 308–10.

Cummins, S., Petticrew, M., Higgins, C., Findlay, A. and Sparks, L. 2005a, 'Large scale food retailing as an intervention for diet and health: Quasi-experimental evaluation of a natural experiment' in *Journal of Epidemiology and Community Health*, vol. 59, no. 12, pp. 1035–40.

Davey Smith, G., Hart, C., Hole, D., MacKinnon, P., Gillies, C., Watt, G., Blane, D. and Hawthorne, V. 1998, 'Education and occupational social class: Which is the more important indicator of mortality risk?' in *Journal of Epidemiology and Community Health*, vol. 52, no. 3, pp. 153–60.

Department of Health (UK) 1996, *Low Income, Food, Nutrition and Health: Strategies for improvement*, London.

Department of Immigration and Multicultural Affairs (DIMIA) 1997, *Immigration Update*, June Quarter 1997, Canberra.

Doljanin, K. and Olaris, K. 2004, 'Subsidised cafe meals program: More than "just a cheap meal"' in *Australian Journal of Primary Health*, vol. 10, no. 23, pp. 54–60.

Elstad, J.L. 2000, *Social Inequities in Health and their Explanations*, Norwegian Social Research, Oslo.

Friel, S. and Conlon, C. 2004, *Food Poverty and Policy*, commissioned by Combat Poverty Agency, Crosscare and the Society of St Vincent De Paul, National University of Ireland, Galway.

Furey, S., Farley, H. and Strugnell, C. 2002, 'An investigation into the availability and economic accessiblity of food items in rural and urban areas of Northern Ireland' in *International Journal of Consumer Studies*, vol. 26, pp. 313–21.

Giskes, K., Turrell, G., van Lenthe, F.J., Brug, J. and Mackenbach, J.P. 2006, 'A multilevel study of socio-economic inequalities in food choice behaviour and dietary intake among the Dutch population: the GLOBE study' in *Public Health Nutrition*, vol. 9, no. 1, pp. 75–83.

Graddy, K. 1997, 'Do fast-food chains discriminate on the race and income characteristics of an area?' in *Journal of Business Economics and Statistics*, vol. 15, pp. 391–401.

Graham, H. 2004, 'Social determinants and their unequal distribution: Clarifying policy understandings' in *The Milbank Quarterly*, vol. 82, no. 1, pp. 101–24.

Harding, A. and Szukalska, A. 2000, *Financial disadvantage in Australia, 1999: The unlucky Australian?*, The Smith Family, Sydney, and National Centre for Social and Economic Modelling, Canberra.

Hitchman, C., Christie, I., Harrison, M. and Lang, T. 2002, *Inconvenience Food: The struggle to eat well on a low income*, Demos, London.

Ireland, G.O. 1997, *National Anti-Poverty Strategy: Sharing in progress*, The Stationary Office, Dublin.

Kumanyika, S. 2006, 'Nutrition and chronic disease prevention: Priorities for US minority groups' in *Nutrition Reviews*, vol. 64, no. 2 (pt 2), pp. S9–14.

Lang, T. and Heasman, M. 2004, *Food Wars: The global battles for mouths, minds and markets*, Earthscan, London.

Lee, A.J., Darcy, A.M. , Leonard, D., Groos, A.D., Stubbs, C.O., Lowson, S.K., Dunn, S.M., Coyne, T. and Riley, M.D. 2002, 'Food availability, cost disparity and improvement in relation to accessibility and remoteness in Queensland' in *Australian and New Zealand Journal of Public Health*, vol. 26, no. 3, pp. 266–72.

Lewis, L.B., Sloane, D.C., Nascimento, L.M., Diamant, A.L., Guinyard, J.J., Yancy, A.K. and Flynn, G. 2005, 'African Americans' access to healthy food options in South Los Angeles restaurants' in *American Journal of Public Health*, vol. 95, no. 4, pp. 668–73.

Macintyre, S., McKay, L., Cummins, S. and Burns, C. 2005, 'Out-of-home food outlets and area deprivation: Case study in Glasgow, UK' in *The International Journal of Behavioral Nutrition and Physical Activity*, vol. 2, p. 16.

Marmot, M. 2005, 'Social determinants of health inequalities' in *Lancet* vol. 365, no. 9464, pp. 1099–104.

McClone, P., Dobson, B., Dowler, E. and Nelson, M. 1999, *Food projects and how they work*, The Joseph Rowntree Foundation, York.

Morland, K., Wing, S. and Diez Roux, A. 2002a, 'The contextual effect of the local food environment on residents' diets: The atherosclerosis risk in communities study' in *American Journal of Public Health*, vol. 92, no. 11, pp. 1761–67.

Morland, K., Wing, S., Diez Roux, A. and Poole, C. 2002b, 'Neighborhood characteristics associated with the location of food stores and food service places' in *American Journal of Preventive Medicine*, vol. 22, no. 1, pp. 23–29.

Nielsen, S.J., Siega-Riz, A.M. and Popkin, B.M. 2002, 'Trends in food locations and sources among adolescents and young adults' in *Preventive Medicine*, vol. 35, no. 2, pp. 107–13.

Parker, H. 1998, *Low Cost but Acceptable: A minimum income standard for the UK; families with young children*, The Policy Press, Bristol.

Prentice, A.M. and Jebb, S.A. 2003, 'Fast foods, energy density and obesity: A possible mechanistic link' in *Obesity Reviews: An official journal of the International Association for the Study of Obesity*, vol. 4, no. 4, pp. 187–94.

Rayner, M. and Scarborough, P. 2005, 'The burden of food related ill health in the UK' in *Journal of Epidemiology And Community Health*, vol. 59, no. 12, pp. 1054–57.

Reidpath, D.D., Burns, C., Garrard, J., Mahoney, M. and Townsend, M., 2002, 'An ecological study of the relationship between social and environmental determinants of obesity' in *Health & Place*, vol. 8, no. 2, pp. 141–45.

Rolls, B.J., Roe, L.S., Kral, T.V., Meengs, J.S. and Wall, D.E. 2004, 'Increasing the portion size of a packaged snack increases energy intake in men and women' in *Appetite*, vol. 42, no. 1, pp. 63–69.

Rose, D. and Richards, R. 2004, 'Food store access and household fruit and vegetable use among participants in the US Food Stamp Program' in *Public Health Nutrition*, vol. 7, no. 8, pp. 1081–88.

Shaw, M., Dorling, D., Gordon, D. and Davey Smith, G. 1999, *The Widening Gap: Health inequalities and policy in Britain*, The Policy Press, Bristol.

Social Exclusion Office (UK) 1998, *Bringing Britain Together: A national strategy for neighbourhood renewal*, HMSO, London.

—— 2003, *Making the Connections: Final report on Transport and Social Exclusion*, Office of the Deputy Prime Minister, HMSO, London.

United Nations (UN) 1995, *Report of World Summit for Social Development Copenhagen, 6–12 March 1995*, Department of Economic and Social Affairs, Gateway to Social Policy and Development, UN.

Veit-Wilson, J. 1994, *Dignity not Poverty: A minimum income standard for the UK*, Institute for Public Policy, London.

VicHealth 2005, *Food for All: Lessons from two community demonstration projects*, The Victorial Health Promotion Foundation, Melbourne.

Victorian Foundation for the Survivors of Torture Inc. (VFST) 2002, *Promoting Refugee Health: A handbook for doctors and other health care providers caring for people from refugee backgrounds*, VFST, Melbourne.

Voss, T. and Begg, S. 1999, *The Victorian Burden of Disease Study: Morbidity*, Public Health Division, Department of Human Services (Victoria), Melbourne.

White, M., Bunting, J., Raybould, S., Adamson, A., Williams, L. and Mathers, J. 2004, *Do Food Deserts Exists? A multi-level, geographical analysis of the relationship between retail food access, socio-economic position and dietary intake; the final report*, The Food Standards Agency (UK), London.

Winkler, E., Turrell, G. and Paterson, C. 2006, 'Does living in a disadvantaged area entail limited opportunities to purchase fresh fruit and vegetables in terms of price, availability and variety?' in *Health & Place*, vol. 12, no. 4, pp. 741–48.

World Bank 2005, *World Development Report 2006: Equity and development*, The World Bank Group, Washington D.C.

World Health Organization (WHO) 2002, *World Health Report: Reducing risks, promoting healthy life*, WHO, Geneva.

Wrigley, N., Warm D. and Margetts, B. 2003, 'Deprivation, diet and food retail access: Findings from the Leeds "food desert" study' in *Environment and Planning A*, vol. 35, pp. 151–88.

Yeatman, H. 1997, *National Review of Food and Nutrition Activities in Local government*, Department of Health and Family Services, Canberra.

Zenk, S.N., Schulz, A.J., Israel, B.A., James, S.A., Bao, S. and Wilson, M.L. 2005, 'Neighborhood racial composition, neighborhood poverty, and the spatial accessibility of supermarkets in metropolitan Detroit' in *American Journal of Public Health*, vol. 95, no. 4, pp. 660–67.

8

Indigenous communities

MALCOLM RILEY
LEISA McCARTHY

The relatively poor health of indigenous minority groups is a very stark demonstration of the importance and power of social determinants of health (Durie 2003a; Foliaki & Pearce 2003; Thomson 2003a). These 'upstream' factors, few of which are under the direct influence of the health sector, are determinants of ill-health, as indicated by reduced life expectancy and increased morbidity. They are beyond the control of individuals, and epitomise the challenges of practising public health. Interventions that seek to influence individuals to adopt specific health-promoting lifestyle behaviours, or to directly address a particular 'downstream' problem (such as poor dietary intake) without acknowledging and addressing upstream determinants, are likely to have limited and passing success at improving health. While generalisation about indigenous people is not likely to hold true in all circumstances, this chapter will attempt two things: first to describe common features regarding the health of indigenous minority groups, particularly as it relates to diet and nutrition; and second to discuss important principles relating to working for improved health for indigenous minority groups.

Indigenous peoples

Indigenous minority populations consist of those peoples descended from the ethnically distinct people living in a defined place prior to the arrival of the current dominant population, although other conceptualisations of the meaning of 'indigenous' are possible (Cunningham & Stanley 2003; Durie 2003a). The total population of indigenous people is estimated to be about 200 million (around 4 per cent of the global population) in up to 5000 indigenous groups (Durie 2003a). Examples of indigenous minority populations are the Inuit of Canada, the Maori of New Zealand, and the Aboriginal and Torres Strait Islanders of Australia. The naming of indigenous people varies from place to place, often group terms for many different and distinct groups of people. In North America, 'First Nations People' is used, and in Australia the term 'Aboriginal and Torres Strait Islander' is acceptable to cover many populations. In New Zealand, the term 'Tangata Whenua' (which translates to 'people of the land') is increasingly preferred to the name Maori (which translates to 'ordinary or common') given by the British colonisers (Cunningham & Stanley 2003). Often, but not always, the determination of whether a person is a member of an indigenous minority group is largely left up to that person. For example, in Australia the census and many other official forms used for population counting ask a specific question regarding indigenous status, allowing a respondent to respond 'Aboriginal', 'Torres Strait Islander', both, or neither. Community acceptance (as an indigenous person) is another important defining factor.

Living circumstances for indigenous people can vary widely. The populations of many Pacific nations are predominantly indigenous people; the indigenous people of New Zealand and Australia are living side by side with the dominant culture to a greater extent than the First Nations People of North America, where a greater proportion live on reservations. Within a country, indigenous people may live with other indigenous people in small groups or communities of many thousands. They may live in large cities, highly integrated with the dominant culture, or in locations relatively remote from cities. They may vary to the extent that they have knowledge of, or follow, the culture and practices of their forebears. Overwhelmingly, they are almost certain to be proud of being indigenous and to value highly the defining characteristics of being indigenous. One important general characteristic of indigenous people is a traditional worldview, which includes a unifying relationship with the natural world (Cunningham & Stanley 2003). Dislocation of indigenous people from the country they belong to, or disruption of their relationship with their natural world through various processes of colonisation or globalisation, has had negative health effects in a broad sense.

In Australia, indigenous people comprised around 2.4 per cent of the total population in 2005 (Australian Indigenous HealthInfoNet 2005). In New Zealand, about 14 per cent of the population is Maori (with about 6 per cent being Pacific Islander and 6 per cent Asian) (McPherson et al. 2003). In Canada, about 3 per cent of the population identify themselves as indigenous (Young 2003).

There may appear to be strong similarities in the living circumstances between indigenous minority groups and other ethnic minority groups. However, there are important differences. Four factors leading to poor health status have been identified as genetic vulnerability, socioeconomic disadvantage, resource alienation and political oppression (Durie 2003a). Despite these factors operating to a different extent in different indigenous groups, the experience of the groups is remarkably similar. Genetic vulnerability to important health issues such as alcohol-related disorders and the development of diabetes have been examined, but are generally regarded to be less important than socioeconomic disadvantage (McDermott 1998). Minority indigenous people have been abruptly removed from their position of being the dominant human culture in a region and subjugated to another culture. Social changes that have taken place over long periods of time in the dominant culture are occurring in a much shorter time in the minority indigenous groups. There is a substantial disempowerment of the groups, with cultural values, practices and law being (intentionally or unintentionally) disregarded or overridden.

Although these issues may seem to current generations to have only historical relevance, they are also critically relevant in the present, and are part of being a numerically dominated cultural group. The sequence of events for indigenous minority groups undergoing colonisation is broadly universal (Durie 2003a) — groups suffer great loss of life from infectious diseases such as measles, typhoid fever, tuberculosis, influenza and smallpox, followed by a rise in the diseases of development, including heart disease, diabetes, obesity, substance abuse, and injury including suicide. Indigenous peoples typically have higher rates than the culturally dominant population of infectious diseases, as well as the diseases of development. The political events also follow a broadly similar sequence, and are typified by the history in Australia (Shannon 2002). Generally, there were four mostly distinct phases — direct conflict, paternalism, assimilation, and self-determination. Conflict occurred during the early parts of the European invasion and expansion. There was substantial loss of life for indigenous people through the spread of new diseases, fatal injuries sustained through fighting, and dispossession of the land to which they belonged. This caused a massive disruption to the culture of indigenous groups due to too few remaining people with knowledge to conduct important activities, or disruption to the land/people relationship. The paternalistic phase recognised the disaster that European occupation had been for indigenous people, and attempted to provide protection for them. This protection included providing reserves, housing and other material goods. It was thought that the indigenous people would die out, and the protectionist policies would only be required for a relatively short time. It was described at the time as a policy of 'smoothing the dying pillow' (Shannon 2002).

One effect of the protectionist policies was to institute a great deal of control over the lives of indigenous people — they could not travel freely, or live anywhere they wished. To a large extent, control of their own affairs had been taken from them and taken over by the government and the church. These circumstances meant that they could not maintain some aspects of their culture. Following this period, the view was formed that the best result for the indigenous population was that it be completely assimilated by the dominant European population — it was determined that indigenous people should eventually live according to the same customs, beliefs and values as all 'Australians'. During this period, consistent with government policy, many hundreds of children were taken from their indigenous parents to be brought up away from indigenous influences. This damaging period for indigenous people was followed by the current orientation towards self-determination and self-management. In Australia, indigenous people were first counted in the national census in 1967, when they were recognised as citizens and allowed to vote. This decision was taken after a referendum on the matter, which occurred 189 years after the first permanent European settlement in Australia, and 66 years after Australia became a nation. In effect, self-determination means that indigenous people would be involved in decisions concerning themselves.

Health status of indigenous people in Australia

There are substantial difficulties in providing accurate quantitative health statistics for indigenous people because of different practices of indigenous person identification and enumeration, and change in practices over time (Durie 2003a). For this reason, health information is often extrapolated from indigenous groups that are not necessarily representative of the total indigenous population; for example, there is much less health information available on Australian indigenous people living in urban centres in the southeast of the country than in the northern parts, despite larger numbers of indigenous people living in the southeastern part of the country. Although, there is some doubt as to the magnitude of the health indicator estimates among groups of minority indigenous people, there is a similarity of health experience — the health status of indigenous minority groups is worse than the dominant culture groups in their country. Health statistics are broadly worse for all conditions and diseases, but much of the excess mortality is due to diseases of development, or diseases of affluence. These are the diseases that result when people become affluent enough to access an abundant industrialised food supply and are able to be largely sedentary in their work. It is ironic that indigenous minority populations, in unwillingly becoming part of more economically advanced nations, generally suffer the ill effects of low socioeconomic status within that nation, as well as a disproportionate burden of the diseases of affluence, such as diabetes, obesity, hypertension and other cardiovascular diseases.

While universally minority indigenous groups have poorer health than the dominant culture, they differ in the magnitude of their poor health. In 1990–94, the average all-causes mortality rate for indigenous people in Western Australia and the Northern Territory was 1.9 times the Maori rate (but comparable to Maori rates in the early 1970s), 2.4 times the US indigenous rate, and 3.15 times the all-Australian rate (Ring & Firman 1998). Life expectancy for an indigenous baby born in the period 1996–2001 was 59.4 years for males and 64.8 years for females (Australian Bureau of Statistics 2005). This is about 17 years less than the figure for all Australian babies – 76.6 years for males and 82.0 years for females. The life expectancy for indigenous males in Australia in 2001 is similar to males born in 2001 in Gambia, Ghana, Papua New Guinea and Yemen, and to that for the total Australian male population in the period 1910–15 (Thomson 2003b). The life expectancy for a Maori baby born in 2001 was 69 years for a male and 73 years for a female (Ministry of Health 2006). This compares with a life expectancy at birth in New Zealand in 2001 of 77 years for non-Maori males, and 82 years for non-Maori females. While it is unacceptable for any population group to have a life expectancy eight years lower than the majority population, it is apparent that the mortality experience of Australian indigenous people is much worse than Maori people, while the majority populations from both Australia and New Zealand have an almost identical life expectancy.

There are some grounds for optimism. In North America and New Zealand, indigenous people experienced an improvement in health and life expectancy at the end of the last century (Ring & Firman 1998). There appeared to be a trend for lower mortality for indigenous people in Western Australia, South Australia and the Northern Territory (accounting for 32 per cent of the Australian indigenous population) over the period 1991–2002, particularly for mortality from circulatory disease (Australian Bureau of Statistics 2005).

In some regions and towns, particularly in the northern and central parts of Australia, indigenous people make up the largest percentage of the population; for example, of the total population of the Northern Territory, about one-quarter are indigenous people. Despite this, and due to the geographic concentration of the Australian population, most indigenous Australians live in the southern and eastern parts of Australia. Of the areas where indigenous Australian populations reside, indigenous people are more likely to live outside of urban areas than are non-indigenous people. In Australia, 70 per cent of indigenous people recognise their homeland or traditional country, 54 per cent identify with their clan, tribal or language group, and 21 per cent speak one or more indigenous languages (Australian Bureau of Statistics 2005). There are parts of Australia (mainly remote areas) where access to non-indigenous Australians is restricted, and there are laws that differentiate between people on the basis of their indigenous status; for example, some animals are only allowed to be hunted by indigenous people.

The age structure of the indigenous population of Australia is young compared to non-indigenous Australians. In 1996, nearly 40 per cent of the indigenous population was less than fifteen years old compared to 21 per cent of the total Australian population. About 3 per cent of the indigenous population was aged above 65 years compared to about 10 per cent of the total Australian population (Australian Indigenous HealthInfoNet 2005). One reason for this difference in age structure is the higher mortality rate experienced by the indigenous population, coupled with the higher birthrate of the indigenous Australian population compared to the overall Australian population.

Indigenous Australians have a higher burden of disease and die at a younger age for almost every disease and condition for which information is available. In 2002, Australian indigenous people were at least twice as likely as non-indigenous people to have a profound or severe core activity limitation (disability) (Australian Bureau of Statistics 2005). Indigenous people are more than twice as likely to be hospitalised as non-indigenous people, with most of the difference due to potentially preventable chronic conditions (Australian Bureau of Statistics 2005).

The all-causes mortality rate for indigenous Australians is almost three times that for non-indigenous Australians (Australian Bureau of Statistics 2005), with the mortality rates for almost all conditions being many times higher for indigenous people than for non-indigenous people (see Table 8.1). Excess deaths are those deaths in excess of the number expected if the reference mortality rate (in this case, that for the total Australian population) were applied to the indigenous population. Table 8.1 indicates that there were 2737 excess male deaths and 2022 excess female deaths in the indigenous population over the period 1999 to 2003 for four Australian states. These are deaths that would not have occurred if mortality rates for indigenous Australians were at least the same as non-indigenous Australians. Four broad categories — circulatory conditions (mainly ischaemic heart disease and stroke), injury and poisoning (mostly transport accidents, homicide and suicide), respiratory conditions, and endocrine conditions (mainly diabetes) — account for about 65 per cent of the excess deaths (see Figure 8.1) (Australian Bureau of Statistics 2005). While the standardised mortality rate for most causes in the Australian indigenous population is substantially higher than the corresponding rate in the non-indigenous population, it may seem paradoxical that major chronic diseases, such as diseases of the circulatory system and neoplasms, cause a lower proportion of total deaths in indigenous people (27.3 per cent and 14.8 per cent respectively) than in non-indigenous people (38.2 per cent and 29.3 per cent). The explanation for this is the different population age structure (indigenous people are younger and die at a younger age), and competing causes of mortality. It should be

Table 8.1 Australian indigenous deaths—main causes 1999–2003*

	Males			Females		
	Observed deaths	Expected deaths	SMR†	Observed deaths	Expected deaths	SMR
Diseases of the circulatory condition	1134	388	2.9	882	347	2.5
External causes	842	306	2.7	356	111	3.2
Neoplasms	592	407	1.5	502	345	1.5
Endocrine, nutritional and metabolic diseases	303	41	7.5	372	35	10.5
Diseases of the respiratory system	368	92	4.0	269	76	3.5
Diseases of the digestive system	208	42	4.9	152	36	4.3
Diseases of the genitourinary system	87	16	5.3	139	19	7.3
Symptoms, signs and ill-defined conditions	136	24	5.8	88	15	5.7
Certain conditions originating in the perinatal period	124	43	2.9	88	35	2.5
Diseases of the nervous system and sense organs	111	41	2.7	70	41	1.7
Certain infectious and parasitic diseases	97	20	5.0	80	14	5.8
Mental and behavioural disorders	122	22	5.5	52	24	2.2
All causes	**4222**	**1485**	**2.8**	**3165**	**1143**	**2.8**

Source: Australian Bureau of Statistics 2005

* Data for Queensland, South Australia, Western Australia and the Northern Territory combined — deaths are based on year of occurrence of death for 1999–2002, and year of registration of death for 2003
† Standardised mortality rate

clearly understood that, despite the difference in proportion of total deaths, the major causes of death for non-indigenous Australians affect indigenous Australians at substantially higher rates (see Table 8.1). External causes (injury, homicide, suicide) caused 16.2 per cent of the total deaths in the indigenous population compared to 6.5 per cent in the non-indigenous population, diabetes caused 8.2 per cent of total deaths in the indigenous population compared to 2.2 per cent in the non-indigenous population, and chronic kidney disease caused 3.7 per cent of total deaths in the indigenous population compared to 1.7 per cent in the non-indigenous population (Australian Bureau of Statistics 2005).

For most of the main causes of death (for example, diseases of the circulatory system, neoplasms, respiratory diseases, diabetes and chronic renal disease), the mortality rate increases with age for each sex. Generally, indigenous Australians die from these causes at a younger age than non-indigenous Australians. For deaths from external causes, the mortality rate does not increase with age. In the indigenous Australian group, the mortality rate was particularly high for 25- to 44-year-old males. Suicide accounted for 34 per cent of the total deaths from this cause in the indigenous population (Australian Bureau of Statistics 2005).

In the Maori, using slightly different definitions of conditions, the five major causes of death in the period 2000 were, for men, ischaemic heart disease, lung cancer, diabetes, chronic obstructive pulmonary disease, other heart disease; for women, ischaemic heart disease, lung cancer, chronic obstructive pulmonary disease, cerebrovascular disease, and diabetes (Ministry of Health 2006).

The relative health disadvantage of indigenous people starts at the beginning of life – in Australia, babies born to indigenous women in 2002 weighed on average 2.13 kilograms less than babies born to non-indigenous women, and were more than twice as likely to be defined as 'low birthweight' (birthweight less than 2.5 kilograms) (Australian Indigenous HealthInfoNet 2005). Contributing to low birthweight are a high smoking rate and possibly earlier delivery, in addition to nutritional factors. Indigenous babies were also about two to three times more likely to die in their first year of life when compared with non-indigenous babies (Australian Indigenous HealthInfoNet 2005). For the Maori, there was no difference in the prevalence of low birthweight in 2000–02; however, the infant mortality rate was about 1.5 times the rate of the non-Maori in New Zealand (Ministry of Health 2006).

Dietary and nutrition issues
Poor health in indigenous populations would not be resolved solely by improving nutrition of indigenous people. Nor is it practicable to adequately address many

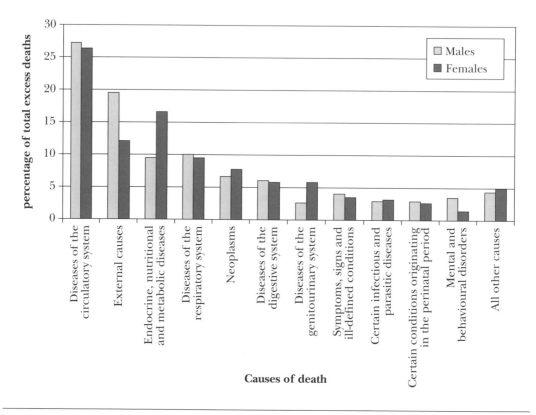

Figure 8.1 Main causes of excess Australian Indigenous Deaths 1999–2003*

Source: Australian Bureau of Statistics 2005

* Data for Queensland, South Australia, Western Australia and the Northern Territory combined – deaths are based on year of occurrence of death for 1999–2002, and year of registration of death for 2003

health issues without focusing on issues relevant to nutrition and diet.

Poor diet is a contributory factor to poor growth in children, the severity of infectious disease, and to the high incidence and mortality rates of chronic diseases such as heart disease, diabetes and cancers. Dietary intake is relevant to the capacity to undertake work, and the ability to have and raise children. It is likely that poor health resulting partly from substandard nutrition leads to intergenerational effects on health – effects that reach generations yet to be born.

Food and dietary intake and customs are an important expression of the culture of a people – they identify and affirm people as belonging to a group. Food beliefs and practices are strongly held and therefore resistant to change.

Breakdown in culture and values will be reflected in what food is eaten, by whom, and how it is prepared. Enforced changes in food intake, such as has occurred in indigenous minority populations, raise issues of whether new and unfamiliar foods are incorporated into traditional food culture, or whether they are treated outside the system contributing to cultural breakdown (Stacey 1975). An understanding of the 'web of influence' on food practices, including food culture, is a prerequisite to promoting beneficial population dietary change for a free-living population.

In contrast to traditional diet, the contemporary diets of indigenous people tend to be high in energy and sugar and low in unrefined carbohydrate and dietary fibre (Guest & O'Dea 1993; Lee 1996; Kuhnlein et al. 2004). In an examination of community diet in six remote Aboriginal communities in the Northern Territory of Australia (Lee et al. 1994), more than half the apparent dietary energy was provided by sugar, white flour, bread and meat. Fatty meats contributed almost 40 per cent of the total fat intake in northern coastal communities, and more than 60 per cent in central desert communities. White sugar contributed about 60 per cent of the total sugars consumed. Compared to data for the Australian population, more than six times the amount of white sugar, up to three times the amount of carbonated drinks, less than one-quarter of the amount of fruit and less than one-fifth of the amount of vegetables were apparently consumed per head of population (Lee et al. 1994).

A nutritional dimension can be identified for most of the causes of premature mortality identified as being prominent for indigenous people, but rarely is dietary intake the only relevant factor. For example, it is well-recognised that particular dietary components are associated with circulatory disease and many cancers; however, other risk factors and protective factors are also important and relevant to the situation of indigenous people. Low birthweight is influenced by smoking during pregnancy, and gestational age at delivery; sub-optimal childhood growth is strongly associated with childhood illnesses.

Iron deficiency anaemia
Rates of iron deficiency in children and pregnant women appear to be substantially higher in indigenous Australians based on the limited data available (National Health and Medical Research Council 2000). Iron deficiency may cause developmental delay and poor mental performance in children, and decreased work productivity in adults.

Dental health

Dental health can be an important influence on dietary intake, by determining the types of food that a person is able to easily manage. In contrast to Australian non-indigenous children, the rate of caries in deciduous teeth of Australian indigenous children appears to be increasing (Thomson 2003a). In older indigenous people, the experience of tooth loss and periodontal disease is worse than the general Australian population.

The rate of missing or filled teeth for Maori children was greater than the New Zealand average in 2003, and Maori adults were less likely to have visited a dentist over the past year than non-Maori adults (Ministry of Health 2006).

Issues that affect food intake and nutritional status

Illness and disease

Poor living conditions can lead to diarrhoeal disease, intestinal parasites, respiratory tract infections, urinary tract infections, skin infections, and eye disease. In young children, these conditions may be an important contributory cause of malnutrition, growth faltering, retarded mental development, and permanent stunting. Infections affect nutritional status by increasing energy and nutrient requirements while influencing food intake, potentially nutrient digestion and absorption, and nutrient losses. Malnutrition may have a negative affect on the immune system, setting up a vicious cycle where infection is more common and more severe because of the effects of previous infection. The high burden of disease and disability in indigenous communities can decrease mobility for food collection and preparation, influence dietary requirements, increase poverty due to decreased capacity to work and diversion of resources to manage the disease or disability. The excess mortality rate in indigenous popuations results in a relatively young age structure — older people who may traditionally have been involved in the care of children are under-represented in the population.

Remoteness

The geographic isolation from markets of some indigenous communities results in a limited range of foods being relatively infrequently delivered to some community food stores. Invariably, distance from market and the need for transportation increases food costs. For people from the dominant culture living in remote areas, there may be a salary inducement that covers extra food costs. Within large cities, due to their low socioeconomic status, indigenous people may live in areas distant from large food stores. Even a relatively short distance will be reason for people to go to smaller stores, which are more expensive and have less variety of food. This problem is accentuated for people with poor mobility because of physical illness or lack of transport.

Low socioeconomic status is often associated with poverty

This affects the resources available to buy food, and the equipment to store and cook food. Limited storage and cooking equipment influences the types of food bought. Low socioeconomic status may be associated with poor and over-crowded housing, leading to domestic instability, and contributing to family and cultural breakdown. There may be a resulting reliance on takeaway or convenience foods, with the associated poor nutritional value.

Removal of traditional food sources, or access to them

Traditional foods may not have the same availability under the current living circumstances as it did during traditional times (see following section). The skills to collect and prepare traditional foods may have been lost, particularly where a new food system or practices have replaced the traditional system, making some skills no longer relevant.

Loss of traditional food culture and practices

Many traditional practices are reduced or ceased under circumstances of living with larger mainstream cultures. The central importance of food means that the redundancy and loss of some of these practices will influence food intake and nutritional status. For example, among the indigenous people of North East Arnhem Land, food hunting would be undertaken by men, and food collection by women accompanied by children, where some food collected would be eaten. Toddlers and babies were left at the camp under the care of grandmoth-ers. There they would be fed small amounts of leftover traditional foods (the only food available). The breakdown of traditional food collection, the avail-ability of foods of low nutritional quality and the culturally based autonomy of children has meant that young children are likely to eat what they desire – often sweet, energy dense foods.

Difference in worldview

This is an important reason for the misunderstandings between indigenous minority groups and the dominant culture. Much of the information that an indigenous minority group learns about food and diet (and other aspects of the dominant culture) is disseminated by mass media broadcasts targeted mainly at the dominant culture. Members of the dominant culture recognise the selling intent of television, print and radio advertising, and generally have a raised level of distrust for the messages delivered from the producers and sellers of food. Members of an indigenous minority group may not have this sophisticated view, and have a limited understanding of how content of advertising in mass media is controlled – it may be considered to make little sense that advertising would be allowed for food that does not promote health.

Substance abuse

High rates of tobacco, alcohol and other substance use and misuse in indigenous communities has many different effects on food intake. People who misuse substances are unable to contribute to activities that might increase food availability or care for people they might otherwise be responsible for, and may neglect appropriate food intake for themselves. Substance abusers may cause disruption to the community and their families, distracting them from productive activity. Money used for procuring substances is diverted away from food purchase.

Lack of need for physical activity

In many developed populations, the need for physical activity has decreased with increasing labour-saving devices and easier ways of doing things. For indigenous people, the changing lifestyle from traditional times has meant a large decrease in the physical activity necessary to accomplish basic living requirements, such as the search for food and shelter. In some indigenous communities of Australia, where western-style employment for indigenous people is scarce, a large proportion of the population receive government social security payments, which is known as 'sit-down money', acknowledging that it requires no physical activity to obtain.

Traditional foods

Traditional diet of indigenous people was varied and nutrient dense (Lee et al. 1994). In general, many components of the diet were seasonal, and the preparation of foods involved little processing and wasn't generally stored for significant periods of time. The hunting, growing or collection of food required substantial energy expenditure and skill. With the development of a westernised lifestyle, for most indigenous people the amount of traditional food eaten has greatly decreased – the 'development diet' is energy dense, substantially refined, high in fat and sugar. Food can be obtained with far less energy expenditure than traditional times. Traditional foods are less available for a range of reasons, including areas around settlements being 'hunted out' due to the large number of people living there, neglect of land-management practices that previously led to increased food production (or different land-management practices by the dominant culture), legal restriction in some areas on particular traditional food production activities, changes in land ownership, the relatively low prestige accorded traditional food resulting from dominant culture attitudes, and the limited resources of indigenous people due to their low socioeconomic status.

Traditional foods are strongly associated with health – their declining use is correlated with increasing westernisation and associated poor health (Lakos 2001; Kuhnlein et al. 2004). The classic study of O'Dea (1984) conducted more than two decades ago showed that returning a small group of indigenous Australians to their traditional lifestyle, including food collection and consumption practices, for a few weeks greatly improved subjective and objective measures of their health status. In a northern coastal Australian Aboriginal community, it has been estimated that traditional foods provided less than 8 per cent of the total energy intake for the dry season, with less than half this amount during the peak of the wet season (Lee et al. 1994). In the more populated southern and eastern areas of Australia, traditional foods would be a much less common part of the diet of indigenous people. In 44 indigenous communities in the Arctic, it was estimated that between 10 and 36 per cent of total dietary energy came from traditional food sources in the 1990s, with older people eating a greater proportion than younger people (Kuhnlein et al. 2004). It is no more practicable for indigenous people to permanently return to traditional food production practices than it is for any population of a developed nation to return to labour-intensive, non-globalised methods of food production. However, understanding of the justification for dietary intervention can be improved by appropriate reference to traditional food knowledge. For example, Lee and colleagues (1994) recommend that indigenous people 'eat store foods that are most like traditional foods', meaning foods that are minimally processed.

Health education in traditionally oriented indigenous communities

The following information has been provided from various sources (Stacey 1975; Harris 1984; Trudgen 2000) relating to Australian indigenous communities in the Northern Territory. It is intended to provide insight into the issues that a public health practitioner might experience when taking a 'teaching' role in an indigenous community, and to demonstrate the extent of cultural understanding that is necessary to work effectively in indigenous communities.

Teaching

There is no indigenous concept of a 'teacher' — although some semiformal instruction occurs from a teaching figure, its role is minimal in comparison to learning by observation and by trial and error. Knowledge isn't necessarily public and open to all, but available only to those with 'the right to know'. In Australian indigenous culture, the line of authority is through kinship — the closest equivalence for an outsider is a 'personal relationship'. Verbal instruction is always conducted in a meaningful real-life context, and is almost always supplementary to learning by other means. The present-time orientation of indigenous people may thwart teaching that attempts to use hypothetical situations. Verbal instruction usually occurs from a close older relative who has the authority to give that instruction. Learning is much more person-oriented than information-oriented. For a person from outside the culture to teach through verbal instruction, they need to:

- be patient enough to wait for shared experience with the students to increase earned authority as a teacher figure
- pay close attention to the relevant rules of interpersonal communication as sufficient rapport is developed to be able to teach the students without offence
- try to make sure that the learning context is meaningful and real-life (Harris 1984).

A person is not judged for their suitability as a teacher by their qualifications, knowledge or experience, but by displaying appropriate behaviour at all times. This requires understanding what constitutes culturally appropriate behaviour. If offence is caused to a person, particularly an older person, it is likely to also cause offence to his extended relations, with implications for community workers.

Mutually inconsistent understandings may be held at the same time, such as the dominant culture versus the indigenous culture view of a health relationship. It may be noticed that people will cooperate with particular people, but not with everybody — this is a function of kinship relationships. This is relevant to group educational activities and to group working situations.

The paradox of appropriate cultural interaction and working toward the goals of a dominant culture worldview is captured by the experience of one health worker of many years experience from a dominant culture:

As health workers we establish a rapport or build a relationship so we can teach some aspect of health. The goal is improved health, and the relationship is largely seen by us as the means to that end. The Aboriginal people participate in programmes, retain knowledge and sometimes apply it so they can build a relationship. By relationship I mean interaction. To Aborigines interaction is an end in itself and, by contrast with our views, not a means to an end. The goal is the relationship itself . . . I have found that as my relationships have developed my ability to function as a teacher has decreased (Stacey 1975).

Elements of verbal communication

Talking is used more as a facilitator for social relationships than for transferring information and organising activities. The talk interaction is more interesting than the message – thus repetition is not considered odd or unusual. When talking is used as an agent of drive and organisation, it is extremely tiring and intimidating for indigenous people. Questions never demand an answer, and people who ask a question never assume they have the right to an answer – it is culturally acceptable to ignore or evade questions. Questioners tend to leave the assessment of the reasonableness of a request to the person being asked (in contrast to dominant Australian culture, where a request is expected to be reasonable before it is asked), and the asker is not normally offended by refusal to a request. In the dominant Australian culture, people may be offended if their questions are seemly ignored. While non-response may be misunderstood, responses to questions may also be misinterpreted. A request for assistance that is met by a genuine response from a dominant culture person, such as 'I'll do it later', may be taken as a euphemistic refusal to the request by an indigenous person.

In personal interaction, the proportion of silence to talk may be different to what a practitioner is used to. The length of silence before response may be elongated, and a demand for a quick response is considered rude. Outsiders may interpret this as awkward silence or as meaning that their presence is not welcome. This is not necessarily the case. Personal names are not used as freely or as frequently, and conversations take place with much less eye contact. Exchanging greetings, making introductions and making small talk with strangers is much less formalised than in the dominant Australian culture – these social conventions may not occur.

A verbal commitment may not be kept – planning and promising about future activities often bear little resemblance to what happens when the time arrives. The subsequent action may not occur because the person said what he thought was wanted to be heard, or because his attitude to time and urgency is different, and because not keeping a verbal commitment does not have the same negative moral connotation; for example, to the dominant Australian concept of keeping a promise. There is no expression of thanks in traditional culture – people do things because they want to, or because they have cultural obligations to specific relations. The notion of humanism or public spiritedness (not uncommon for people working in public health) may not be well understood.

Direct talk of a disciplinary or critical nature is interpreted as an expression of anger and personal animosity, and regarded as an act of hostility. Indigenous people tend to avoid direct verbal confrontation; for example, they may agree with something they do not in fact agree with, or say what they think others want to hear. Questions seeking a personal motive ('why did you . . ?'), or questions of a hypothetical nature may cause misunderstanding and offence. Often questions concerning others may be ignored, since people do not like becoming involved in the affairs of others.

Kinship relationships directly influence communication, the names of recently dead people should be avoided, and it is preferable not to ask a person their own name. These factors can lead to apparent rambling conversations, which can be confusing to outsiders. In general, people are accorded the right to speak, but not to be listened to. Conversely, listeners reserve the right to ignore the speaker, but acknowledge their right to speak. In a public speaking situation, audience restlessness and apparent inattention is typical and doesn't constitute rudeness. On the other hand, a capable indigenous speaker may be unnerved by the intense, continuous attention and direct eye contact of an interested dominant culture audience, and, as a result, be unable to perform a speaking task.

A practitioner should carefully reflect on the aims and purposes of their educational work with indigenous communities, and be realistic about what is possible. The health worker quoted previously, who was frustrated at her increasing cultural competency but decreasing effectiveness as an educator, turns from her own personal effectiveness to how benefit might be achieved for indigenous communities:

> Unless the community defines the need, any attempt to conduct a program will be an imposition, and chances of persistant behaviour change are minimal . . . The aim of any education program is not to solve all problems. Problems are never solved: an intolerable set of problems are replaced by a tolerable set. An educator should, by working through the expressed needs of a community, bring people to a capacity where they can determine their own problems and create their own methods to alleviate them. Unless this occurs the program is not educational but causes the client to become dependent. In order for the program to have its desired effect, the educator must have a thorough knowledge of the communities with

which she is working. She must learn from them how they see the world. Only then can she achieve her aims and help her clients to perceive alternatives. Effective communication can only be achieved by working from the present knowledge and values of the clients (Stacey 1975).

Working as a public health nutrition practitioner with indigenous groups

Working as a public health nutrition practitioner for indigenous communities presents considerable challenges; however, with perhaps the exception of the challenge of working with an unfamiliar cultural group, they are broadly similar in concept to all work in public health nutrition.

Change to community health status is generally expected to be slow. The reasons for this are that indigenous people generally have relatively poor access to healthcare services, and such services and programmes may be culturally insensitive or inappropriate. The coordination and priorities of healthcare services can also be inappropriate for indigenous people. They may have an understanding of disease that obstructs early detection, decisions about treatment, and personal assessment of risk factors. Bad experience with the health sector may result in people presenting with disease late (if at all), and many of the determinants of health for indigenous people are external to the health sector, including issues such as housing, access to land, racism, self-esteem, and culture. Practitioners should be prepared to be patient with the slow rate of change at any level.

Understanding and adapting to the culture of the group you are working with is likely to be critical to the work you do. By necessity, this means learning from the community you are working with, and this will be at least a daily activity and should use indigenous learning styles as far as possible. Undertaking this learning activity quickly changes the relationship with community members to a partnership arrangement of mutual respect: it empowers community members and demonstrates intent to understand their worldview and fit in with it. It also makes it much more likely that you will be able to provide sustainable benefit to the community. Failure to adapt to the culture of the group you are working with suggests that you expect them to work according to your cultural values. You could expect considerable resistance to expectations of cultural assimilation at any level with its unfortunate and inherent racist overtones.

Undertake your work activities in a culturally safe manner. The principle of 'cultural safety' requires health professionals to reflect on their own cultural background and the nature of power relations in the provision of service to a minority culture from a dominant culture (Hughes & Gray 2003). Providers acknowledge their own culture as different from the groups they serve, to ensure they don't impose their beliefs on the minority communities. Cultural safety also requires providers from the dominant culture to challenge their own stereotyped views of a minority culture, thus promoting positive recognition of diversity.

Reflect on your practice — what you do and why you do it, including examination of the reasons for doing something, the assumptions you have made and the methods you use (Harbottle 1999). It is important to provide the learning from your work to other people — particularly efforts that were apparently unsuccessful. By appropriately writing and talking about your work, other people working with indigenous groups will benefit from your experience.

Be aware of the critical importance and dominance of upstream determinants of health for indigenous people. Accept that many factors contributing to the problems as you understand them are outside your control. While you may feel powerless as an individual to effect change in areas outside your professional discipline, your experience will give you a powerful basis for advocacy for change to other sectors. You may recognise the importance of working directly on upstream factors operating in the community such as factors effecting food access. You may also find that the highest priority of the community at a particular time is not related to food, or nutrition.

CASE STUDY 8.1

THE NATIONAL ABORIGINAL AND TORRES STRAIT ISLANDER NUTRITION STRATEGY AND ACTION PLAN

The National Aboriginal and Torres Strait Islander Nutrition Strategy and Action Plan (NATSINSAP) is the indigenous component of the Australian national public health nutrition strategy, 'Eat Well Australia'. The development of both strategies was undertaken by the Strategic Inter-Governmental Nutrition Alliance for the National Public Health Partnership to cover a ten-year period from 2000 to 2010. The purpose of the strategy is to ensure national coordination and cooperation across the country, and to build on existing efforts to make healthy food choices easier for Aboriginal and Torres Strait Islander peoples, irrespective of where they live. The seven key priority areas for action identified in the strategy and action plan are:

1. food supply in remote and rural communities
2. food security and socioeconomic status
3. family focused nutrition promotion
4. nutrition issues in urban areas
5. the environment and household infrastructure

6.   Aboriginal and Torres Strait Islander nutrition workforce
7.   national food and nutrition information systems.

It is acknowledged that each of the action areas requires the active cooperation and support of a range of sectors other than health.
  Six guiding principles underpin the NATSINSAP. They are:

1.   Aboriginal and Torres Strait Islander self-determination and community-control
2.   open consultation and an ongoing commitment to working together
3.   Aboriginal and Torres Strait Islander community and family relationships
4.   support of the principles and goals of the National Aboriginal Health Strategy, which promotes an holistic approach to healthcare and an Aboriginal and Torres Strait Islander definition of health
5.   build and complement existing state and territory food and nutrition policies and plans for Aboriginal and Torres Strait Islander peoples, in addition to other key indigenous health strategies
6.   long-term commitment and resources to improve the health of Aboriginal and Torres Strait Islander peoples.

NATSINSAP was clearly developed within a public health nutrition framework. It recognises the need for broad-ranging activities that strengthen and empower indigenous communities while addressing a priority range of upstream determinants of poor nutritional status. The strategy and action plan builds in sustainability using capacity building activities such as indigenous workforce development and insisting on community control and self-determination. The strategy and action plan is also developed as a learning and evolutionary plan, in that it emphasises the need for monitoring and evaluation to contribute to the evidence base to guide future programmes and strategies. In recognition of the importance of strengthening community and family relationships, the family is made a central priority of the strategy and action plan. While this is somewhat different to Eat Well Australia, which attempts to define specific population sub-groups for particular attention, it is in keeping with an indigenous worldview.
  While Eat Well Australia was developed as a strategic framework, the developers of the NATSINSAP component were pointed in naming it a strategy and action plan. This was perhaps in frustrated reaction to too much talk of working to improve indigenous health through better nutrition and too little action. Without denigrating the very good work of the Working Party, and the achievements in the area of nutrition for indigenous peoples in Australia over the past ten years, it is apparent that the hopes for action expressed in the NATSINSAP (and indeed in the Eat Well Australia framework) have not yet been met. Perhaps the largest disappointment has been the struggle to find resources for national coordinating activities and partnership development.

Source: National Aboriginal and Torres Strait Islander Nutrition Working Party 2001

Case Study 8.2

FoodNorth: Food for health in north Australia

FoodNorth addresses food supply issues in North Australia, with particular focus on remote indigenous communities. The food supply had been identified for many years as an important factor influencing the capacity to consume a healthy diet in remote communities. It has been broadly recognised that food prices are high, and food availability limited, particularly for healthier options such as fruit, vegetables and wholemeal foods. These problems are exacerbated by the relatively low level of income for most indigenous people living in remote communities.

In 2003, the Office of Aboriginal Health of the Department of Health in Western Australia funded a short project to articulate the critical food supply issues in remote communities, and to recommend what could be done to improve the situation. The stated rationale for improving the food supply was so that 'indigenous people in remote communities in North Australia will be able to purchase the food they need to be healthy, on a consistent basis, from their stores and takeaway food outlets, at a price they can afford'. Four recommendations were made for immediate action, and a number of leverage points identified for effective action. The recommendations were:

1. **Establish a high level 'whole-of-government' approach to resolve issues of food supply:** This recommendation recognises that the issues important to food supply involved many agencies across a number of jurisdictions. The state jurisdictions involved (Queensland, Northern Territory and Western Australia) had been involved in the issues of food supply, but a collaborative and coordinated approach is required that also engages national agencies and involves all levels of government.

2. **Secure funding to implement a north Australia Food Supply Project:** The funding required was estimated to be about $250,000 over eighteen months, and would enable progress to be made on those leverage points where the health sector has a direct influence.

3. **Establish a monitoring and evaluation system:** It was envisaged that standard measurements be made across the remote communities of the northern region of Australia of indicators of food supply (availability and cost), nutrition status and health status.

4. **Include nutrition as a core component in the new national Aboriginal Health Worker Training package:** Work to improve health through nutrition in indigenous communities currently relies heavily on non-indigenous nutritionists. It is recognised that sustained improvements in the

nutrition and health of Aboriginal and Torres Strait Islander people requires the critical step of empowering and building capacity within the community. The FoodNorth project provides the opportunity to restate this.

Leverage points were identified under the following headings:

- store governance and purpose issues
- best retail practice
- stocking healthy food (store level)
- stocking healthy food (funding and other agencies)
- subsidies
- freight
- local production of fresh fruit and vegetables
- banking and credit
- takeaway food
- increasing demand for healthy food
- training and workforce
- monitoring and evaluation (food supply)
- monitoring and evaluation (health and nutrition).

Source: Leonard 2003

CASE STUDY 8.3

THE WHARE TAPA WHA MODEL OF HEALTH

This Maori perspective of health is visualised as a four-sided house (McPherson et al. 2003), where each side is required for health. The link between the four constructs is fundamental – each one must be secure. If any one is moved, however slightly, the person may become unwell. The four sides are:

1. *Taha Wairua* (spiritual) – capacity for faith and wider communion
2. *Taha Hinengaro* (mind) – capacity to communicate, think, and feel
3. *Taha Tinana* (physical) – capacity for physical growth and development
4. *Taha Whanau* (extended family) – capacity to belong, to care, and to share.

The Maori health strategy is *He Korowai Oranga*. Its overall aim is *whanau ora* – Maori families supported to achieve their maximum health and wellbeing. The health strategy is built on three principles:

1.   partnership—working together to develop strategies for Maori health gain and appropriate health and disability services
2.   participation—involving Maori at all levels of the sector in decision making, planning, development and delivery of health and disability services
3.   protection—working to ensure Maori have at least the same level of health as non-Maori and safeguarding Maori cultural concepts, values and practices.

Source: http://www.maorihealth.govt.nz

Conclusion

There is general agreement about the direction to move for sustainable health improvement in indigenous groups (Cunningham & Stanley 2003; Foliaki & Pearce 2003; Ring & Brown 2003; Thomson 2003a), and the case studies in this chapter are consistent with this direction. The way ahead includes the following elements.

* Indigenous people are substantially disadvantaged with respect to health and other aspects of their lives. The historical factors and colonial experiences leading to this situation should be acknowledged, and appropriate needs-based resources to address the issues made available.
* Primary healthcare services for indigenous people should be community controlled, take an holistic approach, and be adequate for the prevention, early detection and treatment of the high levels of illness already present. The most significant contribution of community controlled health services is improved access to services, earlier intervention, more energetic outreach, higher levels of compliance, and a greater sense of community participation and ownership (Durie 2003b).
* Indigenous people should be in control of the planning, implementation and evaluation of their own healthcare programmes at the local, national and international level. In this way, the traditions, attitudes, customs and beliefs of indigenous people will be fully acknowledged.
* Most of the social and environmental factors relating to health lie upstream, outside the direct responsibility of the health sector. Many of these issues require socioeconomic, political and legislative change. The sharing of global experience in improving health for minority indigenous groups is likely to be helpful. Substantial gain is unlikely to occur without improvements to the upstream determinants.

- Appropriate infrastructure (housing, water supply, education, income) should be provided recognising the importance of the links of indigenous people with nature (land and sea, etc.).
- Human resource capacity should be developed by increased training of indigenous health professionals as well as culturally competent non-indigenous practitioners.
- Research and appropriate programme evaluation, and the dissemination of the learning from these will assist in strengthening healthcare.

REFERENCES

Australian Bureau of Statistics (ABS) 2005, *The Health and Welfare of Australia's Aboriginal and Torres Strait Islander Peoples*, publication no. 4704.0, ABS, Canberra.

Australian Indigenous HealthInfoNet 2005, 'Summary of Australian Indigenous health, November 2005' cited <http://www.healthinfonet.ecu.edu.au/ html/html_keyfacts/keyfacts_plain_lang_summary.htm> on March 2006.

Cunningham, C. and Stanley, F. 2003, 'Indigenous by definition, experience, or world view' in *British Medical Journal*, vol. 327, pp. 403–04.

Durie, M.H. 2003a, 'The health of indigenous peoples' in *British Medical Journal*, vol. 326, pp. 511–12.

—— 2003b, 'Providing health services to indigenous peoples' in *British Medical Journal*, vol. 327, pp. 408–09.

Foliaki, S. and Pearce, N. 2003, 'Changing pattern of ill health for Indigenous people' in *British Medical Journal*, vol. 327, pp. 406–07.

Guest, C. and O'Dea, K. 1993, 'Food habits in Aborigines and persons of European descent of south-eastern Australia' in *Australian Journal of Public Health* vol. 17, pp. 321–24.

Harbottle, L. 1999, 'Beyond cultural sensitivity: Employing ethnographic techniques to improve the effectiveness and outcomes of community nutrition surveys' in *Public Health and Nutrition: The challenge*, Kohler B.M. (ed.), Sigma, Berlin, pp. 218–27.

Harris, S. 1984, *Culture and Learning: Tradition and education in North East Arnhem Land*, Australian Institute of Aboriginal Studies, Canberra.

Hughes, F.A. and Gray, N.J. 2003, 'Cultural safety and the health of adolescents' in *British Medical Journal*, vol. 327, p. 457.

Kuhnlein, H.V., Receveur, O., Soueida, R. and Egeland, G.M. 2004, 'Artic indigenous peoples experience the nutrition transition with changing dietary patterns and obesity' in *Journal of Nutrition*, vol. 124, pp. 1447–53.

Lakos, J.V. 2001, 'Dietary trends and diabetes: Its association among indigenous Fijians 1952 to 1994' in *Asia Pacific Journal of Clinical Nutrition*, vol. 10, pp. 183–87.

Lee, A., 1996, 'Transition of Australian Aboriginal diet and nutritional health' in *World Review of Nutrition and Dietetics*, vol. 79, pp. 1–52.

Lee, A., O'Dea, K. and Mathews, J. 1994, 'Apparent dietary intake in remote Aboriginal communities' in *Australian Journal of Public Health*, vol. 18, pp. 190–7.

Leonard, D. 2003, *FoodNorth: Food for health in north Australia*, North Australia Nutrition Group (NANG), Population Health Division, Health Department of Western Australia.

Maori Health cited at <www.maorihealth.govt.nz> on April 2006.

McDermott, R., 1998, 'Ethics, epidemiology and the thrifty gene: Biological determinism as a health hazard' in *Social Science Medicine*, vol. 47, pp. 1189–95.

McPherson, K.M., Harwood, M. and McNaughton, H.K. 2003, 'Ethnicity, equity, and quality: Lessons from New Zealand' in *British Medical Journal*, vol. 327, pp. 443–44.

Ministry of Health (NZ) 2006, *Tatau Kahukura: Maori Health Chart Book*', Public Health Intelligence Monitoring Report no. 5, Ministry of Health, Wellington.

National Aboriginal and Torres Strait Islander Nutrition Working Party 2001, *National Aboriginal and Torres Strait Islander Nutrition Strategy and Action Plan*, National Public Health Partnership, Canberra.

National Health and Medical Research Council 2000, *Nutrition in Aboriginal and Torres Strait Islander peoples: An information paper*, Commonwealth of Australia, Canberra.

O'Dea, K. 1984, 'Marked improvement in carbohydrate and lipid metabolism in diabetic Australian Aborigines after temporary reversion to a traditional lifestyle' in *Diabetes*, vol. 33, pp. 596–603.

Ring, I. and Brown, N. 2003, 'The health of Indigenous peoples and others' in *British Medical Journal*, vol. 327, pp. 404–05.

Ring, I.T. and Firman, D. 1998, 'Reducing indigenous mortality in Australia: Lessons from other countries' in *Medical Journal of Australia*, vol. 169, pp. 528–33.

Shannon, C. 2002, 'Acculturation: Aboriginal and Torres Strait Islander nutrition' in *Asia Pacific Journal of Clinical Nutrition*, vol. 11, pp. S576–78.

Stacey, S. 1975, 'Nutritional integration of the Aborigine' in *Food and Nutrition Notes and Reviews*, vol. 32, pp. 163–68.

Thomson, N. (ed.) 2003a, *The Health of Indigenous Australians*, Oxford University Press, Melbourne.

— 2003b, 'Responding to our "spectacular failure"' in *The Health of Indigenous Australians*, N. Thomson (ed.), Oxford University Press, Melbourne, p. 489.

Trudgen, R. 2000, *Why Warriors Lie Down and Die*, Aboriginal Resource and Development Services, Darwin.

Young, T.K. 2003, 'Review of research on aboriginal populations in Canada: Relevance to their health needs' in *British Medical Journal*, vol. 327, pp. 419–22.

9

Obesity prevention

BOYD SWINBURN
COLIN BELL

Substantial increases in obesity prevalence occurred in many countries from about the 1970s and '80s, in high and low middle-income countries alike (WHO 2000). However, there was little public or political attention paid to this rising epidemic until the number of media stories began to rise steeply from the early 2000s (International Food Information Council 2006). This has created a focus, particularly from governments, on what can be done about the problem. Globally, obesity is one of the biggest health challenges of the early twenty-first century, and this makes it an important public health nutrition case study – examining the problems and the solutions, the evidence and the practice, and the local to the global responses.

The obesity problem

The obesity epidemic, or more correctly pandemic, follows several discernable patterns as it moves through the populations of the world. For obesity prevalence to increase, a country needs to be wealthy enough to have obesogenic products like energy dense foods, cars, labour-saving devices, television and electronic games available to at least a proportion of the population. It is therefore not surprising that the first sub-populations to show an increase in obesity in the early stages of the epidemic tend to be middle-aged, wealthier, urban dwellers, and often women have a higher prevalence compared to men (WHO 2000; Monteiro et al. 2004). With time, overweight and obesity become ever more prevalent at younger ages, men catch up and overtake women, and the relationship with socioeconomic status flips, as do the rural/urban patterns. In wealthy countries, therefore, the common pattern is:

• highest prevalence in middle-aged people, but increasingly affecting more children and adolescents
• more men classified as overweight or obese than women
• higher prevalence in low-income groups
• slightly higher prevalence in rural compared to urban areas (WHO 2000).

It is uncertain how the future patterns will evolve over time as obesity awareness increases and prevention programmes take hold. Based on the experience from the evolution of other epidemics, it is likely that the higher-income, higher-educated groups will be the first to show attenuation then decreases in obesity prevalence because of their greater future orientation and capacity to make changes in eating and physical activity patterns. Women will probably show improvements before men because of their greater health awareness, and it is possible that children and adolescents will also show earlier improvements than adults because that is where the majority of obesity intervention programs are likely to focus.

The consequences of obesity

The health consequences of obesity are well documented in terms of relative risks (WHO 2000). There are several diseases, such as type 2 diabetes and sleep apnoea, for which obesity is the dominant cause, and therefore a reduction in the prevalence of obesity would markedly reduce these diseases. The relative risks conferred by excess weight for type 2 diabetes in particular are very high indeed (Colditz et al. 1995). For other diseases, such as cardiovascular diseases, some cancers, and arthritis, obesity is one of many contributing factors (some known, some unknown), so that even the elimination of obesity would only have a partial effect on their occurrence.

Coronary heart disease is an interesting case in point because, in many wealthy countries, the incidence and mortality rates have been declining markedly since the 1970s, and continue to do so even though obesity prevalence increased at the same time. Part of the explanation has been the declines in other risk factors that are largely unrelated to obesity, such as smoking and LDL cholesterol levels, but to probably a greater extent, it reflects the advances in the medical and surgical treatment of heart disease (Hunink et al. 1997).

There has been a strengthening of the evidence of the effect of obesity on a variety of cancers (WHO 2003), particularly post-menopausal breast cancer and colon cancer. The impact of obesity on total mortality is hotly debated (Mokdad et al. 2004) and this will vary enormously according to rates of competing causes of death.

The impact of obesity and other risk factors that contribute to the total burden of disease has been modelled at a global level (Ezzati 2004a; Ezzati 2004b). Similar modelling has been done for Australia, and the combined impact of obesity and physical inactivity exceeded the impact of smoking (Mathers et al. 2000). This has been powerful evidence for the need for action. The psychological and social effects of obesity, especially in children and adolescents, are also important (Lobstein et al. 2004), but have not been accounted for in these modelling exercises. For example, the quality of life in children and adolescents with obesity is significantly reduced (Williams et al. 2005), and since the likelihood of obese children becoming obese adults is high (Magarey et al. 2003), this would add substantially to the lifetime burden of obesity.

Concepts in obesity prevention

The obesity epidemiological triad

Identifying all the determinants of obesity and their relationships results in a complex depiction of the web of causation (Kumanyika et al. 2002), which even then is probably a simplification. An alternative model is the simplified epidemiological triad of host, vector and environment, which has been used as a guide to the etiology and to action for various epidemics from infectious diseases to road injuries (Egger et al. 2003) (see Figure 9.1).

The host factors include unmodifiable components (such as gender, age and genetic makeup), modifiable components (such as behaviours and attitudes), and more dynamic, responsive factors (such as hormones and physiological adjustments to weight change). The vectors for energy intake are predominantly energy density and serving size (the product of which is total energy intake), but other factors directly related to the food or beverage product (such as packaging, labels, monosodium glutamate content) also affect energy intake. The vectors for energy expenditure are essentially machines, almost all of which are obesogenic, such as cars and computers. A few machines are designed to expend energy, such as bicycles and exercise equipment, but in general, machines are obesogenic. The environmental factors can be present in micro-environments (in settings such as schools or workplaces) or in larger sectors

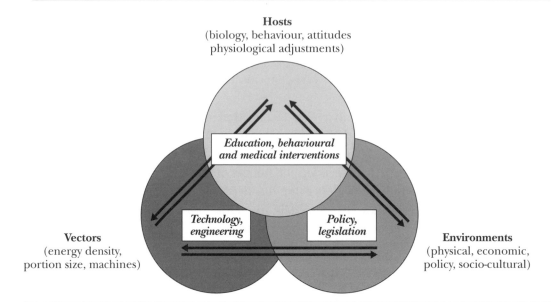

Figure 9.1 The epidemiological triad for obesity prevention

Source: Egger et al. 2003

(such as the health system, the food industry, or the government). A helpful classification of the types of environmental factors is contained in the ANGELO Framework (analysis grid for elements linked to obesity), which identifies the physical environment (what is or is not available), the economic environment (what are the financial factors), the policy environment (what are the rules), and the sociocultural environment (what are the attitudes, beliefs, practices, values and perceptions) (Swinburn et al. 1999).

Influencing hosts, vectors and environments

The epidemiological triad clumps the determinants into these three main areas of influence, and of course this is an oversimplification; however, it does also point to the general strategies for intervention. The main avenues for influencing the hosts at the population level are mainly through education and social marketing — relatively weak strategies by themselves. Since obesity is not caused by a knowledge deficit, it is unlikely that an education-based approach will be successful. Social marketing, when done well and linked closely to activities on the ground, can change behaviours, and it does this by motivating and selling the benefits rather than by filling in knowledge gaps (Donovan & Henley 2003).

Changing vectors can often be achieved through a technical approach, and reducing the fat and energy content of certain foods and drinks is a classic example. Unfortunately, an over-reliance on vector-based solutions leads to 'magic bullet' thinking, and the wave of new functional foods and the promises that go with them illustrate this point.

The strengths of changing environments have been well documented (Swinburn & Egger 2002) and include sustainability, cost-effectiveness, ability to influence the hard-to-reach populations, and, in the case of obesity prevention, a reduced risk of accentuating disordered eating patterns and stigmatisation of obesity. While the ANGELO Framework identifies the four types of environments, when it comes to interventions, changes in the policy environment are often needed to create changes in the physical, economic, and even sociocultural environments. For example, the introduction of taxes and or subsidies to influence the food supply and thus consumption, would need a policy decision that would then drive the changes in the economic environment. The same would be true for changes in the built environment and transport systems to encourage physical activity and reduce car use. Even changes in the sociocultural environment are greatly influenced by policy changes, and one only needs to think of the case of smoke-free environments legislation accelerating the public attitudes towards the new norm of expecting that indoor areas are smoke-free.

Solutions-oriented research

In a classic paper, Robinson and Sirard (2005) put forward a cogent argument for research in obesity to become more solutions-focused. They pointed out the dominant paradigm in obesity research comes from the biomedical, reductionist approach that is more problem-oriented — finding out what to blame rather than what to do. Knowing the determinants of obesity may help with finding the solutions, but not always. For example, knowing some of the genetic markers for obesity or knowing that sedentary occupations are an increasing cause of physical inactivity might be interesting, but because they are largely unchangeable, they are not helpful in creating solutions. Similarly, cross-sectional or longitudinal studies will not find that an absence of dance is a cause of obesity, yet a dance programme may be an important part of the solution for adolescent girls.

The evidence base for obesity prevention

Achieving action

Public health action is often inhibited by a 'mismatch between the magnitude and importance of a public health problem, and the adequacy of evidence on potential interventions to address the problem' (Rychetnik et al. 2004), and this is now the case for obesity. While children and adolescents are considered priority age groups for prevention efforts (Lobstein et al. 2004), there is little in the way of specific effectiveness evidence to clearly guide the way, and this is a major impediment to action. Systematic reviews on obesity prevention clearly highlight this gap (Summerbell et al. 2005; Doak et al. 2006). The obesity epidemic is a current and urgent public health problem, and reflects other contemporary public health nutrition issues in having a multiple, layered etiology, including many social, cultural and economic determinants. Its control will therefore demand a multifactorial approach across many settings and sectors, and involving a mix of policy, environmental, educational, and social marketing approaches (Swinburn and Egger 2002).

International Obesity Task Force framework

The International Obesity Task Force (IOTF) has published a framework for an evidence-based approach to obesity prevention (Figure 9.2). This framework identifies the key issues and the different types of evidence needed to address them (Swinburn et al. 2005). Some of the issues are very contextual, such as the burden for a particular population (issue 1), the main determinants of unhealthy weight in that population (issue 2) and, especially, the final decisions about what should be done (issue 5). Other issues tend to be somewhat more universal, such as the framework of settings and strategies for action (issue 3) and the range of possible interventions (issue 4). For example, Tonga, Texas and Taiwan will all have very different burdens of obesity, but there will be a degree of commonality in the driving forces across those populations, such as dependence on cars, availability and promotion of energy dense foods and drinks, and availability of labour-saving devices. There will probably be more commonalities in the broad strategic plans to reduce childhood obesity because all would involve schools and preschool settings, address healthy eating and physical activity, and identify social marketing, policies, curriculum, programmes, and environmental changes as the key strategies. The possible range of specific interventions is also somewhat universal, but the process of determining a final portfolio of actions is highly contextual, so the selection of actions that might work well in Tonga may not apply at all in Texas or Taiwan.

There is good evidence to address issues 1 and 2, and many governments can readily achieve a broad framework for action (issue 3) that includes all the main implementation areas (that is, appropriate settings and sectors) and support actions (for example, monitoring, capacity building, research, and social marketing) (National Obesity TaskForce 2003).

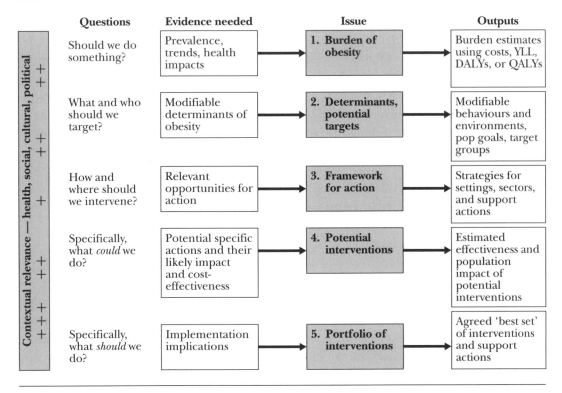

Figure 9.2 The International Obesity Task Force framework for obesity prevention

Source: Swinburn & Kumanyika 2005

Issues 4 and 5 in the IOTF framework, however, are much more challenging — what are the concrete programmes, policies and actions that *could* be initiated and, of those, which ones *should* be done to provide the best investments for reducing obesity? It is here that the lack of effectiveness evidence is proving to be a barrier to action. Even the few programmes with evidence of success, such as the one in Singapore (Toh et al. 2002), are not necessarily transferable to other cultures and countries.

Practice-based evidence

Evidence is not sufficient by itself to guide appropriate decision-making (Green 2001) and true evidence-based policymaking is probably quite rare (Marmot 2004). Therefore, getting the process right and engaging decision-makers from the start moves towards practice-based evidence (Marmot 2004) that is more relevant than the classical evidence-based practice approach. An obesity prevention plan based only on the limited published trials available would be patchy and probably ineffective.

Therefore, achieving a broad portfolio of promising interventions for obesity prevention requires both an assessment of the likely impact of those interventions (as far as can be estimated from the available evidence) and a process by which to engage the key stakeholders in all decisions. Working with the key stakeholders to derive a plan of action increases the relevance, ownership and the likelihood of the recommendations being implemented but, as always, political considerations, funding limitations and extraneous events play a major role in what finally gets supported.

Obesity prevention in communities

Evidence from trials

Reviews of trials to prevent obesity in children show that they have mainly been conducted in primary schools, and that they have usually not been successful (Story 1999; Glenny et al. 1997; Campbell et al. 2002). More recently, however, there have been calls to broaden the definition of what constitutes evidence of effectiveness in obesity prevention (Swinburn et al. 2005), and a subsequent review, using broader inclusion criteria for interventions and programmes, paints a more optimistic picture (Doak et al. 2006). Inclusion criteria for the Doak and colleagues review were that the study must focus on school-aged children (six to nineteen years), anthropometric measures must have been taken at baseline, and follow-up must have included an intervention on diet, physical activity or both, and the evaluation must have been documented. They found that 68 per cent of the interventions (17 out of 25) were effective, based on a significant reduction in body mass index or skinfolds at some point in time in the intervention group (or a sub-group). While it was hard to tease out exactly what it was about the effective interventions that made them effective, there were some interesting differences between effective and non-effective interventions. A tension between intervention dose and sustainability was highlighted, such that effective interventions tended to focus more resources onto fewer components. Physical education at school and reducing television viewing appeared to be particularly effective components. Effective interventions also had fewer schools but larger numbers of students as their target population. Their response rates were also lower (83 per cent versus 71 per cent) and they were of shorter duration.

This review suggests that a range of diet and physical activity strategies, whether individual or multi-component, are likely to work if they are implemented in the right way. Ineffective studies, for example, may have diluted their intervention dose by overemphasising the scientific rigour of the evaluation methods (that is, the time and energy boosting response rates). They may also have spread themselves too thin by applying limited resources across too many components, or across a heterogenous target population. Another potential trap was an over-emphasis on the educational components of an intervention and an under-emphasis on environmental changes that support the behavioural change being sought. The authors of the review reasoned that the effective interventions provided a sufficient foundation for action on a larger scale, and gave directions for future action and research on obesity prevention (Doak et al. 2006), in keeping with the solution-based research paradigm of Robinson and Sirard (2005).

Whole-of-community programmes

Whole-of-community demonstration areas have been recognised as an integral part of the national strategic approach to obesity prevention in Australia (National Obesity TaskForce 2003). The advantage of whole-of-community programmes is that they provide a context in which scientific evidence can be produced in a solution-orientated way, and where multiple strategies can be implemented in multiple settings. Successful aspects of the school-based programmes described above can be implemented alongside advocacy for change at a local and a national level. Also, they can be a vehicle for piloting national policies and programmes.

Several of these whole-of-community projects have been established in Australia across a range of age and cultural groups. The Colac Be Active, Eat Well (BAEW) was the first of these (established in mid-2002) and is described in Case study 9.1 to paint the picture of a multi-setting, multi-strategy intervention.

CASE STUDY 9.1
THE COLAC BE ACTIVE EAT WELL

Based in Colac, a small (population 11 000) rural town in the Barwon southwest region of Victoria, the programme aims to improve the health and wellbeing of children aged two to twelve years, and to strengthen the local community through the promotion of healthy eating and physical activity. The community developed an action plan using a facilitated process in a two-day workshop. The workshop used the ANGELO Framework (Swinburn et al. 1999) described above to identify potential behaviours, knowledge and skill gaps, and environmental barriers to target and then prioritise them into a plan of

---

action. The action plan had objectives focused around behaviour changes (supported by environmental changes and social marketing), increasing community capacity, and testing some innovative programmes.

Baseline surveys done in early 2003 included measurements of anthropometry, behaviours, environments, and community capacity. A representative sample from the wider Barwon southwest region was measured as a comparison group. Follow-up surveys will take place after the first three years of intervention. A mid-intervention point assessment was conducted to assess penetration of the programme into families and settings. It consisted of telephone interviews with a random selection of 30 participating families, along with several key stakeholders. Families and stakeholders were aware of key project messages, and this awareness was closely related to the 'intervention dose'; for example, when the survey was conducted, no specific message had been delivered discouraging television viewing. Consequently, awareness of messages promoting less screen time was low (approximately 29 per cent). Both parents and stakeholders saw the benefits of the programme for themselves and the wider community. In response to BAEW, most families reported limiting the consumption of sweet drinks (68.2 per cent), participating in an after-school activity programme (67.9 per cent), and providing healthier lunch box foods (57.1 per cent). Interestingly, 32 per cent of respondents said they had made no changes because they considered their family to be healthy already.

Schools reported increased availability of healthy foods at the school canteen, the introduction of fruit breaks during class where only fruit or vegetable sticks can be consumed, and increased physical activity through increased class physical activity time. Sporting clubs confirmed that large numbers of children had been participating in the after-school activity programme, and reported that many children had subsequently joined the clubs as members. It was clear from the comments that good partnerships had been established between the target population, stakeholders and the project team, and that the capacity of the Colac community to promote healthy eating and physical activity had increased through training and reorientation of services.

Separate evaluations of specific initiatives add to the picture of the impact of the overall programme in Case study 9.1. A television 'Power-Down' week, based on curriculum material developed in the United States as part of Planet Health (Gortmaker et al. 1999), was run through primary schools. Telephone interviews with families after the event showed a high awareness (71 per cent) and 95 per cent of the parents surveyed reported that their children watched less than two hours of television on school nights during Power-Down week.

These reported behavioural changes are encouraging, but effectiveness can only be judged by changes in anthropometric measurements compared to controls.

The evaluations of these whole-of-community programmes may need to extend for many years. It takes several years to gather sufficient momentum to achieve a high enough dose of intervention. Programmes need to be established, social marketing needs to get through, community attitudes and expectations about healthy choices need to change, and many organisations need to reorient towards the overall programmes goals. This all takes time. A hint of just how long it takes can be seen from the Fleaurbaix-Laventie Ville Sante programme in the north of France. Interventions were running for eight years in these two small villages before the prevalence of overweight and obesity began to decline (Borys 2005).

Obesity prevention at a national level

Learning from other epidemics

As governments gear up to tackle the epidemic of obesity in children, they will be able to draw on the types of strategies, policies and programmes that have worked to control other epidemics. The usual comparison epidemic is smoking (Chopra & Darnton-Hill 2004), and while critics state that the comparison is unfair because food is needed for life but tobacco isn't, there are many parallels in relation to the approaches taken by governments, the public and private-vested interests. The most powerful interventions for tobacco control have been taxation and legislation, supported by prominent, ongoing social marketing campaigns and Quitlines. We have seen countries and states leap-frog each other with these initiatives, with each lead jurisdiction setting the height of the bar for others to match or surpass. The Republic of Ireland is a leader in Europe, having introduced smoke-free legislation for all public places and workplaces, including bars, in 2004 (Howell 2005). In the United States, with lawsuits, and Australia, with smoke-free legislation, we have seen the leap-frogging occur at a state level.

There are common lessons from the control of epidemics other than tobacco, such as road injuries, HIV/AIDS, skin cancer and cardiovascular diseases (Swinburn 2002). If the prevention approach is dominated by a medical approach (for example, screening and treatment or secondary prevention), then it can become very costly. Healthcare services, drugs and operations are expensive and have greatly pushed up the cost of preventing coronary heart disease and cervical cancer. Immunisations, on the other hand, are very cost-effective.

Another lesson is that, in general, education-dominated strategies are generally weak compared to policy/legislative approaches, environmental change, or fiscal instruments (Casswell 1997). This is because most of the risk behaviours (such as, not exercising enough, drink-driving, speeding, eating high-fat foods, unsafe sex, smoking) are not occurring because of a knowledge deficit. Therefore, adding more knowledge is unlikely to change those risk behaviours unless it is backed by other strategies (for example, speed cameras, random breath tests, smoke-free legislation, conducive environments for healthy choices). An example of an exception to the impact of a knowledge-based approach has been the success of the cot death campaigns, putting babies on their backs to sleep and reducing their exposure to second-hand smoke. Here there was a knowledge deficit, the behaviour change is easy and the potential benefits are very high.

Components of a national strategy for obesity prevention

Several countries have developed national plans of action that incorporate existing knowledge and activities, and recognise current policies, systems and capacities. A comprehensive framework for action would ensure that all the main implementation areas (that is, appropriate settings and sectors) and support actions (for example, monitoring, capacity building, research and social marketing) are included, and that the main strategy options (such as, policies, curriculum, parent support, regulations) are identified. The policy context for obesity prevention may vary from country to country – some may be stand-alone obesity-prevention plans (National Obesity TaskForce 2003), part of non-communicable diseases reduction plans (Ministry of Health Tonga 2003), included in a nutrition and physical activity plan of action (Ministry of Health New Zealand 2002), or part of a Healthy Cities or Healthy Islands framework. In general, countries can get to this stage relatively easily – it is the implementation of the plan that is the problem. Most countries have not turned general plans into specific actions that are backed by the necessary funding and policies, and the only one with any track record in this area is Singapore (see Case study 9.2).

Much better evaluation of the Singapore programme is needed, especially using standardised definitions and assessing any negative consequences such as increased stigmatisation of obese children who are selected for added exercise classes. It is also likely that Singapore-style approaches to obesity prevention will be less acceptable in countries with a less authoritarian culture.

CASE STUDY 9.2
THE SINGAPORE EXAMPLE OF A NATIONAL STRATEGY

In response to data based on national weight-for-height standards that showed a steady increase in obesity prevalence (greater than 120 per cent of median weight-for-height) from 2 per cent in 1976 to 15 per cent in 1992, the Ministry of Education, in close collaboration with the Health Promotion Board (Ministry of Health), established the Trim and Fit (TAF) programme to increase physical fitness and reduce obesity among school children (Toh et al. 2002). TAF was part of a National Healthy Lifestyle programme implemented nationwide that backed up a multi-sectoral and multi-pronged approach to lowering the population's risk of non-communicable disease with political commitment and support. At the school level, TAF integrated nutrition education into the school curriculum, controlled the types of foods and beverages available at school, conducted annual fitness tests, and boosted opportunities for physical activity (for example, lunchtime workouts and friendly sports matches between staff and students).

In Singapore, schools have several vendors contributing to the food available at the tuckshop. Thus, information and guidelines were supplied to vendors that encouraged healthier options. For example, snacks like fishballs and crabsticks were boiled rather than fried, and coconut milk was replaced with evaporated milk in curry dishes.

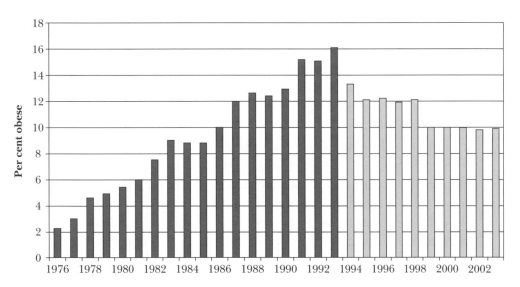

Prevalence of obesity among Singaporean school children aged six to eighteen years.

Source: Toh et al. 2002

Information was also supplied to parents and students. A unique feature of TAF were the Special School Nutrition Clinics available to children who were very overweight (greater than 140 per cent of median weight-for-height). Based at schools, the clinics were designed to pass on weight management strategies to students and parents, they gave children access to a multidisciplinary team of health professionals, and the children participated in special physical exercise programmes.

Surveillance of children's weights and heights over subsequent years has shown declines in the prevalence of obesity. Between 1992 and 2000, obesity declined among eleven- to twelve-year-olds from 16.6 to 14.6 per cent and among fifteen- to sixteen-year-olds from 15.5 to 13.1 per cent (Toh et al. 2002). The figure on the previous page shows that these declines have been maintained in recent years, although it should be noted that the definitions of childhood obesity changed in 1994.

Promising state/national school initiatives

Mandating the quality of food provided in schools is an obvious target for intervention. In many countries, school food is provided and it represents a significant proportion of children's energy intake, whereas in countries like Australia most food is brought from home, and school canteens provide only about two to three per cent of children's total annual energy intake (Bell & Swinburn 2004). Nevertheless, even in Australia, food sold at schools should set the standard for a healthy diet so that the message is clear to both children and parents (Bell & Swinburn 2005). Policies are now in place in New South Wales and Queensland that use a 'traffic light' system to categorise the healthiness of all foods and thus place restrictions on the sales of 'red' foods and some 'amber' foods in schools (The New South Wales School Canteen Association 2004).

Schools will continue to be a priority setting for obesity prevention in children and adolescents. Other strategies include bans on soft drinks in schools, as has recently occurred in schools in Victoria, mandating and increasing physical education time; strengthening curriculum on healthy eating and physical activity (Newell et al. 2004); linked in-school and after-school activities with sport and recreation clubs; and social marketing of healthy eating to parents.

Media campaigns

Media campaigns and other information or education programmes can be developed quickly and they have high visibility. This makes them attractive actions for politicians, and may explain why they are springing up early in response to calls for action. The 'We Can!' from the National Heart Lung and Blood Institute in the United States is one such example. It is designed as a one-stop resource for parents and caregivers interested in practical tools to help children aged from eight to thirteen years stay at a healthy weight (Department of Health and Human Services 2006). The effectiveness of such strategies is likely to remain low in the absence of policy and environmental changes to make the healthy choices the easy choices.

Food marketing to children

This is a touchstone issue for action on reducing childhood obesity because the debate is highly polarised and attracts a lot of media attention. Marketing obesogenic foods (energy dense, micronutrient-poor foods and beverages) directly to children is huge business. For food companies, it clearly increases sales of the products (specific brands and food categories), whereas for parents and the public it undermines healthy eating messages and makes the job of parents providing healthy foods so much harder. Major reviews of the area (Hastings et al. 2003; McKinnis et al. 2006) have recommended substantial tightening of the regulations on marketing to children. The food and beverage industries are acutely aware of the pressures on them to respond to the obesity epidemic, and they are taking multiple actions to try to avoid the imposition of tighter regulations on marketing to children. Their main strategies at the moment include offering more healthy choices (for example, salads at fast-food outlets); promoting their less obesogenic products (such as diet or 'zero sugar' soft drinks); running their own health promotion activities (for instance sponsoring sport and active recreation, educational information on healthy eating and physical activity, advertising campaigns promoting 'balance, media education); voluntary withdrawals of marketing to young children; and reviewing and altering the composition and portion sizes of products, packaging fresh food and nutrition 'signposting' (such as highlighting the healthier choice of their range, trademark signposts like 'Treatwise' to legitimise a positive 'special' status for confectionary). At this stage, it is very difficult to discern how much of this activity is good public relations or good public health.

Advocacy — shaping public opinion

Governments respond to pressure. Much of that pressure comes from the lobby force of industry, but also the advocacy work of health professional groups, and the voice of the public can have a major impact. Shaping the public voice, provoking the debates, and ultimately changing social attitudes and norms related to physical activity and healthy eating is the role of grassroots advocacy groups. On the childhood obesity debate, parents (and, in some cases, the children themselves) can be the best advocates for change. They are not only the guardians of the future generations, but also voters with credibility.

There are emerging examples of groups advocating change in support of obesity prevention that are shaping public opinion and creating political pressure. An example is the Parents Jury (http://www. parentsjury.org.au). The Australian version (borrowed from the United Kingdom) is a web-based network of parents who wish to improve the food and physical activity environments for children in Australia. It started in 2004 with the foundation jury of twelve parents, and within two years had a membership of more than 1200, and had run several public campaigns. Parents voice their views on children's food and physical activity issues, and collectively advocate for the improvement of children's food and physical activity environments (for example, reduced marketing targeted at young children, more healthy choices for school canteens, and making neighbourhoods safer and more child-friendly). Awards for the worst and best in television advertisements aimed at children, surveys of confectionery in supermarket checkout aisles, and membership polls generate substantial media coverage and maintain the visibility of the issue. For example, one membership poll found that more than 70 per cent of parents would consider changing where they shopped if a rival supermarket offered confectionery-free checkouts. The publicity is followed up where possible by direct contact with the decision-makers relevant to the issue (for example, supermarket managers, food companies, politicians).

Another group that has successfully advocated for change is Fight the Obesity Epidemic (FOE). FOE is a voluntary organisation (consisting of individuals and organisations) in New Zealand that advocates for policy interventions to reduce obesity, particularly restrictions on television advertising to children (as exists in Sweden) and soft drinks tax (as occurs in some states in the United States). Apart from media activities to drive the advocacy, FOE has also commissioned a review of how a fat tax may help to fight obesity (Sinner and Davies 2004).

Global action on obesity prevention

Trade and agriculture
Trade agreements, agricultural subsidies and tariffs, and other agricultural policies and regulations, greatly influence the food supply of countries (Guo et al. 1999). For example, countries in the European Union operate under the Common

Agricultural Policy (see http://europa.eu.int/pol/agr/index_en.htm), and the subsidies for sugar, vegetable oil and meat production ensure that the price of fat and sugar are low, whereas production policies are structured to maintain high prices for fruit and vegetables. In general, the cost per kilojoule of energy dense foods is low because added fat and sugar is cheap and the cost per kilojoule for fruit and vegetables is high (Drewnowski & Darmon 2005). This means that the economic drivers for food favour a higher consumption of obesogenic foods.

Countries with a heavy reliance on imported foods, such as the Pacific Island nations, are even more at the mercy of these economic drivers (Evans et al. 2001). High-fat products such as mutton flaps (belly strips) and turkey tails have been exported to the Pacific countries for many years, especially from New Zealand and the United States (Lawrence 2002a). Attempts by these island nations to restrict these imports is met with opposition from the exporting countries, and as the Pacific countries move to accede to the World Trade Organization, any such trade-restrictive practices (such as quotas on fatty meat imports) are frowned upon (Lawrence 2002b).

Trade and agricultural policies, tariffs and subsidies are driven by economic and political considerations, and the health consequences are rarely considered. Health (or specifically, obesity) impact assessments are needed to estimate the potential influences of these practices on population health. The modelling and methodologies for such obesity impact assessments are in their very early stages of development and it will take some time before they are included in the decision mix alongside the usual economic or political considerations.

Transnational regulations on food and marketing

As with agriculture, there are increasingly transnational regulations on food such as labelling, claims, definitions and fortification. Many of these have an impact on food purchasing and therefore nutrient and energy intake. The food industries will generally oppose regulations that may put their food products in a bad light to consumers (such as having to disclose the saturated fat content or the presence of genetically modified products) and lobby hard for the regulations that might give its products a competitive edge (such as health claims and fortification). The national and transnational regulatory authorities have to continuously weigh up the pros and cons of new regulations in the population's interest. However, the ground is often heavily contested and it is important to note that the weight of lobby power strongly favours the food industry over public health advocates.

Another area of contested ground, as previously noted, is in that of food marketing to children. In places like Europe, this is a transnational as well as a national issue. Sweden, which bans advertising to children on television, has little control over cable and satellite television broadcasts that enter Sweden, and thus the national regulation is circumvented by activities over its borders. The European Union is considering EU-wide regulations, and this will be the subject of fierce lobbying on both sides (Mason 2002), reminiscent of the wars over tobacco advertising.

Global health organisations

The World Health Organization is progressing its Global Strategy on Diet, Physical Activity and Health as its major platform for combating obesity. The WHO went through many processes of gathering the evidence and support in the lead-up to the launch of this strategy. The most controversial of these was the consultation and publication of the Technical Report 916 on Diet, Nutrition, and the Prevention of Chronic Diseases (WHO 2003). In this report, issues beyond specific nutrients and behaviours were included in the assessment and recommendations. Environments, such as the heavy marketing of energy dense foods, were identified as probable contributors to obesity (Swinburn et al. 2004) and therefore candidates for interventions. In addition, there was a recommendation that a population's added sugar intake should be less than ten per cent of energy because of the role that sugars, especially in sugar drinks, have on promoting dental diseases (caries and enamel erosion) and obesity. The furore and lobbying from the sugar industry was enormous and nearly scuttled the agreement at the 2004 World Health Assembly on the Global Strategy on Diet, Physical Activity, and Health. The United States and other sugar-producing countries were greatly influenced by the sugar industry lobby, and the US Secretary of Health even openly criticised WHO and the science behind the recommendations for the Global Strategy (see Case study 18.1). The WHO still has some distance to go to create global support for the national and transnational action needed to combat obesity.

Several diseases are linked through obesity, and a Global Alliance for the Prevention of Obesity and Chronic Diseases has been established by the International Association of Societies on Obesity (which includes the International Obesity Task Force), the World Heart Federation, the International Diabetes Federation, International Pediatric Association, and the International Union of Nutritional Sciences. This Alliance has the potential to stimulate important global action to accelerate the global and national action on obesity prevention.

Conclusions

Obesity prevention research and action is poised to expand enormously over the next twenty years in an effort to attenuate, then turn around, the rising epidemic that is affecting almost every country. Whole-of-community projects that are able to achieve a high dose of intervention and can be sustained over time will provide the evidence about what works and what does not work at a community level. Research will hopefully become more solutions-oriented and work closely with stakeholders to fill the knowledge gaps so that obesity prevention actions can be as evidence-based as possible. There will need to be improvements in modelling methodologies to estimate population impacts and cost-effectiveness until empirical data can provide clearer answers. At a state/national level, there should be ongoing funding of programmes and policy changes to promote the healthy choices, but to ensure this sustained level of funding and political support, advocacy groups like the Parents Jury and FOE will need to remain active and effective. Policies that promote healthy environments and healthy choices will be the most sustainable actions that governments can create, but many of these will face stiff opposition from the food and advertising industries. It is likely that in the future, the targeting of children to market foods that are known to be obesogenic will be considered unethical, and that over time, such marketing will be reduced by the food and advertising industries' own actions or (more likely) by government regulations. The transnational reforms needed to promote a healthier food supply and reduce marketing to children are probably going to take a longer time because of the huge economic and political investments in the status quo and the sheer inertia of these large, complex issues.

Despite the obstacles, history tells us that this epidemic will come under control (albeit unevenly) like the other epidemics we have faced. The solutions will not be limited by a lack of human ingenuity or care and concern for our children, but will undoubtedly be slowed by the lack of political will and vested commercial interests.

REFERENCES

Bell, A.C. and Swinburn, B.A. 2004, 'What are the key food groups to target for preventing obesity and improving nutrition in schools?' in *European Journal of Clinical Nutrition*, vol. 58, no. 2, pp. 258–63.
—— 2005, 'School canteens: Using ripples to create a wave of healthy eating' in *Medical Journal of Australia*, vol. 183, no. 1, pp. 5–6.
Borys, J.M. 2005 'A successful way of preventing childhood obesity: The Fleurbaix-Laventie Study' in proceedings of the 18th International Congress of Nutrition: Nutrition safari for innovative solutions, Karger, Durban, South Africa, 19–23 September.

Campbell, K., Waters, E., O'Meara, S. and Summerbell, C. 2001, 'Interventions for preventing obesity in childhood: A systematic review' in *Obesity Review*, vol. 2, no. 3, pp. 149–57.

Campbell, K., Waters, E., O'Meara, S., Kelly, S. and Summerbell, C. 2002, 'Interventions for preventing obesity in children' in *Cochrane Data Base System Review*, no. 2, CD001871.

Casswell, S. 1997, 'Population level policies on alcohol: Are they still appropriate given that "alcohol is good for the heart?"' in *Addiction*, vol. 92, pp. S81–90.

Chopra, M. and Darnton-Hill, I. 2004, 'Tobacco and obesity epidemics: Not so different after all?' in *British Medical Journal*, vol. 328, no. 7455, pp. 1558–60.

Colditz, G.A., Willett, W.C., Rotnitzky, A. and Manson, J.E. 1995, 'Weight gain as a risk factor for clinical diabetes mellitus in women' in *Annals of Internal Medicine*, vol. 122, no. 1, pp. 481–86.

Department of Health and Human Services (US) 2006, 'We Can! Ways to enhance children's activity & nutrition', National Institutes of Health (US), cited at <http://www.nhlbi.nih.gov/health/public/heart/obesity/wecan/> on 1 November.

Doak, C.M., Visscher, T.L., Renders, C.M. and Seidell, J.C. 2006, 'The prevention of overweight and obesity in children and adolescents: A review of interventions and programmes' in *Obesity Review*, vol. 7, no. 1, pp. 111–36.

Donovan, R. and Henley, N. 2003, *Social Marketing: Principles and Practice*, IP Communications, Melbourne.

Drewnowski, A. and Darmon, N. 2005, 'The economics of obesity: Dietary energy density and energy cost' in *American Journal of Clinical Nutrition*, vol. 82, no. 1, pp. S265S–73.

Egger, G., Swinburn, B. and Rossner, S. 2003, 'Dusting off the epidemiological triad: Could it work with obesity?', *Obesity Review*, vol. 4, no. 2, pp. 115–9.

Evans, M., Sinclair, R.C., Fusimalohi, C. and Liava'a, V. 2001, 'Globalization, diet, and health: An example from Tonga', *Bulletin of World Health Organisation*, vol. 79, no. 9, pp. 856–62.

Ezzati, M., Lopez, A.D., Rodgers, A., Murray, C.J.L. (eds) 2004a, *Comparative quantification of health risks: Global and regional burden of disease attributable to selected major risk factors*, vol. 1, World Health Organization (WHO), Geneva.

—— 2004b, *Comparative quantification of health risks: Global and regional burden of disease attributable to selected major risk factors*, vol. 2, World Health Organization (WHO), Geneva.

Fight the Obesity Epidemic (NZ) 2006, 'Stop our children developing type 2 diabetes', cited at <http://www.foe.org.nz/> in August, Wellington.

Glenny, A.M., O'Meara, S., Melville, A., Sheldon, T. and Wilson, C. 1997, 'The treatment and prevention of obesity: A systematic review of the literature' in *International Journal of Obesity*, vol. 21, pp. 715–37.

Gortmaker, S.L., Peterson, K., Wiecha, J., Sobol, A.M., Dixit, S., Fox, M.K. and Laird, N. 1999, 'Reducing obesity via a school-based interdisciplinary intervention among youth: Planet Health' in *Archives Pediatric Adolescent Medicine*, vol. 153, no. 4, pp. 409–18.

Green, L. 2001, 'From research to "best practices" in other settings and populations' in *American Journal of Health Behavior*, vol. 25, pp. 165–78.

Guo, X., Popkin, B.M., Mroz, T.A. and Zhai, F. 1999, 'Food price policy can favorably alter macronutrient intake in China' in *Journal of Nutrition*, vol. 129, no. 5, pp. 994–1001.

Hastings, G., Stead, M., McDermott, L., Forsyth, A., MacKintosh, A., Raynor, M., Godfrey, C.,

Caraher, M. and Angus, K. 2003, *Review of the research on the effects of food promotion to children*, Centre for Social Marketing, University of Strathclyde, Glasgow.

Howell, F. 2005, 'Smoke-free bars in Ireland: A runaway success' in *Tobacco Control*, vol. 14, pp. 73–74.

Hunink, M.G.M., Goldman, L., Tosteson, A.N.A., Mittleman, M.A., Goldman, P.A., Williams, L.W., Tsevat, J. and Weinstein, M.C. 1997, 'The recent decline in mortality from coronary heart disease, 1980–1990: The effect of secular trends in risk factors and treatment' in *Journal of American Medical Association*, vol. 277, no. 7, pp. 535–42.

International Food Information Council 2006, 'Trends in obesity related media coverage', cited at <http://www.ific.org/research/obesitytrends.cfm> in August.

Kumanyika, S., Jeffery, R.W., Morabia, A., Ritenbaugh, C. and Antipatis, V.J. 2002, 'Obesity prevention: The case for action' in *International Journal of Obesity and Related Metabolism Disorder*, vol. 26, no. 3, pp. 425-36.

Lawrence, M. 2002a, 'An analysis of the appropriateness, acceptability and implications of regulatory approaches to control the flow of fatty foods in Pacific Island countries' (Background paper), Food and Agriculture Organisation/Secretariat of the Pacific Community (FAO/SPC), World Health Organization (WHO), Pacific Islands Food Safety and Quality Consultation, Nadi, Fiji.

— 2002b, *Using domestic law in the fight against obesity: An introductory guide for the Pacific*, Deakin University, Melbourne.

Lobstein, T., Baur, L. and Uauy, R. 2004, 'Obesity in children and young people: A crisis in public health' in *Obesity Review*, vol. 5, pp. S4–104.

Magarey, A.M., Daniels, L.A., Boulton, T.J. and Cockington, R.A. 2003, 'Predicting obesity in early adulthood from childhood and parental obesity' in *International Journal of Obesity and Related Metabolism Disorders*, vol. 27, no. 4, pp. 505–13.

Marmot, M.G. 2004, 'Evidence based policy or policy based evidence? in *British Medical Journal*, vol. 328, no. 7445, pp. 906–07.

Mason, T. 2002, 'Snack attack: The next ad ban? Pressure groups and a threat of changes to European law have brought the issue of marketing food to kids to the fore' in *Marketing*, February 7, pp. 13.

Mathers, C.D., Vos, E.T., Stevenson, C.E. and Begg, S.J. 2000, 'The Australian Burden of Disease Study: Measuring the loss of health from diseases, injuries and risk factors' in *Medical Journal of Australia*, vol. 172, no. 12, pp. 592–96.

McGinnis, J.M., Gootman, J.A., Kraak, V.I. (eds) 2006, *Food Marketing to Children and Youth: Threat or opportunity?*, Institute of Medicine, The National Academic Press, Washington.

Ministry of Health New Zealand 2002, *Healthy Eating–Healthy Action* (Oranga Pumau–Oranga Kai), Wellington.

Ministry of Health Tonga 2003, *A National Strategy to Prevent and Control Non-Communicable Diseases in Tonga*, Nuku'alofa, Tonga.

Mokdad, A.H., Marks, J.S., Stroup, D.F. and Gerberding, J.L. 2004, 'Actual causes of death in the United States, 2000' in *Journal of American Medical Association*, vol. 291, no. 10, pp. 1238–45.

Monteiro, C.A., Conde, W.L., Lu, B. and Popkin, B.M. 2004, 'Obesity and inequities in health in the developing world' in *International Journal of Obesity and Related Metabolism Disorders*, vol. 28, no. 9, pp. 1181–86.

National Obesity TaskForce 2003, *Healthy Weight 2008" Australia's Future*, Department of Health and Ageing, Canberra.

Newell, S.A., Huddy, A.D., Adams, J.K., Miller, M., Holden, L. and Dietrich, U.C. 2004, 'The tooty fruity vegie project: Changing knowledge and attitudes about fruits and vegetables' in *Australian and New Zealand Journal of Public Health*, vol. 28, no. 3, pp. 288–95.

Robinson, T.N. and Sirard, J.R. 2005, 'Preventing childhood obesity: A solution-oriented research paradigm' in *American Journal of Preventative Medicine*, vol. 28, no. 2, pp. 194–201.

Rychetnik, L., Hawe, P., Waters, E., Barratt, A. and Frommer, M. 2004, 'A glossary for evidence based public health' in *Journal of Epidemiology Community Health*, vol. 58, no. 7, pp. 538–45.

Sinner, J. and Davies, S. 2004, 'Cutting the fat: How a fat tax can help fight obesity' in *Diabetes New Zealand*, Fight the Obesity Epidemic, Wellington.

Story, M. 1999, 'School-based approaches for preventing and treating obesity' in *International Journal of Obesity*, vol. 23, pp. S43–51.

Summerbell, C., Waters, E., Edmunds, L., Kelly, S., Brown, T. and Campbell, K. 2005, 'Interventions for preventing obesity in children' in *Cochrane Data Base System Review*, no. 3, CD001871.

Swinburn, B. 2002, 'Sustaining dietary changes for preventing obesity and diabetes: Lessons learned from the successes of other epidemic control programs' in *Asia Pacific Journal of Clinical Nutrition*, vol. 11, pp. S598–606.

Swinburn, B. and Egger, G. 2002, 'Preventive strategies against weight gain and obesity' in *Obesity Review*, vol. 3, no. 4, pp. 289–301.

Swinburn, B., Caterson, I., Seidell, J.C. and James, W.P. 2004, 'Diet, nutrition and the prevention of excess weight gain and obesity' in *Public Health Nutrition*, vol. 7, no. 1A, pp. 123–46.

Swinburn, B., Egger, G. and Raza, F. 1999, 'Dissecting obesogenic environments: The development and application of a framework for identifying and prioritizing environmental interventions for obesity' in *Preventative Medicine*, vol. 29, no. 6 (pt 1), pp. 563–70.

Swinburn, B., Gill, T. and Kumanyika, S. 2005, 'Obesity prevention: a proposed framework for translating evidence into action' in *Obesity Review*, vol. 6, no. 1, pp. 23–33.

The New South Wales School Canteen Association 2004, 'Healthy Canteens' cited at <http://www.schoolcanteens.org.au>.

Toh, C.M., Cutter, J. and Chew, S.K. 2002, 'School based intervention has reduced obesity in Singapore' in *British Medical Journal*, vol. 324, no. 427.

Williams, J., Wake, M., Hesketh, K., Maher, E. and Waters, E. 2005, 'Health-related quality of life of overweight and obese children' in *Journal of American Medical Association*, vol. 293, no. 1, pp. 70–76.

World Health Organization (WHO) 2000, 'Obesity: Preventing and managing the global epidemic', report of a WHO consultation, Geneva.

—— 2003, 'Diet, nutrition and the prevention of chronic diseases', report of a joint Food and Agriculture Organization/WHO expert consultation, Technical Report Series no. 916, WHO, Geneva.

—— 2004, 'Global strategy on diet, physical activity, and health' cited at <http://www.who.int/dietphysicalactivity/goals/en> in August.

10

International nutrition

IAN DARNTON-HILL
MICKEY CHOPRA

Malnutrition increasingly involves both undernutrition, especially in infants and children, and overnutrition, especially in adults, and they not infrequently occur in the same communities, and even families. Although the mechanisms are not the same and are affected by many other factors, there is some optimism that addressing maternal nutrition and antenatal care, and infant and young child feeding practices and care, will help to address both problems (WHO 2006), but this is likely to be unduly optimistic in communities living in poverty. Undernutrition includes vitamin and mineral deficiencies (micronutrient malnutrition), maternal undernutrition and low birthweight. Overnutrition is used imprecisely to refer to the current overweight and obesity global epidemic, and the dramatic increase in the diet-related chronic diseases (WHO 2003). Both are over-represented in the more disadvantaged and poorer strata of societies, although overnutrition remains relatively rare in the poorest countries. A further common link is that infants who suffer undernutrition antenatally are likely to be at greater risk from noncommunicable diseases such as obesity, diabetes and hypertension later in life (Darnton-Hill et al. 2004). There is now considerable support for the concept that economic development and a nation's health will not improve without progress in reducing malnutrition (United Nations Development Programme 2003; World Bank 2006).

Extent of problem

Undernutrition

Undernutrition is continuing to worsen in some countries (UNICEF 2006). Micronutrient deficiencies are widespread globally (Mason et al. 2005). There are 146 million (or one in four) underweight children in the developing world (UNICEF 2006). Of the more than eleven million under-five-year-old children dying unnecessarily each year (Black et al. 2003), more than half, or almost six million children, die every year because they are undernourished. Underweight prevalence varies according to region from almost half (46 per cent) of all under-five children in South Asia being underweight, and almost a third (29 per cent) in Sub-Saharan Africa, where rates are not improving (UNICEF 2006) (see Figure 10.1). As well as these figures for failure to grow and thrive are the huge numbers, especially of women and children, who are suffering from deficiencies of micronutrients; almost one in three people suffering from iron and other anaemia deficiencies, vitamin A deficiency, iodine deficiency disorders, zinc deficiency, and other, often multiple, deficiencies.

A recent report by UNICEF notes that broad overall averages for regions or, indeed for individual countries, inevitably tend to hide disparities (UNICEF 2006). A country with a low prevalence of underweight children on average can have significant pockets of undernutrition in a particular area or among certain

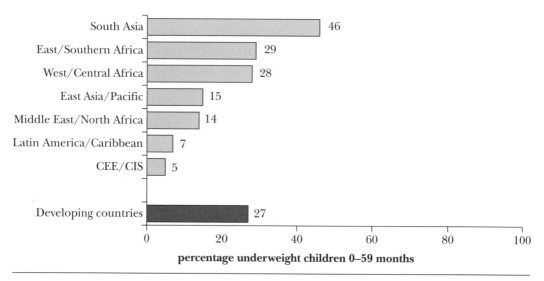

Figure 10.1 Percentage of children underweight

Source: UNICEF 2006

subgroups of the population. Disaggregated data in the same report show large disparities existing between the underweight prevalence of urban and rural children in the developing world. On average, underweight prevalence among children in rural areas is almost double that of children in urban areas (UNICEF 2006). Other specific studies in some of the developing world's rapidly growing cities, however, show this trend may be reversing in the very disadvantaged urban poor (Bloem et al. 2004), so that high underweight prevalence in urban slums in many developing countries still gives cause for concern, as these settings are the same ones where, later in life, overweight and obesity are becoming rampant.

Significant disparities also exist with household income and, on average, children living in the poorest households are twice as likely to be underweight as children living in the relatively richest households (UNICEF 2006). The greatest disparities between rich and poor are found in Latin America/Caribbean, where children living in the poorest households are over three-and-a-half times more likely to suffer from undernutrition than children from the richest households. The lowest disparities are found in East Asia/Pacific, followed by Sub-Saharan Africa and Central European countries. In terms of gender disparities, boys and girls have a similar underweight prevalence in every region except South Asia, where a larger proportion of girls (47 per cent) are underweight than boys (44 per cent).

Iodine-deficient populations suffer sub-optimal brain development, leading to poor school performance, reduced intellectual ability and impaired work capacity. Iron deficiency anaemia, when severe and prolonged in the first two years of life, also causes compromised intellectual development, as well as being a major cause of maternal mortality and a major cause of economic loss to countries. The UN Standing Committee on Nutrition (SCN) has estimated that the economic costs of anaemia in Bangladesh, for example, amount to 7.9 per cent of gross domestic productivity (WHO 2004). Approximately 100 to 140 million children are vitamin A deficient. Most of these children live in the least developed areas of South Asia and Sub-Saharan Africa (WHO 2004). Recent estimates show that, in the absence of adequate action, more than 43 million children in Sub-Saharan Africa are at risk of vitamin A deficiency (Aguayo & Baker 2006), and hence at an increased risk of dying from infectious disease. Other micronutrients of public health significance include zinc, folate, vitamin B12 and, in some settings, thiamin and vitamin D.

Failing to exclusively breastfeed can also be considered a form of preventable malnutrition, given that human milk is the ideal nourishment for infants' optimal survival, growth and development. Exclusive breastfeeding in the first six months of life protects babies from diarrhoea and acute respiratory infections — two of the major causes of infant mortality in the developing world — and stimulates infants' immune system and response to vaccination, and may offer protection against later development of diet-related chronic diseases and obesity. Yet, only around one-third (36 per cent) of all infants in the developing world are exclusively breast-fed for the first six months of life. Considerable variation exists with the highest rates found in East Asia/Pacific (43 per cent) and Eastern/Southern Africa (41 per cent) and the lowest in West/Central Africa (20 per cent) and the Central and East European countries (22 per cent) (UNICEF 2006). Appropriate complementary feeding is also critical in the first two years of life — identified as the most effective window of opportunity to make up for low birthweight, avoid stunting, and as a basis for adequate growth and cognitive development (World Bank 2006).

More than 20 million, or 17 per cent, of the infants born each year in the developing world are of low birthweight, which is more than twice the level in industrialised countries (7 per cent) (UNICEF/WHO 2004). Infants born with low birthweight are at higher risk of subsequent death (Lawn et al. 2005). Those who survive are liable to be stunted, to have an impaired immune system and an increased risk of disease, and may suffer a higher incidence of chronic diseases such as diabetes and heart disease in later life (Darnton-Hill et al. 2004). More than 96 per cent of low-weight births occur in the developing world, reflecting the higher likelihood of low birthweight babies born to women living in poor socioeconomic conditions, their earlier own sub-optimal growth, inadequate weight gain antenatally, poor diet, and the likelihood of doing physically demanding work during pregnancy (UNICEF/WHO 2004).

There is significant variation in the incidence of low birthweight across the regions of the developing world (see Figure 10.2). South Asia has the highest incidence, with nearly one-third (31 per cent) of all infants born with low birthweight, while East Asia/Pacific has the lowest (7 per cent). India alone is home to nearly 40 per cent of all the babies born with low birthweight in the developing world. Nearly one in every seven infants in Sub-Saharan Africa (14 per cent) and Middle East/North Africa (15 per cent) are also born with low birthweight (UNICEF 2006). Reliable monitoring of this vital indicator of low birthweight is difficult, however, given that more than half (58 per cent) of all infants in the developing world are not weighed at birth. Limited trend data indicates that the incidence of low birthweight has remained roughly constant between 1990 and 2000 in both Sub-Saharan Africa and Asia (UNICEF/WHO 2004).

There is increased risk of undernutrition in emergencies, further increasing children's risk of disease and death. This is of particular concern as emergencies are increasing globally (Shetty 2006; Webb 2006). In most cases, the

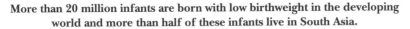

More than 20 million infants are born with low birthweight in the developing world and more than half of these infants live in South Asia.

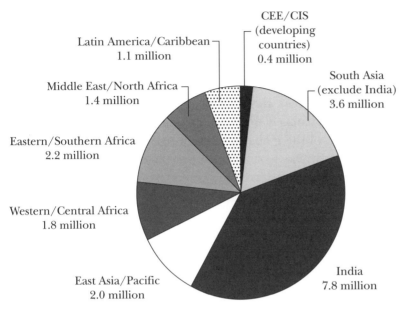

Figure 10.2 Distribution of low birthweight infants
Source: UNICEF/WHO 2004

children's baseline nutrition is poor even before the crisis worsens the underlying undernutrition due to food insecurity, limited access to essential health services, unhealthy environments, and poor feeding and care practices for children and their mothers. Micronutrient deficiencies, particularly in iron, vitamin A and iodine, are frequently a major public health threat in emergencies (Webb 2006). Emergencies can be acute, those which hit the headlines, often too late to avoid the consequences even though there have often been warning signs and calls for attention months before the acute emergency starts starving populations, such as in Niger in the mid 2000s. There are also chronic or slow emergencies in which levels of undernutrition, especially stunting (low height for age), occur in over a third of all the children in a community but are not recognised, or at least not addressed, until things deteriorate in the light of new circumstances, such as a drought or a man-made disaster (Lancet 2006). One could argue that populations with high prevalence of HIV/AIDS infection represent a slow emergency, whereby other factors contributing to undernutrition are aggravated by the epidemic, loss of adults to produce food and as teachers, and increases in numbers of children affected by AIDS (Chopra & Sanders 2004; Shetty 2006).

Overnutrition

At the same time, there is a global epidemic of increasing obesity, diabetes, and other diet-related chronic noncommunicable diseases, especially in low-income and transitional economies, and in the less affluent within these, as well as in the developed countries where those most socioeconomically disadvantaged are most at risk. It has been calculated that, in 2001 chronic diseases contributed approximately 46 per cent of the global burden of disease and this is expected to increase to 57 per cent by the year 2020, at enormous healthcare and other costs for societies and governments (WHO/FAO 2003). Already, 79 per cent of deaths attributable to chronic or noncommunicable diseases are occurring in developing (low-income and transitional) countries, predominantly in middle-aged men (Darnton-Hill et al. 2004). Transitional economies such as those in Latin America, East Europe, and Asia and the Pacific are seeing massive increases in all the diet-related chronic diseases as a result of the nutrition transition, and all the accelerating causes of that (Popkin et al. 2001; Monteiro et al. 2004). All evidence shows the epidemic continuing to increase, and even accelerate (WHO/FAO 2003). In the more affluent countries such as Australia, United Kingdom and United States, up to a third or more of children are overweight or obese (Waters & Baur 2003) and adults may have two thirds of their populations overweight and obese (WHO 2003). This is resulting in, amongst other things, increasing numbers of children and adolescents being diagnosed as having type 2 (previously known as 'adult-onset') diabetes (WHO/FAO 2003). More than a billion adults worldwide are overweight, of whom 300 million are obese (WHO/FAO 2003; WHO 2006). Obesity is itself a cause of early mortality and a separate risk factor for many of the other diet-related chronic diseases such as diabetes, hypertension, and cardiovascular diseases.

Overlap

At the same time, there has been an increase in communities and households that have coincident under- and over-nutrition (Boutayeb 2006). With all the problems of two billion people estimated to have micronutrient deficiencies and 800 million people with inadequate diets, childhood obesity is still becoming a recognised problem even in some low-income countries. As noted, while undernutrition increases risk of death in early life, it also leads to a high risk of disease and death in later life. This combination is increasingly being referred to as the double burden of malnutrition (WHO 2006; Boutayeb 2006). As noted by the SCN, 'these issues are still perceived to be separate [when in] reality both are often rooted in poverty and co-exist in communities, and even the same households, in most countries' (WHO 2006). The SCN and many others contend that this double burden has common causes – inadequate foetal and child undernutrition followed by exposure to an excess of unhealthy energy dense, nutrient-poor processed foods and lack of physical activity (WHO 2006). The trends in obesity seen in the most affluent countries are now being seen in Eastern Europe and Latin America (Chopra & Darnton-Hill 2004), and even in women in poor populations in countries such as Mauritania and South Africa (World Bank 2006). In Brazil, for example, there were almost two cases of underweight to every one case of obesity in 1975, whereas twenty years later there were more than two cases of obesity to one case of underweight, and it had become the low-income women, who still had undernourished children in their households, who were at greatest risk (Monteiro et al. 2004).

Causes and factors

Factors leading to undernutrition and to some extent overnutrition, can be categorised as immediate, underlying and basic causes, as seen in the Figure 10.3 an update of the UNICEF framework. Such a conceptual framework is essential in understanding the paradox of the poor progress towards reducing levels of undernutrition in many parts of the world, even though this poor progress has coincided with the greatest expansion in crop and food production in human history.

With the doubling in food production over the past 40 years, there is now more than enough food to feed everybody on the planet (Chopra & Sanders 2004; Shetty 2006). The global value of trading in food grew from $224 billion in 1972 to $438 billion in 1998; food now constitutes 11 per cent of global trade, a percentage higher than fuel. Globally, food prices have fallen by 50 per cent and are at an all-time low. However, it is clear that many millions of people are not sharing in the benefits of this increased production and lower food prices. Nowhere is this currently more important than in Africa (Chopra & Darnton-Hill 2006). A public health nutrition response can use the same conceptual framework to analyse the causes leading to the design of effective responses.

Basic causes

In less than four decades, Sub-Saharan Africa has been transformed from a continent that was a net exporter of food to one that is now heavily dependent on food imports. Africa accounted for 18 per cent of world imports in 2001 (up from 8 per cent just fifteen years previously) (FAO 2004). This has occurred

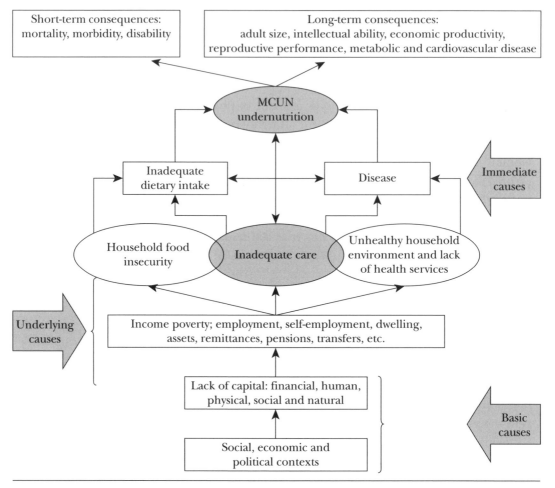

Figure 10.3 UNICEF framework of the relationship linking poverty, food insecurity and other underlying and intermediate causes of child and maternal undernutrition

Source: UNICEF 1998, modified by Morris et al. 2006

partly because of a decline in agricultural and rural investment in Africa, leading to a decline in agricultural productivity. Agricultural productivity per worker for the region as a whole has fallen by about 12 per cent from US$424 in 1980 to an estimated US$365 per worker (constant: 1995 US$) in the late 1990s. Growth in agricultural output has arisen mostly from expansion in the area under cultivation.

Significantly, the yields of most important food grains, tubers and legumes (maize, millet, sorghum, yams, cassava and groundnuts) in most African countries are no higher today than in 1980. This compares with a 14 per cent increase in Latin America and the Caribbean, a region with similar population densities and resource endowments (Chopra & Sanders 2004). Fertiliser application is 15 per cent lower today than in 1980. The number of tractors per worker is 25 per cent lower than in 1980, and the lowest in the world. Africa's share of total world agricultural trade fell from 8 per cent in 1965 to 3 per cent in 1996 (Chopra & Sanders 2004). The environmental impacts of deforestation and drought, floods and the loss of topsoil are being compounded by the lack of investment. Only about 4.2 per cent of land under cultivation in Africa is irrigated. Similarly, in China, where rates of undernutrition have been a main driver in improved averages of the numbers of undernourished children in Asia, the environmental impact will be unsustainable (Brown 2005).

For years, public investment in agriculture has been falling, not rising. In countries where 20 to 35 per cent of the population is defined as food insecure, agricultural spending averaged 7.6 per cent in 1992 and 5.2 per cent in 1998. For countries with more than 35 per cent of their population suffering food insecurity, agricultural spending in 1992 was 6.8 per cent, declining to 4.9 per cent in 1996, the last year for which data are available (International Food Policy Research Institute 2004).

The shift of resources away from rural areas and agriculture noted above can be traced to the increasing role of food aid in the 1960s. This provided cheap cereals and encouraged national governments to focus investment on large-scale industrial developments. Through the Public Law 480, the United States was able to export wheat to developing countries at concession prices. Wheat exports grew 250 per cent between 1950 and 1970, with the share of developing nations increasing from 19 per cent in the late 1950s to 66 per cent in the late 1960s (Friedland 1994). More recently, this process has been accelerated by the undermining of the prices of agricultural commodities and products because of the massive farming subsidises in the developed countries. In the European Union, the average European dairy cow has a bigger annual income than most people in the world (Chopra & Sanders 2004). In the United States, the 2002 Farm Bill recently authorised the paying out of US$180 billion over a ten-year period as 'emergency measures', mainly in support of staple cereal crops (Institute for Agriculture and Trading Policy 2004). The Institute for Agriculture and Trade Policy (IATP 2004) has calculated that United States subsidies mean that major crops are put on the international market at well below their production costs: wheat by an average of 43 per cent below the cost of production, soyabeans at 25 per cent below, cotton at 61 per cent below, and rice at 35 per cent below (Institute for Agriculture and Trading Policy 2004). This depression of commodity prices is having a devastating effect on farmers in developing countries. Research by the International Food Policy Research Institute has clearly demonstrated that subsidies to farming in the Organisation for Economic Cooperation and Development (OECD) countries, which totalled US$311 billion in 2001 (or US$850 million per day), displaces farming in the developing countries, costing the world's poor countries about US$24 billion per year in lost agricultural and agro-industrial income (International Food Policy Research Institute 2004).

Intermediate causes

Poor food security or poverty alone do not explain why many countries and populations have managed significant reductions in undernutrition before there were similar reductions in poverty. For example, in a comparison between Indonesia, the Philippines, Sri Lanka and Thailand, Sri Lanka and Thailand showed rapid improvement in nutrition in the 1980s to '90s. Indonesia showed slower but consistent improvement, and the Philippines little progress (Mason 2001). At a regional level, malnutrition in Latin America decreased from an estimated 21 per cent in 1970 to 7.2 per cent in 1997, while the rate of poverty (measured by income level) decreased only slightly over the past three decades, from 45 per cent in 1970 to 44 per cent in 1997 (Figure 10.4). These trends show that the reduction of malnutrition is not solely dependent on increases in income. In Latin America, the gains in reducing malnutrition are attributed, at the underlying level, to good care practices (such as improved complementary feeding) and access to basic health services, including family planning, and

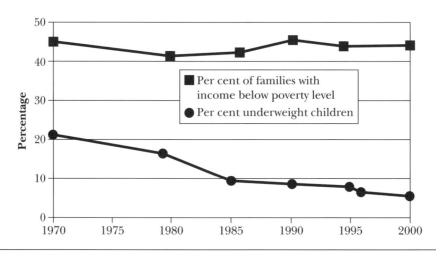

Figure 10.4 Changes in malnutrition and poverty in Latin America 1970–2000

Source: UNICEF 1998

[232]

water/sanitation services; and, at the basic level, to women's empowerment in terms of their education and the cash resources they control (UNICEF 1998).

Immediate causes

Poor diets, high infectious disease loads, and poor healthcare and systems are the immediate causes of malnutrition, complicated by such factors as discriminatory intrahousehold distribution, poverty that does not allow even available food to be accessible, and sometimes lack of knowledge; for example, not giving colostrums to newborns. The poor are more likely to be born with low birthweight to mothers who are undernourished (Gillespie et al. 2003), and are less likely to receive energy rich complementary food or iodised salt (UNICEF 1998). The only advantage they have, and this is only in poorer countries, is that infants are more likely to be breastfed, and for longer, than their richer counterparts. However, the exploitation and uncertainty around the risk of transmitting HIV through breast milk is now eroding this tendency in some regions, although evidence is accumulating that exclusive breastfeeding remains the best option in resource-poor environments. Poorer children are also less likely to live in households with safe water or sanitation, and more likely to be exposed to indoor air pollution (Chopra & Sanders 2004).

Addressing malnutrition

This section looks at the current understanding of how to address malnutrition, but especially from a perspective of low birthweight and undernutrition, with the expectation that this would address some aspects of later nutritionally related chronic disease. The current picture of addressing overnutrition in childhood is even less encouraging than the low success rate in adults (Ebbeling et al. 2002; Waters & Baur 2003), and is not covered further here. It would seem that there is a particular biological window of opportunity from conception to the first two years of life (Shrimpton et al. 2001; World Bank 2006), both to prevent undernutrition and to allow catch-up growth (Gillespie et al. 2003). After that, stunting is likely to be lifelong, so that any weight gain is likely to lead to later obesity and, in adulthood, nutritionally related chronic disease. Nevertheless, a lifestyle approach is recommended as a means for both primary and secondary prevention of the diet-related chronic diseases (Darnton-Hill et al. 2004). A national intervention programme in Singapore was able to reduce some of these factors and stabilised the prevalence of obesity and diabetes mellitus (Cutter et al. 2001).

Public health nutrition responses

Understanding the multiple causes of poor nutrition as they relate to the different socio-political levels thus allows an outline of possible responses. In particular, it draws attention to the fact that, while it is important to address proximal causes – such as diet, care, health systems and agriculture – distal factors such as women's education and global trade agreements must also be addressed. The following not only emphasises the prevention of low birthweight and undernutrition, but looks at it in an holistic way, addressing many sectors and all levels of governance, which mirrors the approach above on causes.

Public policy responses

There is a growing literature on how to address undernutrition. There was a major push in the 1970s and '80s to address undernutrition, with some notable successes. However, these improvements were usually either not scaled up to national programmes, or were not sustained. The latter was occasionally because progress was slow, or expensive, or relied on external funding, or was based on overly complex national nutrition programmes. These either did not have the backing of planning and finance ministries, or were so complex that they sometimes just collapsed under their own weight.

There seems to be growing evidence that the lack of sustainability, or scaling up, was due to a failure to address the fact that interventions need to be widely based, with all levels reinforcing activities at each level. For example, it is possible to have a successful community intervention (often heavily supported by external funding), but if this is not adequately supported at the district and national levels, it is unlikely to be sustained when funding stops, or when capacity of both human and financial resources are inadequate for sustainability. It is also likely that the human capacity needed has been underestimated. There has been a mass emigration of trained health personnel both to the cities, and also to richer countries. Looking at how to address the problem therefore requires a mutually supportive framework that addresses global, national, district and communities, including families. Another likely factor for past lack of success was that nutrition interventions, while including commodities (availability and accessibility to food, vitamin A and other micronutrients) directed inadequate resources to the equally important behaviour-change aspects (increasing rates of exclusive breastfeeding and appropriate complementary feeding and other care and sanitation practices).

Global

The proven practices as outlined, and subsequent costings, of the Bellagio Child Survival Study Group, quite specifically noted that they were addressing Health

Systems interventions (Black et al. 2003). However, these systems, in most situations where child mortality rates are highest, are often dysfunctional at best (UN Millennium Project 2005). This can be due to a variety of reasons, but there is increasing acceptance that the factors are also global. Inequitable trade practices are one such factor that make it impossible for countries to escape from being resource-poor; for example, cotton farmers in West Africa trying to compete with heavily subsidised US-based cotton farmers. Another is the failure of many western countries to adequately train their own health workers and instead to actively recruit in poor countries that are already short of staff. Funding is another factor, and while there is debate on how well these funds have been used, they are also often directed at the 'easier', more vertical programmes, such as micronutrients, or commodity-based interventions, for instance impregnated bednets. The evidence is convincing that the pressure from donor countries and the World Bank on recipient countries to move towards economic rationalisation in the late 1980s and '90s, whereby, among other things, health services (and education) were to be paid for by the recipients of those services, led to worsened health, nutrition and educational levels, especially among the rural poor.

National

There were, and are, often distinct external pressures on national governments to, or not to fund, specific health and nutrition areas that may be the main national problems, but not donor priorities; the national governments themselves have often been less committed to funding adequately social goods such as health, nutrition, education and so on, compared with infrastructure building in big cities. Another recurring problem has been the lack of good governance, including corruption. National (and sometimes regional) action is necessary in the areas of facilitative legislation – for example, for iodisation of salt – but resource-poor governments rarely have the funds or capacity to ensure such legislation and provisions are enforced.

Policies providing for female education, social safety nets, affordable food and public health services have been clearly identified to have contributed to the improvements in undernutrition rates, even with minimal changes in poverty levels. The impact on child nutrition and survival of widespread female education in Sri Lanka and the Indian state of Kerala is well documented, with 77 per cent of married women in Sri Lanka now having above primary schooling. Drèze and Sen (1989) also highlight the establishment of social safety nets, especially the free or heavily subsidised distribution of rice, providing a minimum consumption floor for the poor, as important reasons for the impressive performance of Sri Lanka. In a more recent review for Save the Children UK, Chopra and Sanders

(2004) emphasise the provision of a universal, equitable and efficient public health system as an important reason for the low levels of maternal and child mortality in this country. Studies on women's status and childhood nutritional status have concluded that there is good evidence to show that a woman's status and her education level affect the nutritional status of her child. Educated girls and women have fewer children, seek medical attention sooner for themselves and their children, and provide better care and nutrition for their children (Darnton-Hill et al. 2005).

An interesting feature of the often-quoted success in Thailand in reducing undernutrition was the incorporation of nutrition as an important part of the National Economic and Social Development Plan. This led to the establishment of an extensive community-based network of village health communicators and volunteers who became incorporated into existing village committees and their leaders. The focus of these groups was the fulfilment of basic needs such as optimal nutrition (as measured by community-based growth monitoring and promotion) and education (Tontisirin & Winichagoon 1997).

Further evidence of the importance of public policy comes from the work of Wagstaff and Watanabe (2001), who calculated the level of inequality in the distribution of stunting, and plotted it against the general inequities in income for twenty countries. Not surprisingly, countries with unequal income distributions also tend to have unequal distributions of malnutrition. Unequal distribution of purchasing power, *prima facie*, leads to an unequal distribution of food spending (intake), health spending and utilisation of health services, and consequently unequal health outcomes. But the authors go on to point out that what is more interesting, perhaps, is the fact that the fit of the bivariate regressions is fairly bad – there are, in other words, many countries that buck the trend. Nepal and Peru, for example, have roughly the same level of income inequality, and yet Nepal has far lower levels of inequality in stunting and underweight than Peru. This implies that there must be some form of mechanism in these countries that breaks the link between poverty and malnutrition (Wagstaff & Watanabe 2000). They go on to comment on the case of Egypt, which tends to positively deviate from the mainstream trend, and the need to explore what factors, given the level of consumption inequality, contribute to the relatively low inequalities in malnutrition.

District level

Where district services do not specifically budget for health interventions, including supplies and personnel, health and nutrition have suffered. Effective interventions are known, especially those using a health systems approach

(Jones et al. 2003), and have a good evidence base, but will require greater resources and a decrease in inequities (UN Millennium Project 2005). In addition to the increasing body of knowledge of the importance of poverty reduction and broader social policies in reducing levels of malnutrition, there is also this increasing evidence base of the efficacy of primary healthcare interventions. There is now a fair body of evidence illustrating the impact – sometimes sustained and sometimes ephemeral – of large-scale health interventions in improving child health and nutrition outcomes.

Communities and families

Whereas progress has often been demonstrated at this level, it has often also been donor-driven, externally funded, but not sustainably, nor necessarily reflecting community identified needs, and has often failed to build up local capacity. The poorer communities are more often not empowered to make the changes necessary, nor do they have the resources, or sometimes, the knowledge. Changes at this level are also not infrequently about behaviour change, which takes longer and may be less often supported compared with, for example, 'social marketing', which reflects a certain economic viewpoint and is not always appropriate, especially for the very poor. There have been several studies recently showing the successful scaling up of behaviour change, in this case of exclusive breastfeeding, with an impact on child survival rates (Quinn et al. 2005).

Success factors for large-scale programmes

Public health programmes that are planned, implemented and assessed well can make a difference. Reviews of successful large-scale nutrition programmes enable us to outline a few key 'success factors' that were common across these successful programmes.

Programme relevance

Successful programmes identified the immediate and underlying causes of malnutrition and ways in which they interact. This was followed by the formulation of interventions at different parts of the conceptual framework. So, for example, in a nutrition programme, any intervention around dietary inadequacy (immediate level of causation) should also address household food insecurity (underlying level of causation). Thus, the choice of a food supplement should be based both on its nutrient value and on its availability, cost and ability to be either cultivated and/or purchased, as well as being culturally appropriate.

The careful choice of an appropriate food supplement should be reinforced as an educational action to influence positively food habits and feeding practices. This principle of linking curative or rehabilitative (feeding), preventive (nutrition education), and promotive actions (to achieve improved household food security) could, and should, be applied to health programmes other than nutrition.

Coverage, targeting, resources and intensity

Even effective programmes only improve the health and nutrition of those they reach. Therefore, achieving as complete a coverage as possible of those at risk is a major determinant of the impact. Programmes tend to target specific areas and biological groups – generally women and children – but mainly do not give priority to poorer or less healthy communities. Indeed, the policy is often to aim for complete coverage within the participating areas, and to add new sites until the entire country, region or selected areas are included. Relatively untargeted expansion to universal coverage may be at the expense of establishing adequate resources and quality in the areas initially covered. In at least one case (Thailand), having achieved broad coverage and reduced malnutrition, the programme was then specifically targeted at areas where progress was lagging. Once sufficient coverage has been achieved, there must be sufficient contact between the beneficiaries and trained local workers (with supervision, supplies, etc.). Thus, the intensity measure of community based workers per mother–child, and supervision ratios, are very relevant. The suggested norms, originating from the Thailand experience with community-based communicators and facilitators focusing upon nutrition, are about 1:100 for both these, depending upon the complexity of the intervention (Tontisirin & Winichapoon 1997).

Programme management and monitoring and evaluation

The challenge of good management is to establish a structure that promotes transparency, that defines roles and responsibilities clearly, that permits quick response (to information from a good monitoring system) and limits bureaucratic red tape, but at the same time is able to check misuse of programme resources and is also not inordinately time-consuming.

All programme planners agree that monitoring and evaluation is an essential component of good programme design. Yet few programmes make provision for adequate monitoring and evaluation. The information provided by a programme's monitoring and evaluation system is largely of little interest to communities. What they need is a system to monitor their own progress towards achieving their own specific developmental goals. For this, it is recommended that community groups be encouraged and helped to establish a simple system of participatory monitoring that relates closely to their own identified priorities and activities.

Progress towards the goal of reducing malnutrition

Undernutrition

Partly because it has been a public health problem of greater magnitude for a much longer time, and hence with more experience in addressing it, especially at sub-national level, undernutrition has received more attention. The fact that it is a target of the first Millennium Development Goal (MDG) has also meant more attention, as for example in the recent Progress for Children report on which much of the following is based, along with assessments by UNDP, WHO and the World Bank in 2005.

One of the positive advances has been the relative unanimity and adoption of the eight MDGs (UNDP 2003). Where there has been some criticism that they may present another manifestation of donor values, they have certainly acted as a major engine for development, even if the promises of increased resources by the wealthier countries have not always materialised (UNDP 2003). However, even here there have been some real progress, for example the recent debt forgiveness of nineteen of the most poor countries (Balls 2005). Criticisms of the MDGs, from a nutritional perspective, is the use of the vaguely defined 'hunger' as opposed to undernutrition, the absence of specific mention of the micronutrients and the absence of a goal directed at the current epidemic of nutritionally related chronic diseases, especially obesity and diabetes, which, as we have seen, is increasingly affecting the same most disadvantaged populations, especially in the transitional economies such as East Asia and Latin America (Popkin et al. 2001; Monteiro et al. 2004; Darnton-Hill et al. 2004).

The MDGs were agreed to in 2000, and recent evaluations five years into the fifteen-year target period have generally been only relatively encouraging; for example, the recent report on nutrition looking at progress towards the nutritional target of the first MDG (UNICEF 2006). The MDG1 has two targets, one addressing income poverty and the other hunger as a non-income measure of poverty. Progress towards the poverty target has been reasonable, although it looks better than it is due to averaging across regions; for example, China distorting the lack of progress in countries such as Cambodia. The second target has received much less attention and is the one addressed towards hunger, at which progress is less encouraging and even more uneven. The target has two indicators: underweight as expressed by weight for age, and hunger as expressed by calculated lack of energy (calories), a broad-stroke indicator of hunger, which, however, among other problems, reflects supposed availability of food and loses the accessibility aspect and the inequities of hunger of the very poor in countries with wide disparities of income. The UNICEF report looks at progress towards the undernutrition indicator across regions while addressing countries that are lagging, or indeed, appear to have no chance of reaching the goal (UNICEF 2006). Even this does not address inequities within countries, which in most cases appear to be worsening, including in the most affluent countries, such as Australia and the United States. The report also states that it is important to note that tracking progress toward this goal, which has a 1990 baseline, is limited by the fact that many countries did not have data for underweight prevalence in the early 1990s, although data became more widely available in the mid 1990s.

Despite an overall improvement between 1990 and 2004 (Figure 10.5), the present rate of decline in the proportion of underweight children in the developing world will not be sufficient to reach the MDG target of reducing by half the proportion of people who suffer from hunger. The report uses the self-explanatory average annual rate of reduction, which is currently 1.7 per cent. The report notes that, 'unless that rate improves, 50 million children whose lives could have benefited from adequate nutrition by 2015 will miss out, their very lives at stake' (UNICEF 2006).

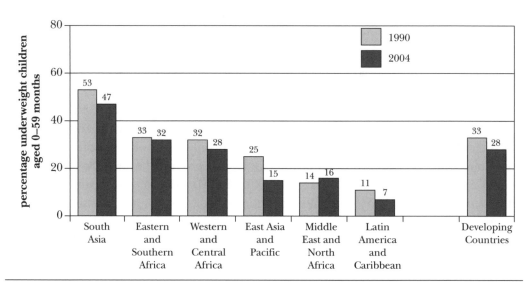

Figure 10.5 Trends in prevalence of underweight children in low-income countries

Source: UNICEF 2006

A brief synopsis of the report shows that the regions of Latin America/ Caribbean and East Asia/Pacific, with average rates of reduction of 3.9 and 3.7 per cent per year respectively, are on track to reach the target. In fact, East Asia/Pacific has already achieved the goal of reducing the 1990 levels by half; again, the region's progress is primarily driven by China, where underweight prevalence declined from 19 per cent in 1990 to 8 in 2002. Both West/Central Africa and South Asia have made progress, but not sufficient to reach the target. In the Middle East/North Africa, the rate has actually deteriorated (–1.6 per cent), mainly attributable to three countries, Iraq, Sudan and Yemen, all of which have large populations and have been affected by conflict or natural disasters.

The Eastern/Southern Africa region as a whole, far from making progress towards the MDG goal of reducing hunger by half, has shown no improvement at all since 1990 in the proportion of children that are underweight, due mainly to the declines in agricultural productivity, recurring food crises during drought and conflict, and increasing levels of poverty. At the same time, HIV/AIDS, especially when coupled with the drought-related food crises, has posed serious challenges to nutrition development, slowing or reversing progress since the early 1990s, particularly in six southern African countries. As a result, the absolute number of underweight children has actually increased in the region over the last fifteen years. Of the eighteen countries in this region with sufficient trend data to assess progress toward the MDGs, only Botswana is on track to reach the target, and ten countries are showing either no change or are getting worse.

On the other hand, a positive trend is the increased incidence of exclusive breastfeeding in the first six months of life, which has improved since 1990, although it continues to be low across the developing world. Between 1990 and 2004, exclusive breastfeeding rates rose from 34 to 41 per cent in the developing world — based on 37 countries for which there are trend data (UNICEF 2006). Significant improvements were made in Sub-Saharan Africa, where rates more than doubled over the same period, rising from 15 to 32 per cent, and where Eastern/Southern Africa has, at 41 per cent, a higher rate of exclusive breastfeeding than any other region except East Asia/Pacific.

As a result of the campaign to eliminate iodine deficiency through universal salt iodisation, more than two-thirds (69 per cent) of households in the developing world consume adequately iodised salt, and 82 million newborns are now being protected every year from learning disabilities caused by iodine deficiency disorder. Yet large differences exist in the consumption of adequately iodised salt among regions of the developing world, from around 85 per cent in Latin America/Caribbean and East Asia/Pacific, to 64 per cent in Sub-Saharan Africa (almost two-thirds of households), to the lowest levels in the Central European countries, at 47 per cent, although progress has recently been made. The provision of high-dose vitamin A supplements every four to six months is presumed to have had a dramatic impact on the health of young children, reducing the risk of mortality by up to 23 per cent, with an overall coverage rate of supplementation to children between six and 59 months in the developing world (excluding China) standing at 61 per cent in 2003. In general, supplementation coverage is higher than average in the least developed countries (76 per cent), where the need is greatest. Iron supplementation reduces iron-deficiency anaemia in pregnant and lactating women, but pro-grammes have been largely unsuccessful so far, not least because they have tended to reach women too late in their pregnancy. As a result, there has been no evidence of significant improvement in the global incidence of anaemia over the past fifteen years. In the low-income countries, anaemia remains a major threat, with unacceptable rates of anaemia in children and their mothers, reflecting the need for large-scale interventions for anaemia control in children and women that integrate the control of micronutrient deficiencies, malaria infection and intestinal parasitic infestation.

Overnutrition

There is less evidence of both the extent of the diet-related chronic disease problem and the experience with successful interventions, which is quite limited (Ebbeling et al. 2002; Waters & Baur 2003). On a national level, Singapore is perhaps the only country with a national programme to show results in the reduc-tion of childhood overweight and obesity (Cutter et al. 2001). Major western countries, Australia, France, United Kingdom and United States among others, as well as East Asian countries, China, Korea and Japan, have all recently devoted more attention and resources to halt the epidemic of overweight, obesity and diet-related chronic diseases. However, the trends are mainly up and accelerating for obesity and diabetes, although countries have shown success in reducing coronary heart disease death rates in countries such as Australia, Singapore and the United States (WHO/FAO 2003). It is likely the problem will need to be addressed at the same four levels as undernutrition: at the family and community level by culturally appropriate nutrition and health education and behaviour change; at the subnational level by measures to increase physical activity and improve diets, for instance by removing soft drink dispensers from schools; at the national level by ameliorating the obesogenic environment by abolishing advertising for unhealthy foods to very young children and by examining options such as taxing some foods (Caraher & Cowburn 2005); and, finally, at a global level, whereby trade legislation considers the public health implications of free trade, particularly in low-income countries (Hawkes 2005).

Conclusions

Food availability is often cited as potentially sufficient on a global basis, but the access by many is inadequate, leading to food insecurity at both family and community levels. Both socioeconomic and gender discrimination may play a role, as may culture and habit, but overwhelmingly poverty and inequity are the main causes of inadequate diets and health. Conversely, there is now overwhelming evidence that poverty is, in itself, a cause in the failure of some countries to develop economically. Other factors include geography, water, international trade laws and debt. Nevertheless, there has been a global response, one of which is the endorsement of all countries of the Millennium Development Goals, the first of which addresses poverty, hunger and undernutrition. At the same time, the evidence based on factors affecting child and maternal survival has increased the recognition that we do know what should be done. However, the interventions presume functioning health systems and adequate staffing, not to mention adequate supplies and infrastructure, and progress has been made with proven strategies.

Improvements in equity and gender equality will improve children's nutritional status. Women's education and women's status relative to men are the second and third main factors after food availability in child nutrition. Vitamin A supplementation programmes, for example, saved the lives of more than 350 000 children in 2003 alone. The global campaign to iodise salt is protecting 82 million newborns from iodine deficiency every year. The promotion by UNICEF and others of exclusive breastfeeding until the child reaches six months of age, and complementary feeding thereafter, has saved more than a million lives since 1990. In the meantime, as painfully slow progress is made in reducing undernutrition, another global epidemic, that of obesity, diabetes and other diet-related diseases, is adding another public health nutrition burden to those already most disadvantaged. This is a double burden that will tax individuals, health systems and governments increasingly. There needs to be a clear understanding of the problem, with governments willing to take strong measures to tackle it, and strong partnerships between civil society, community groups, and appropriate corporate sectors, to decrease global and national inequities and, above all, through the education and empowerment of families and communities so that they have the means to properly feed and care for their children and themselves.

REFERENCES

Aguayo, V.M., Baker, S.K. 2006, 'Vitamin A Deficiency and Child Survival in sub-Saharan Africa: A reappraisal of challenges and opportunities' in *Food Nutrition Bulletion*, vol. 26, pp. 348–55.

Balls, A. 2005, 'IMF approves debt relief for poorest countries' in *Financial Times*, 22 December, cited at <http://news.ft.com/cms/s/48388ce4-7279-11da-9ff7-0000779e2340. html> on 22 December.

Black, R., Morris, S. and Bryce, J. 2003, 'Where and why are 10 million children dying every year?' in *Lancet*, vol.361, pp. 2226–34.

Bloem, M.W., de Pee, S. and Darnton-Hill, I. 2004, 'Micronutrient deficiencies: first link in the chain of nutritional and health events in economic crises' in *Preventive Nutrition (vol 2): Primary and Secondary Preventive Nutrition* (2nd edition), Humana Press, Totowa, NJ.

Boutayeb, A. 2006, 'The double burden of communicable and non-communicable diseases in developing countries' in *Transactions of the Royal Society of Tropical Medicine and Hygiene*, vol. 100, pp. 191–9.

Brown, L.R. 2005, *Outgrowing the Earth: The food security challenge in an age of falling water tables and rising temperatures*, Earth Policy Institute, WW Norton & Co. New York, pp. 177–94.

Bryce, J. Arifeen, S. Bhutta, Z.A., Black, R.E., Claeson, M., Gillespie, D., Gwatkin, D.R., Habicht, J.P., Jones, G. Lanata, G.F., Morris, S.S., Mshina, N., Pariyo, G., Perkin, G., Schellenberg, J.A., Steketee, R.W., Trudsson, H. and Victora, G.G. 2006, 'Getting it right for children: A review of UNICEF joint health and nutrition strategy for 2006–15' in *Lancet*, vol. 368, pp. 817–19.

Caraher, M. and Cowburn, g. 2005, 'Taxing food: Implications for public health nutrition' in *Public Health Nutrition*, vol. 8, pp. 1242–49.

Chopra, M. and Darnton-Hill, I. 2006, 'Responding to the crisis in Sub-Saharan Africa: The role of nutrition' in *Public Health Nutrition* (in press).

Chopra, M. and Sanders, D. 2004, 'Child health and poverty', Save the Children CHIP Report No. 10, Child Poverty Research and Policy Centre, pp. 1–61.

Chopra, M., Darnton-Hill, I. 2004, 'Tobacco and obesity epidemics: Not so different after all?' in *British Medical Journal*, vol. 328, pp. 1558–60.

Cutter, J., Tan, B.Y. and Chew, S.K. 2001, 'Levels of cardiovascular disease risk factors in Singapore following a national intervention programme' in *Bulletin of World Health Organisation*, vol. 79, pp. 908–15.

Darnton-Hill, I., Nishida, C. and James, W.P.T. 2004, 'A life course approach to diet, nutrition and the prevention of chronic diseases' in *Public Health Nutrition*, vol. 7, pp. 101–21.

Darnton-Hill, I., Webb, P., Harvey, P.W.J., Hunt, J.M., Dalmiya, N., Chopra, M., Ball, M.J., Bloem, M.W., de Benoist, B. and Dalmiya, N. 2005, 'Micronutrient deficiencies and gender: Social and economic costs' in *American Journal of Clinical Nutrition*, vol. 819, pp. S1198–205.

Drèze, J. and Sen, A. 1989, *Hunger and Public Action*, Oxford University Press, Oxford.

—— 2002, *India: Participation and democracy*, Oxford University Press, Oxford.

Ebbeling, C.B., Pawlak, D.B. and Ludwig, D.S. 2002, 'Childhood obesity: Public-health crisis, commonsense cure' in *The Lancet*, vol. 360, pp. 473–82.

Editorial, 'A global famine' in *The Lancet*, p. 367.

Food and Agriculture Organization (FAO), *FAOSTAT 2004*, FAO of the United Nations, Rome, cited at <http://www.fao.org>.

Friedland, W.H. 1994, 'The new globalisation: The case of fresh produce' in Bonnano, A., Busch, L. and Friedland, W.H. (eds) 1994, *From Columbus to ConAgra: The globalisation of agriculture and food*, Kansas University Press, Lawrence.

Gillespie, S., McLachlan, M. and Shrimpton, R. 2003, *Combating Malnutrition: Time to act*, UNICEF, World Bank Washington, D.C.

Hawkes, C. 2005, 'The role of foreign direct investment in the nutrition transition' in *Public Health Nutrition*, vol. 8, pp. 357–65.

Institute for Agriculture and Trade Policy (US) 2004, *US dumping on world agricultural markets*, Institute for Agriculture and Trade Policy, Minnesota.

International Food Policy Research Institute (IFPRI) 2006, cited at <http://www.ifpri.org/>.

Jones, G., Steketee, R., Bhutta, Z. and Morris, S. and the Bellagio Child Survival Study Group 2006, 'How many child deaths can we prevent this year?' in *Lancet*, vol. 362, pp. 65–71.

Lawn, J.E., Cousens, S. and Zupan, J. for the Lancet Neonatal Survival Steering Team 2005, '4 million neonatal deaths: When? Where? Why?' in *The Lancet*, cited at <http://image.thelancet.com/extras/05art1073web.pdf>.

Mason, J. 2001, *Measuring Hunger and Malnutrition*, Tulane School of Public Health and Tropical Medicine, New Orleans.

Mason, J., Rivers, J. and Helwig, C. 2005, 'Recent trends in malnutrition in developing regions: Vitamin A deficiency, anemia, iodine deficiency, and child underweight' in *Food Nutrition Bulletin*, vol. 26, pp. 57–162.

Monteiro, C.A., Conde, W.L. and Popkin, B.M. 2004, 'The burden of disease from undernutrition and overnutrition in countries undergoing rapid nutrition transition: A view from Brazil' in *American Journal of Public Health*, vol. 94, pp. 433–34.

Popkin, B.M., Horton, S.H. and Kim, S. 2001, 'The nutrition transition and prevention of diet-related diseases in Asia and the Pacific' in *Food Nutrition Bulletin*, vol. 22, pp. S3–58.

Quinn, V.J., Guyon, A.B., Schubert, J.W., Stone-Jimenez, M., Hainsworth, M.D. and Martin, L.H. 2005, 'Improving breastfeeding practices on a broad scale at the community level: Success stories from Africa and Latin America' in *Journal of Human Lactation*, vol. 21, pp. 345–54.

Shetty, P. 2006, 'Achieving the goal of halving global hunger by 2015' in *Nutrition Society*, vol. 65, pp. 7–18.

Shrimpton, R., Victora, C.G., de Onis, M., Costa Lima, R., Blössner, M. and Clugston, G. 2001, 'Worldwide timing of growth faltering: implications for nutritional interventions' in *Paediatric*, vol. 107, pp. e75–82.

Tontisirin, K. and Winichagoon, P. 1997, 'Community-based programmes: Success factors for public nutrition derived from the experience of Thailand' in *Food Nutrition Bulletin*, vol. 20, pp. 323–35.

UNICEF, 1998, *Nutrition. State of the World's Children*, UNICEF, New York.

— 2006, *Progress for Children: A report card on nutrition*, UNICEF, New York, no. 4, pp. 1–33.

UNICEF/World Health Organization (WHO) 2004, *Low Birthweight: Country, regional and global estimates*, UNICEF, New York, WHO, Geneva.

United Nations Development Programme (UNDP) 2003, 'Millennium Development Goals: A compact among nations to end human poverty', Human Development Report, UNDP, New York.

United Nations Millennium Project, 2005, 'Who's got the power? Transforming health systems for women and children', Summary version of the report of the Task Force on Child Health and Maternal Health, UNDP, New York.

Wagstaff, A. and Watanabe, N. 2000, *Socioeconomic Inequality in Child Malnutrition in the Developing World: Health and population poverty* (working paper no. 2434), The World Bank, Washington, D.C.

Waters, E.B. and Baur, L.A. 2003, 'Childhood obesity: Modernity's scourge' in *Medical Journal of Australia*, vol. 178, pp. 422–3.

Webb, P. 2006, *World program nutrition policy papers*, World Food Program of the United Nations, Rome in *Food Nutrition Bulletin,* vol. 27, pp. 46–75, cited at <http://www.wfp.org/policies>.

World Bank 2006, 'Repositioning nutrition as central to development: A strategy for large-scale action', The World Bank/The International Bank for Reconstruction and Development, Directions in Development, Washington, D.C.

World Health Organization (WHO) 2003, *Obesity and overweight*, WHO, Geneva, cited at <http://www.who.int/met/obs.htm> on 13 April 2006.

— 2004, *5th report on the World Nutrition Situation*, The UN System Standing Committee on Nutrition, WHO, Geneva.

— 2006, *The double burden of malnutrition: A global agenda* (draft report), The UN System Standing Committee on Nutrition, 33rd Annual Session, WHO, Geneva, cited at <http://www.unsystem.org/scn/ Publications/AnnualMeeting/SCN33/33rd_ sessionagenda.htm> on 2 April.

World Health Organization (WHO)/Food and Agriculture Organization (FAO) 2003, *Diet, Nutrition and the Prevention of Chronic Diseases: Report of a Joint WHO/FAO Expert Consultation*, WHO Technical Report no.?916, WHO, Geneva.

11

Global developments in the food system

PHILIP MCMICHAEL

The twenty-first century is already marked by growing political tensions over the organisation of food provisioning. A central divide looms between localised systems of food provisioning and the ongoing construction of a 'world agriculture' of large-scale industrial monocultures of crops and livestock production managed by transnational corporations. While localised systems have the potential to remain embedded in local biological cycles that replenish soil by maintaining biotic diversity, and to connect with consumers, the global food system separates producers and consumers, reformulating agriculture as an input–output process abstracted from locality, increasingly dependent on chemical inputs and bio-engineered seeds, and vertically integrated through extensive global supply chains. This ecologically-disruptive system[1] yields a cornucopia of year-round food products, rendered durable to survive the 'food miles' to distant markets. However, it provisions only the 25 to 30 per cent of the world's population that can afford to purchase such relatively high-value food.

Local systems centre on questions of social and ecological sustainability, whereas the global system centres on questions of power and profitability. As such, the relationship between these two systems is increasingly adversarial. To the extent that the global food system represents a set of corporate empires, its trajectory involves the appropriation and/or incorporation of land, seeds, circuits of food, and farming knowledge as it brings more of the world's agri-culture under its control. In this context, small farming is experiencing a sustained crisis, symbolised by farmer suicides, and represented in extensive displacement of rural populations, new migrant labour circuits, and growing agrarian resistance movements. The latter resistances crystallise around the discourse of 'food sovereignty', which, in asserting the rights of farmers, citizens and nations to manage their food needs, challenges the corporate reconstruction and control of agricultures in the name of global food security. In short, global developments in the food system include significant social, political and ecological implications.

Food system globalisation

Food system globalisation is not a late-twentieth-century novelty. European expansion to the Orient and the Americas in the fifteenth century followed the pepper trade, anticipating the 'Columbian exchange', wherein Columbus brought wheat to the New World, and American maize and tomatoes and the Andean potato returned to Europe, which then introduced the potato into Africa and India. Today, Indians routinely dine on the potato as a staple, the tomato defines southern Italian pasta sauces, and their respective cuisines feature New World chillies and capsicums. Meanwhile, sugar circulated from Polynesia to Asia, to the Mediterranean, and back to the West Indies with Columbus. In the twentieth century, East Asia soyabean exports supplied expanding global needs for cooking oil and protein for livestock and vegetarians alike. Thus many diets and cuisines across the world are at one and the same time local and global.

Initially, the fruits of empire, as it were, included those well-known 'articles of pleasure' – the stimulants, tobacco, coffee, tea and sugar. As Mimi Sheller notes in *Consuming the Caribbean*, 'Contrary to the assumption that it was only the pursuit of gold and other precious metals that drove European exploration, it was as much the desire to acquire new edible, pleasurable, and pharmaceutical substances, things that had direct and powerful effects on the bodies of those empowered to consume them' (2003). Sheller quotes the Liverpool Maritime Museum: 'Much of the social life of Western Europe in the Eighteenth Century depended on the products of slave labour. In homes and coffee-houses, people met over coffee, chocolate, or tea, sweetened with Caribbean sugar.' She concludes: 'In consuming the Caribbean . . . Europe was itself transformed' (Sheller 2003).

In this way, the modern (western) diet depended historically on a (racialised) platform of monoculture, which became the model for agro-industrialisation, now organising the global food system. The globalisation of monoculture is perhaps best represented in the expansion of the beef culture.

The introduction of European cattle to the New World anticipated an agribusiness complex that now links specialised soyabean producers, feed-corn farmers, and lot-fed cattle across the world. The global beef complex is embedded in a series of commodity chains supplying animal protein to affluent consumers. Beef followed the lead of sugar, a formerly aristocratic food whose modern availability to the emerging European proletariat depended on a global system of slave plantations. In the nineteenth century, beef moved down the social scale from the aristocracy to the swelling urban classes who dined 'up' the food chain, consuming North American beef financed by British investors (Rifkin 1992). By the mid twentieth century, mass consumption subdivided the beef industry into lot-fed, high-value beef cuts, and grass-fed cattle supplying the cheaper, lean meat for the global fast-food industry. In this sense, beef has come to symbolise modernity and the representation of its social hierarchy in class-based diets.

The beef complex imposes monocultures on local ecologies, competing with the production of food staples like wheat, rice and beans. In this sense, diets have a political history framed by class, cultural and imperial relations. While animal protein consumption signals affluence and emulation of western diets, it bids resources away from staple, or 'peasant' foods. Movement up the food-chain hierarchy (from starch, to grain, to animal protein and vegetables) signifies modernity. Arguably, this hierarchy is as much a political construct as it is associated, as a 'nutrition transition', with the natural course of modernisation. Beef consumption legitimises political and corporate regimes – as exemplified in the World Bank's current sponsorship of the emerging domestic livestock revolution in China, and previous export strategies encouraged by development agencies in Central America to develop an offshore source of hamburger meat for US consumers in the 1960s to '80s. The food-chain hierarchy is also socially constructed through markets that routinely privilege the supply of affluent, over staple, foods. As wealthy consumers dine up on beef and shrimp, local peasants and fishermen, displaced by cattle pastures, shrimp farms and deteriorating coastal lands and mangroves, must depend on tenuous low-protein starchy diets (see, for example, Hall 2004).

Compounding the class and cultural impacts of globalised food, its technologies override locality with externally introduced inputs, emulating the outsourcing relationship that is endemic in manufacturing and service industries. The 'world steer' is one such globalised food, resembling the 'world car' (fabricated from globally sourced components). The world steer is produced with global inputs (standardised genetic lines and growth patterns) for global sale (standardised packaging).[2] This is a logical extension of mass production, where inputs, processes and outputs are reproducible in multiple locations.

For example, Brahman bulls (or bull semen) are imported into Central America from Florida and Texas, crossed with native *criollo* and fattened with imported African and South American pasture, producing a more pest- and heat-resistant, and beefier steer (Sanderson 1986). The global market is embedded in the life of the steer: animal health and growth depend on medicines, antibiotics, chemical fertilisers and herbicides sourced from elsewhere by transnational corporations, such as International Foods, United Brands and R.J. Reynolds.

While the slaughtered beef supplies a global fast-food industry, Central American peasants lose their hold on their customary mixed farming culture, as (commons) woodland have given way to pastures and *criollo* herds decline, reducing milk and meat supplies, in addition to side products such as tallow, cooking oil and leather for clothing and footwear (Sanderson 1986). In other words, food security for distant consumers in the form of cheap beef is gained at the expense of food sovereignty for local populations. This is now a common worldwide pattern, especially with the very recent supermarket revolution. Thus, the director-general of the Centre for International Forestry Research (CIFOR) noted: 'In the 1970s and the 1980s most of the meat from the Amazon was being produced by small ranchers selling to local slaughterhouses. Very large commercial ranchers linked to supermarkets are now targeting the whole of Brazil and the global market' (quoted in Vidal 2004). Huge ranching operations organised by European supermarkets dominate the beef export market (75 per cent of Brazil's beef exports flow to Europe and the Middle East). According to a 2005 Food and Agriculture Organization report, cattle-ranching is the main cause of deforestation in Latin America (Nierenberg 2005).

The beef complex is subdivided into two branches corresponding to class divisions among modern consumers: extensive cattle grazing for low-value lean meat for hamburgers, and intensive lot feeding for high-value specialty cuts. The latter branch has also globalised as transnational meat-packing firms have consolidated their global empire. Thus, the two largest Japanese meatpackers, Nippon and Itoham Foods, have invested in United States and Australian ranchland, feedlots and meatpacking plants, importing their own processed meat (boxed beef) for Japanese consumption (Tozanli 2005; McMichael 2000). And, while United States and Australian beef exports to Northeast Asia are predominantly high-value, grain-fed, chilled beef cuts, hamburger meat accounts for three-quarters of Australian beef exports to the United States (Pritchard 2006).

Corporate-led factory farming is the new model of development in the food sector — currently targeting Argentina, Brazil, China, India, Mexico, Pakistan, the Philippines, South Africa, Taiwan and Thailand — and accounting for 74 per cent of global poultry products, 50 per cent of pork, 43 per cent of beef and 68 per cent of eggs (Nierenberg 2005). Asia, whose global consumer class outstrips that of North America and Europe combined (French 2004), leads the livestock revolution, driven by the identification of development with animal protein consumption. 'Beefing up' has been a long-standing legacy of the British empire, now reproduced through the corporate empire (Rifkin 1992). Two-thirds of the global expansion of meat consumption is in the global South, sourced with soyabeans from Brazil. As the Chinese middle class emerges, prioritising an animal protein diet, China has transformed from a net exporter of soyabeans to the world's largest importer of whole soyabeans and oils – even Brazilian pastures are converted to soyabean fields, pushing cattle herds deeper into the Amazon (Rohter 2003). Meanwhile, in its recent report, 'Eating up the Amazon,' Greenpeace says that 'Europe buys half the soya exported from the Amazon state of Matto Grosso, where 90 per cent of rainforest soya is grown. Meat reared on rainforest soya finds its way onto supermarket shelves and fast-food counters across Europe' (2006).

Global meatpackers raise animal protein on feedstuffs supplied by their own grain marketing subsidiaries (and often partners for regional influence). For example, the world's largest grain trader, Cargill, with operations in more than 70 countries, established a joint venture with Japan's Nippon Meat Packers, called Sun Valley Thailand, which exports corn-fed poultry to Japanese consumers (Heffernam & Constance 1994). Michael Pollan, who claims factory farming is the progeny of cheap supplies of corn and soyabeans, observes 'a Chicken McNugget is corn upon corn upon corn, beginning with corn-fed chicken all the way through the obscure food additives and the corn starch that holds it together. All the meat at McDonald's is really corn. Chickens have become machines for converting two pounds of corn into one pound of chicken' (Pollan 2002).

Factory farming, depending on its specialised feed inputs, expands its supply chains across the world. Tyson Foods, the largest meat and poultry company in the world, has operations in Argentina, Brazil, China, India, Indonesia, Japan, Mexico, the Netherlands, the Philippines, Russia, Spain, the United Kingdom, and Venezuela (Neirenberg 2005). It partners, for example, with the Japanese firm C. Itoh to produce poultry in Mexico for local consumers and for export to Japan. Smithfield Foods is the largest pig producer and pork processor in the world, with operations in Canada, China, Mexico and Europe (Neirenberg 2005). ConAgra owns more than 50 companies and operates in more than two dozen countries, processing feed and animal protein products in the United States, Canada, Australia, Europe, the Far East, and Latin America (*The Economist* 1995).

The Thai-based Charoen Pokphand (CP) Group dominates the Asian live-stock complex, founded on a lucrative vertically integrated poultry industry, providing inputs (chicks, feed, medicines, credit, and extension services) to farmers under contract and, in turn, processing and marketing poultry products domestically and regionally. Its recently formed Charoen Pokphand Foods focuses on animal feed and livestock products (poultry, pigs, ducks, cattle and shrimp). CP is the world's largest producer of farmed shrimp, which it has expanded through joint ventures into Indonesia, Vietnam, China and India (in part because these are cheaper, and less ecologically problematic, sites), and it produces poultry in Turkey, Vietnam, China, Cambodia, Malaysia, Indonesia, and the United States, as well as animal feed in Indonesia, Vietnam, China and India. In 2001, CP operated 100 feed mills in China, and has integrated forward into fast-food (KFC and now Chester's Grill), and retailing outlets such as 7-Eleven stores in Thailand and Lotus Supermarkets in China (Goss et al. 2000; Burch & Goss 2005).

In transforming the food landscape, corporate-led factory farming deepens a bio-war against the environment (including animals) and the human body.[3] In the United States, for example, 'animal factories produce 1.3 billion tons of manure each year. Laden with chemicals, antibiotics, and hormones, the manure leaches into rivers and water tables, polluting drinking water supplies and causing fish kills in the tens of millions' (Kimbrell 2002). This ecological crisis includes direct impacts on human health: 'animals in cramped conditions easily catch and transmit bacteria, which may then be passed to humans. Farmers routinely use antibiotics to combat infectious diseases, but in so doing may be contributing to growing antibiotic resistance among humans' (Millstone & Lang 2003). The global threat of an avian flu pandemic is deepened by the ecology of rising densities of urban populations and factory farming systems, and transnational human mobility. The spread of factory farming is ironically intensified by East and South-East Asian governments' attempts to control virus outbreaks by culling backyard chicken flocks, privileging corporate chicken factories (GRAIN 2006). 'Although poultry conglomerates claim their industrial farming is impregnable to viral outbreaks and epidemics, factory farming is more likely to maximise the accumulation of viral load and subsequent antigenic drift . . . In an epidemiological sense, the outdoor flocks are the fuse, and the dense factory populations, the explosive charge' (Davis 2005).

Global food retailing trends

Typically, livestock processors have vertically integrated from processing upstream into production of meats and grains, but rarely downstream into retailing (other than producing prepared meals). As relative latecomers, CP, and its neighbour, the Salim Group (Indonesia's largest conglomerate, regionally dominant in instant noodles), counterpoint this trend by controlling retail outlets (and also by integrating horizontally into other sectors, such as telecommunications, real estate, petrochemicals). In other words, these regional conglomerates signal significant shifts in the balance of power in the global food system. On the one hand, horizontal integration involves multi-product conglomerates (the top three being Nestlé, Philip Morris and Unilever) expanding into food products easily duplicated and standardised in emerging markets, such as dairy products, biscuits, baked goods, beer and spirits, and confectionery (Tozanli 2005). On the other hand, global retailing, now dominated by European-based TNCs, Tesco (UK), Ahold (Netherlands) and Carrefour (France), is dramatically remaking food processing and farming practices to meet increasingly private 'quality' standards.

The supermarket revolution is currently playing out in the global South, where small, independent producers, and local 'wet' markets and street vending are incorporated into new corporate circuits of production and marketing. In the 1990s, Latin America experienced an expansion in supermarket retailing at a growth rate five times that in the United States, now accelerating across Asia. In Latin America, Ahold, Carrefour and Wal-Mart account for 70 to 80 per cent of the top-five supermarket chains, centralising procurement from farmers across the region (and their own global processing operations), and serving regional customers (Regmi & Gehlhar 2005). As above, the incorporation of farmers into corporate empires has contradictory consequences. In Guatemala, where supermarkets now control 35 per cent of food retailing, it was reported that 'their sudden appearance has brought unanticipated and daunting challenges to millions of struggling, small farmers' — especially tenuous relations in the absence of binding contractual agreements, rewarded only if they consistently meet new quality standards, but subject to declining prices as retailers have virtually unlimited suppliers (Dugger 2004). Meanwhile, urban diets converge on a narrowing base of staple grains, increasing consumption of animal protein, edible oils, salt and sugar, and declining dietary fibre, as consumption of brand-named processed and store-bought foods rises, contributing to an increasing prevalence of non-communicable (dietary) diseases and obesity (Kennedy et al. 2004). Across the world, North and South, this 'nutrition transition' is contributing to the rising incidence of obesity, described by the World Health Organization as 'one of the greatest neglected public health problems of our time' (quoted in Gardner & Halweil 2000).

The broad patterns in the global consolidation of retailing have been documented as follows: in the early to mid 1990s, much of South America and East

Asia (other than China and Japan), Northern–Central Europe, and South Africa saw the average share of supermarkets in food retailing grow from roughly only 10 to 20 per cent (1990) to 50 to 60 per cent by the early 2000s. (For comparison, in 2005, supermarkets have a 70 to 80 per cent share in food retail in the United States, United Kingdom and France.) Within those regions, in the mid 1990s, a second set of countries, in which super-marketisation reached 50 per cent of food retail, were Costa Rica, Chile, South Korea, the Philippines and Thailand. A 'second wave' incorporated parts of South-East Asia, Central America and Mexico, and Southern–Central Europe, where the share rose from 5 to 10 per cent in 1990 to 30 to 50 per cent by the early 2000s, and then a 'third wave,' reaching 10 to 20 per cent of food retail by 2003, occurred in parts of Africa (especially Kenya), remaining parts of Central and South America and South-East Asia, and China, India and Russia — these last three being the current frontrunner destinations for retail foreign domestic investment (FDI) (Reardon & Timmer 2005).

The supermarket, or retailing, revolution marks an important dimension of food system globalisation, namely, it involves a significant restructuring of domestic food markets (where typically about 85 per cent of food consumption locates). While trade in processed foods such as juice, baked goods, snacks, meats and beverages exploded between 1980 from 18 per cent of global food trade to 34 per cent in 2000 (Regmi & Gehlar 2001), this is 'eclipsed by growth in sales by foreign subsidiaries of developed country firms to consumers in developing countries; for example, local sales by foreign subsidiaries of US processed food firms are five times the exports of processed food from the US to the rest of the world' (Reardon & Timmer 2005).

Distinguishing domestic sales by foreign subsidiaries from internationally traded foods is, however, only to draw attention to the consequences of structural adjustment and liberalisation policies over the past two decades, which have institutionally strengthened the freedom of movement of agribusiness firms across national borders. This has resulted in a flood of FDI in domestic foods: 'in 1980, total FDI was roughly US$1 billion a year into Asia, and the same in Latin America; agrifood investments followed this general pattern for total FDI. By 1990, the amount was roughly US$10 billion a year into each of these two regions that were forerunners in globalisation. By 2000, the figure was US$80 to 90 billion' (Reardom & Timmer 2005). In other words, the World Trade Organisation (WTO) regime has institutionalised and enabled the international consolidation of retailing, whereby global firms acquire local chains. Thus, the Dutch firm, Royal Ahold, now owns 50 per cent of La Fragua supermarkets in Central America (Busch & Bain 2004), and, for example, in 2002 six global retailers (British Tesco,

French Carrefour and Casino, Dutch Ahold and Makro, and Belgian Food Lion) invested US$120 million in Thailand alone, while WalMart invested US$600 million in Mexican supermarket development (Reardon & Timmer 2005).

In addition, supermarkets are not simply consolidating market power, they are reformulating it, by integrating backwards to manage own brand food manufacturing, displacing traditional brand manufacturers (like Heinz, Nestlé) and coordinating 'just-in-time' foods. In the United Kingdom, as the advance guard of this trend, supermarket own brand products comprise about 95 per cent of the market for chilled ready meals. As Burch and Lawrence (2005) note:

> partly in order to control and manage a production and distribution system that is logistically increasingly sophisticated and complex, the supermarkets have reconfigured the supply chains for their own brand lines, by underwriting the establishment of new agri-food manufacturing companies which *are* flexible, adaptable and innovative, and which produce nothing but own brand products for the UK and overseas supermarkets.

Within this shifting balance of power in the global food system, oligopolistic retailers have come to compete less in price terms and more in terms of variety, convenience, quality, and year-round supply (Busch & Bain 2004). In other words, private standards have become a competitive advantage, conferring legitimacy on retailers as 'market-based authorities' (Dixon 2002), and are now a significant new vector in the global food production complex. The WTO regulation of trade relations is increasingly complemented by a far-reaching private regulation of production standards, regarding quality, food safety, packaging and convenience. It is integral to the centralisation of retailing capital, and the dual imperatives of satisfying quality demands of relatively affluent consumers and replacing smallholding by global/factory farms in order to realise those standards (Dolan & Humphrey 2000). Thus, in Kenya, where 90 per cent of horticulture is destined for Europe (especially the United Kingdom), the shift away from smallholder-contract production to centralised employment on farms and in packhouses depends upon an extensive female migrant labour force, performing off-farm labour to maintain their households (Dolan 2004). Similarly, the Mexican *agro-maquila*, producing tomatoes, avocadoes, melons and so on for the North American market, depends on a migrant labour force of indigenous peasant women (Barndt 2002).

The standards revolution marks a change in the conventions of capitalism, whereby 'good agricultural practices' underlie certification schemes within EurepGAP, an association of European supermarket chains concerned with regulating quality, safety, environment and labour standards surpassing publicly required standards (Busch & Bain 2004; Campbell 2005). However, the standards revolution involves selective appropriation by food corporations of social movement demands for environmental, food safety, animal welfare and fair trade relations, with the potential of deepening social inequality globally (at the expense of peasants and poor consumers) as private regulation displaces public responsibilities (Friedmann 2005).

The global food regime

Arguably, the livestock revolution (including factory farming and its specialised feed supply chains) and the retailing revolution are central dynamics in the global food system today. But they depend on important institutional relations, which underlie the global food regime: from the mode of regulating 'green' standards in corporate food supply chains (Friedmann 2005) to the political reconstruction of world agriculture (McMichael 2005).

While the reconstruction of world agriculture includes the standards revolution,[4] it rests on a corporate foundation of agro-industrialisation, enhanced by WTO rules. The WTO's Agreement on Agriculture (1995) outlaws artificial price support via trade restrictions, production controls, and state trading boards. While members from the global South are required to open their farm sectors, those from the global North have been allowed to retain huge subsidies, producing a 'comparative advantage' by generating the lowest prices for (their) farm commodities in history. Decoupling subsidies from prices removes the price floor, effectively establishing a 'world price' for agricultural commodities. Prices for the major commodities in world trade fell 30 per cent or more since 1994, and are at an all-time low for the last century and a half (Ritchie 1999; *The Economist* 1999). This world price engineered through the Quad's (United States, European Union, Canada and Japan) domestic support policies is not considered 'artificial', and yet it threatens all farmers through the global dumping of cheapened foods (Peine & McMichael 2005).

The impact of this lowered world price is enabled by a WTO rule eliminating the right to a national strategy of self-sufficiency. The dumping of food surpluses decimates Southern rural cultures, as small farmers are unable to compete with falling prices for farm products. Meanwhile, 60 per cent of global food stocks are in corporate hands, six of which control 70 per cent of the world's grain trade. The United States accounts for 70 per cent of world corn exports, 70 per cent of which are controlled by two corporations, Cargill, and Archer Daniel Midlands. Thus, in the latter half of the 1990s, food deficit states experienced a 20 per cent rise in food bills, despite record low prices (Murphy 1999). And, for example, after thousands of years of food security based in its original maize culture, Mexico was transformed by North American Free Trade Associaion-style liberalisation into a food-deficit country, importing yellow corn from the United States, at the expense of almost two million *campesinos* (Carlsen 2003), and exporting fruits and vegetables from corporate plantations. Articulating the free-trade version of food security, Cargill's chairman observed: 'There is a mistaken belief that the greatest agricultural need in the developing world is to develop the capacity to grow food for local consumption. This is misguided. Countries should produce what they produce best – and trade' (quoted in Lynas 2001).

This corporate regime rests on the displacement of staple food crops with exports – whether dumped on the world market, or installed locally as a development strategy. Agro-food export strategies typically divide between corporate plantations and small-holder contract farming. The commercial agricultural complex is fast-changing, using information technology and mobile phones to link to commodity markets, and seeking production niches in a volatile global marketplace – where retail markets include a proliferation of specialty products targeted at the new quality standards of the global market (Long & Roberts 2005). Thus, Brazil's Sao Francisco Valley is the site of the 'new agrarian districts', exporting mangoes, grapes, tomatoes, and acerola – 50 per cent overseas (25 per cent under contract with French retail giant, Carrefour), and 50 per cent to corporate retailers in Brazilian cities (Marsden 2003). For Latin America, fruit and vegetables accounted for 27 per cent of its major agricultural exports (oilseeds at 32 per cent) in 2000 (Long & Roberts 2005).

Export platforms are tenuous development strategies in terms of income generation or food security because of global dependencies, as demonstrated in Jasper Goss's (2002) research on the conversion of Thailand to a high-value agro-food export platform for chicken, shrimp, seafood and fresh fruit. Bill Pritchard and David Burch's (2003) fieldwork on Thai contract farming for the international processing tomato industry confirms that long-term volatilities override short-term gains to producers. But the extant producers are not the only ones affected. Within the global shrimp economy, for example, the average shrimp farm provides fifteen jobs on the farm and 50 security jobs around the farm, while shrimp culture displaces 50 000 people through loss of land, traditional fishing and agriculture. One Filipino fisherman observed: 'The shrimp live better than we do. They have electricity, but we don't. The shrimp have clean water, but we don't. The shrimp have lots of food, but we are hungry' (quoted in Tilford 2004).

The point is that agro-exporting, while located increasingly in the global

South, is part of a corporate agricultural complex linked through global supply chains producing high-value 'food from nowhere' (Bové & Defour 2001), often at the expense of rural cultures. And, as trade rules deepen access to cheaper land and labour, it has become profitable for corporations to outsource agriculture – especially when the differential between the value (in US$) of a square metre of New Jersey farmland and that of Brazilian virgin timberland is 1.98 to 0.005, respectively (WorldWatch 2006). Recent Common Agricultural Policy reform, introducing 'multi-functionality' to reward agriculture's non-remunerative services (environment, space, rural habitation, food safety and animal welfare) has generated a movement towards de-localisation of agricultural production to preserve the European environment, while importing food from offshore regions with low wages and weak environmental regulations – which Doux, France and Europe's foremost poultry producer, accomplished by acquiring Frangosul, the fourth-largest poultry producer in Brazil, where production costs undercut those in France by two-thirds (Herman & Kuper 2003).[5] In Chile, the largest supplier of off-season fruits and vegetables to Europe and North America, food cropping in beans, wheat and other staples has declined by more than a third, as plantations controlled by five food corporations have displaced local farmers into the casual labour force. Across Latin America, while 90 per cent of agricultural research was devoted to food crops in the 1980s, during the 1990s export crops commanded 80 per cent of research expenditures (Madeley 2000). Whether squeezed by agro-export promotion policies, or by food dumping, between 20 and 30 million people have lost their land under the impact of trade liberalisation (Madeley 2000). Dispossessed peasants enter new, global circuits where they labour overseas, produce food for spatially and socially distant consumers, or migrate to the cities, looking for work. While 2006 is the tipping point for the world's urban population to exceed its rural population, the United Nations reports that 43 per cent of the population of the global South now lives in urban slums (Vidal 2003).

In this reconfiguration of world agriculture, we might say that the comparative advantage of the global South is its under-consumption, while that of the global North is its over-consumption. In fact, there are now roughly 1.2 billion people malnourished, *either way*, in each region, respectively (Gardner & Halweil 2000). That is, artificially low agricultural commodity prices serve the grain traders who dump surpluses overseas, and the food processors who supersize fast foods. In sum, the global food regime implicates populations across the world in a relationship that produces 'hunger amidst abundance' (Araghi 1999), either pole represented by ill-health.

Conclusion

The paradox of the global food system, in generating foods that reproduce the wealth/poverty relation, is the context for growing contention between agro-industrialisation and the (re)localisation of food systems, championed by the principle of food sovereignty. Food sovereignty movements aspire to an alternative, decentralised understanding of food security in which material want–satisfaction is not subordinated to the market, but embedded in ecological principles of community and environmental sustainability. The food sovereignty principle was first articulated at the World Food Summit in 1996 by the *Via Campesina*, which includes 97 farm organisations representing millions of farming families from 43 countries (Desmarais 2003).

Food sovereignty, in the *Via Campesina* vision, would subordinate trade relations to the question of access to credit, land and fair prices, to be set politically via the rules of fair trade to be negotiated in UN Conference on Trade and Development and not at the WTO, with active participation of farmers' movements in building democratic agricultural and food policies. While the consumer movement discovers that 'eating has become a political act', *Via Campesina* adds: 'producing quality products for our own people has also become a political act . . . this touches our very identities as citizens of this world' (Seattle Declaration 1999). The *Via Campesina* vision is for 'the right of peoples, communities and countries to define their own agricultural, labour, fishing, food and land policies that are ecologically, socially, economically and culturally appropriate to their unique circumstances' (quoted in Ainger 2003).

On the other side of the world, and the class divide, the slow food movement, originating in Italy (but now global), builds on similar principles: localising foodsheds, retaining local cuisines, and protecting food heritage in general. The Slow Food Foundation for Biodiversity was formed in Italy in 2003, to 'know, catalogue and safeguard small quality productions and to guarantee them an economic and commercial future'. In relation to this, COOP-Italia, a consortium with more than 200 consumer cooperatives, coordinates production and sale of quality food products traceable to their socio-spatial origins, with the aim of protecting links between consumers and producers, within a broader ethical engagement that includes supporting fair trade initiatives, water provisioning, and contesting diffusion of genetically-modified organisms (Fonte 2006).

By concluding on a note of optimism, this essay draws attention to the extraordinary social activism emerging around the paradox of the global food system, namely its ability to generate food surpluses, whose content and distribution nevertheless contribute to the growing unsustainability of rural communities and environments. Unless we reduce food miles and relocalise food systems, we surrender stewardship of the natural world to the short-term and predatory perspective of the market. In this sense, Colin Duncan's warning that 'agriculture must become our environmental monitor' (1996) revalues food's role as a vector of sustainability rather than a convenience.

NOTES

1   As Anthony J. McMichael notes: '. . . ongoing trends in agricultural activity may cause more global environmental damage over coming decades than will "new" changes such as global climate change. Already, approximately one-third of the world's fertile soil is moderately or severely damaged by erosion, salination, water-logging, chemicalisation, loss of organic material and compaction. The spread of irrigation typically exacerbates alienation and water-logging. It is also depleting many of the world's great aquifers . . . (2005b).

2   Bill Pritchard points out that the 'world steer' metaphor is complicated by trade politics, quarantine and environmental considerations, and these feature at present in the spectacular rise (and competitive potential) of Brazilian fresh and frozen beef exports, which is related to the opening of the Amazon frontier, depreciation of the Brazilian *real*, and progress in combating foot-and-mouth-disease (2006).

3   For example, 'Fish farming is . . . generally intensive, and incurs a range of health and environmental costs. Fish farms are also subject to blanket use of antibiotics and other growth promoters. Further, it is not in any way a contained system, but enables the flow of excess nutrients, drugs, waste and genes into surrounding water and wild populations' (McMichael 2005a).

4   Future reconstruction of world agriculture is likely to include a deepening of the 'gene revolution'. Genetic engineering of foods, rationalised as essential to global food security, replaces biodiversity with uniformity based on the control of the biology of agronomic species, via corporate intellectual property rights institutionalised in the WTO. The resulting genetic erosion contributes to an ecological crisis: 'the U.S. soy crop, which accounts for 75 per cent of the world's soy, is a monoculture that can be traced back to only six plants brought over from China . . . of the seventy-five kinds of vegetables grown in the United States, 97 per cent of all the varieties have become extinct in less than eighty years agriculture' (Rifkin 1998). Vandana Shiva warns of 'a clear narrowing of the genetic basis of our food supply. Currently, there are only two commercialised staple food crops. In place of hundreds of legumes and beans eaten around the world, there is soybean. In place of diverse varieties of millets, wheats, and rices, there is only corn. In place of the diversity of oil seeds, there is only canola' (2000).

5   Relocation of agriculture is enabled by the phenomenon of 'food miles'. Food transport, the cost of which fell 70 per cent for sea freight between 1980 and 2000 and for air freight falls 3 to 4 per cent annually, 'is one of the fastest-growing sources of greenhouse gas emissions' (Millstone & Lang 2003). National accounting systems do not include emissions resulting from international air and sea freight, and, accordingly, they are absent from the Kyoto Protocol targets. As a result, a damaging amount of 'food swapping' exacerbates the 'food miles'

problem, exemplified in the milk trade: 'Until recently most people consumed milk produced locally, but from 1961 to 1999 there was a five-fold increase in milk exports, with many countries both importing and exporting large quantities, resulting in millions of extra food miles' (Millstone & Lang 2003: 66). Analogous to the extension of the Southern land frontier for offshore food production, is the rising fossil fuel consumption involved in the global fishing industry, especially as fish stocks deteriorate.

REFERENCES

Ainger, K. 2003, 'The New Peasants' Revolt' in *New Internationalist*, no. 353, pp. 9–13.

Araghi, F. 1999, 'The great global enclosure of our times: Peasants and the agrarian question at the end of the twentieth century' in Magdoff F., Foster, J.B. and Buttel, F.H. (eds) 1995, *Hungry for Profit: The agribusiness threat to farmers, food and the environment*, Monthly Review Press, New York, pp. 145–60.

Barndt, D. 2002, *Tangled Routes: Women, work and globalization on the tomato trail*, Garamond Press, Aurora, ON.

Bové, J. and Francois D. 2001, *The World Is Not For Sale*, Verso, London.

Burch, D. and Geoffrey L. 2005, 'Supermarket own brands, supply chains and the transformation of the agri-food system' in *International Journal of Sociology of Agriculture and Food*, vol. 13, no. 1, pp. 1–18.

Burch, D. and Jasper G. 2005, 'Regionalization, globalization, and nultinational agribusiness: A comparative perspective from Southeast Asia' in Rama R. (ed.) 2005, *Multinational Agribusinesses*, Food Products Press, New York, pp. 6, 329.

Busch, L. and Bain, C. 2004, 'New! Improved? The transformation of the global agrifood system' in *Rural Sociology*, vol. 69, no. 3, pp. 321–46.

Campbell, H. 2005, 'The rise and rise of EurepGAP: European (re)invention of colonial rood relations?' in *International Journal of Sociology of Agriculture and Food*, vol. 13, no. 2, pp. 1–19.

Carlsen, L. 2003, 'The Mexican Farmers' Movement: Exposing the myths of free trade' in *Americas Program Policy Report*, Inter-hemispheric Resource Center, Silver City (NM), cited at <http://www.americaspolicy.org>.

Davis, M. 2005, *The Monster at our Door: The global threat of avian flu*, The New Press, New York & London, pp. 107–08.

Desmarais, A.A. 2003, *The Via Campesina: Peasants resisting globalization*, Ph.D. dissertation, University of Calgary, p. 2.

Dixon, J. 2002, *The Changing Chicken: Chooks, cooks and culinary culture*, University of New South Wales Press, Sydney, p. 155.

Dolan, C. 2004, 'On farm and packhouse: Employment at the bottom of a global value chain' in *Rural Sociology*, vol. 69, no. 1, pp. 99–126.

Dolan, C. and Humphrey, J. 2000, 'Governance and trade in fresh vegetables: The impact of UK supermarkets on the African horticulture industry' in *Journal of Development Studies*, vol. 37, pp. 147–76.

Dugger, C.W. 2004, 'Supermarket giants crush Central American farmers' in *The New York Times*, December 28, pp. A1, A10.

Duncan, C. 1996, *The Centrality of Agriculture: Between humankind and the rest of nature*, McGill-Queen's University Press, Montreal & Kingston, p. 44.

Economist, The, 1999, 'A raw deal for commodities', April 15.

Fonte, M. 2006, 'Slow foods presidia: What do small producers do with big retailers?' in *Between the Local and the Global: Confronting complexity in the contemporary agri-food sector*, Marsden, T. and Murdoch, J. (eds) 2006, *Research in Rural Sociology and Development*, vol. 12, Elsevier, Oxford.

French, H. 2004, 'Linking globalization, consumption and governance' in Starke, L. (ed.) 2004, *State of the World 2004: The consumer society*, The WorldWatch Institute, Washington D.C.

Friedmann, H. 2005, 'From colonialism to green capitalism: Social movements and emergence of food regimes' in Buttel, F.H. and McMichael, P. (eds) 2005, *New Directions in the Sociology of Global Development*, Elsevier, Oxford, pp. 229–68.

Gardner, G. and Halweil, B. 2000, *Underfed and Overfed: The global epidemic of malnutrition*, World-watch Paper 150, WorldWatch Institute, Washington, DC, pp. 7, 13.

Goss, J. 2002, 'Fields of inequality: The waning of national developmentalism and the political economy of agribusiness in Siam', Ph.D. Thesis, Griffith University.

Goss, J., Burch, D. and Rickson, R. 2000, 'Agri-Food restructuring and Third World transnationals: Thailand, the CP Group and the global shrimp industry' in *World Development*, vol. 28, no. 3, pp. 513–30.

GRAIN 2006, 'The top-down response to bird flu', cited at <http://www.grain.org/ articles/?id=12> in April.

Greenpeace 2006, '*Eating up the Amazon*', cited at <www.greenpeace.org/international/press/ reports/eating-up-the-amazon>

Hall, D. 2004, 'Explaining the diversity of Southeast Asian shrimp aquaculture' in *Journal of Agrarian Change*, vol. 4, no. 3, pp. 315–35.

Heffernan, W.D. and Constance, D.H. 1994, 'Transnational corporations and the globalization of the food systems' in Bananno, A., Busch, L., Friedland, W., Gonvela, L. and Minigione E. (eds) 1994, *From Columbus to ConAgra: The globalization of agriculture and food*, Press of Kansas, Lawrence.

Herman, P. and Kuper, R. 2003, *Food for Thought: Towards a future for farming*, Pluto Press, London, pp. 21–22.

Kennedy, G., Nantel, G. and Shetty, P. 2004, 'Globalization of food systems in developing countries: a synthesis of country case studies' in *Globalization of food systems in developing countries: Impact on food security and nutrition*, Food and Agriculture Organization (FAO) Food and Nutrition Paper no. 83, FAO, Rome, pp. 1–26.

Kimbrell, A. 2002, *The Fatal Harvest Reader: The tragedy of industrial agriculture*, Island Press, Washington, p. 16.

Long, N. and Roberts, B. 2005, 'Changing rural scenarios and research agendas in Latin America in the new century' in Buttel, F.H. and McMichael P. (eds) 2005, *New Directions in the Sociology of Global Development*, Elsevier, Oxford, pp. 55–89.

Lynas, M. 2001, 'Selling Starvation' in *Corporate Watch*, vol. 7, Spring.

Madeley, J. 2000, *Hungry for Trade*, Zed Books, London & New York, pp. 54–55, 75.

Marsden, T. 2003, *The Condition of Rural Sustainability*, Van Gorcum, Wageningen, pp. 30, 57.

McMichael, A.J. 2005a, 'Meat consumption trends and health: Casting a wider risk assessment net' in *Public Health Nutrition*, vol. 8, no. 4, pp. 341–43.

—— 2005b, 'Integrating nutrition with ecology: Balancing the health of humans and biosphere' in *Public Health Nutrition*, vol. 8, no. 6A, pp. 706–15.

McMichael, P. 2000, 'A global interpretation of the rise of the East Asian food import complex' in *World Development*, vol. 28, no. 3, pp. 409–24.

—— 2005, 'Global development and the corporate food regime' in Buttel F.H. and McMichael, P. 2005, *New Directions in the Sociology of Global Development*, Elsevier, Oxford, pp. 269–303.

Millstone, E. and Lang, T. 2003, *The Atlas of Food*, Earthscan Publications, London.

Murphy, S. 1999, 'WTO, agricultural deregulation and food security' in *Globalization Challenge Initiative 4*, cited at <http://www.foreign policy-infocus.org/briefs/vol4n34wto_ body.html> on 24 December.

Nierenberg, D. 2005, *Happier Meals: Rethinking the global meat industry*, WorldwWatch Paper 171, WorldWatch Institute, Washington, D.C., pp. 12, 58.

Peine, E. and McMichael, P. 2005, 'Globalization and Governance' in Higgins, V. and Lawrence G. (eds) 2005, *Agricultural Regulation*, Routledge, London.

Pollan, M. 2002, 'The life of a steer' in *The New York Times*, 31 March.

Pritchard, B. 2006, 'The political construction of free trade visions: The geo-politics and geo-economics of Australian beef exporting' in *Agriculture and Human Values*, vol. 23, pp. 37–50.

Pritchard, B. and Burch, D. 2003, *Agri-Food Globalization in Perspective: International restructuring in the processing tomato industry*, Ashgate, Aldershot.

Reardon, T. and Timmer, C.P. 2005, 'Transformation of markets for agricultural output in developing countries since 1950: How has thinking changed?' in Evenson, R.E., Pingali, P. and Schultz, T.P. (eds) 2005, *Handbook of Agricultural Economics: Agricultural development; farmers, farm production and farm markets*, Elsevier Press, Oxford, pp. 28, 30, 35–37.

Regmi, A. and Gehlhar, M. 2001, 'Consumer preferences and concerns shape global food trade' in *Food Review*, vol. 24, no. 3, pp. 2–8.

—— 2005, 'Processed Food Trade Pressured by Evolving Global Supply Chains' in *Amber Waves*, Economic Research Service/USDA, vol. 3, no. 1, pp. 12–19.

Rifkin, J. 1992, *Beyond Beef: The rise and fall of the cattle culture*, Penguin, New York.

—— 1998, *The Biotech Century: Harnessing the gene and remaking the world*, Tarcher/Putnam, New York.

Ritchie, M. 1999, 'The World Trade Organization and the Human Right to Food Security', Presentation to the International Cooperative Agriculture Organization General Assembly, Quebec City, 29 August, cited at <http://www.wtowatch.org>.

Rohter, L. 2003, 'Relentless foe of the Amazon jungle: Soybeans' in *New York Times*, 17 September, p. 3.

Sanderson, S. 1986, 'The emergence of the 'World Steer': Internationalization and foreign domination in Latin American cattle production' in Tullis F.L. and Hollist, W.L. (eds) 1986, *Food, the State and International Political Economy*, University of Nebraska Press, Lincoln.

Seattle Declaration 1999, cited at <http://viacampesina.org/main_en/index.php> on 3 September.

Sheller, M. 2003, *Consuming the Caribbean*, Routledge, New York, pp. 71, 81.

Shiva, V. 2000, *Stolen Harvest: The hijacking of the global food supply*, South End Press, Boston, p. 95.

Tilford, D. 2004, 'Behind the scenes: Shrimp' in *State of the World 2004*, WorldWatch Institute, Washington, D.C., p. 93.

Tonzanli, S. 2005, 'The rise of global enterprises in the world's food chain' in Ruth R. (ed.) 2005, *Multinational Agribusinesses*, Food Products Press, New York, pp. 24,16.

Vidal, J. 2003, 'Beyond the city limits' in *Guardian Weekly*, 17–23 September, pp. 17–18.

—— 2004, 'Demand for beef speeds destruction of Amazon forest' in *Guardian Weekly*, April, p. 3.

WorldWatch 2006, 'Valuing the Earth' in WorldWatch, vol. 19, no. 3, p. 32.

SECTION 4: PRACTICES

Overview

ROGER HUGHES

In order to protect, promote and maintain the health of populations, the principles, knowledge, skills and strategies of public health nutrition need to be put into practice. This section focuses on the practical application (hereafter referred to as 'practice') of public health nutrition. The preceding chapters of this book demonstrate that public health nutrition as a field of endeavour covers a broad range of issues in multiple contexts and settings that are underpinned by biological, social, cultural, political and environmental determinants. This means that the practice of public health nutrition is difficult to define in a way that suits all contexts. If, as defined in chapter 1, public health nutrition is the promotion and maintenance of nutrition-related health and wellbeing of populations through the organised efforts and informed choices of society (Barcelona Declaration 2006), then the practice of public health nutrition refers to the organised effort required. This organising is usually taken on by practitioners operating within the health system (the workforce), although it can occur within communities by volunteers or community leaders. The focus here is on the practice of public health nutrition from the perspective of practitioners, those individuals who make up the workforce charged with responsibility for the protection and promotion of health via optimal nutrition and physical activity.

Core function of the public health nutrition workforce

There have been numerous and ongoing attempts worldwide to codify the core functions of the public health workforce in order to focus workforce practices and inform workforce development. While it is logical to assume that the core functions for public health would also represent the core functions of public health nutrition, there is a widespread agreement that public health nutrition is a specialty within public health requiring individual attention. With this perspective in mind, a list of ten core functions for public health nutrition are presented in the table that follows, based on public health nutrition workforce development research conducted in the early 2000s. These serve as a framework for considering the practice of public health nutrition in the chapters that follow in this section. The proposed core functions for public health nutrition are underpinned by the following assumptions:

- public health nutrition functions are defined as those activities (processes, practices, services and programmes) that are undertaken by the workforce in order to promote optimal nutrition, health and wellbeing in populations
- core public health nutrition functions are those functions that are regarded as absolutely necessary, without which would imply gaps in public health capacity
- the relative importance of functions may vary, depending on the jurisdiction or workforce level
- core functions are interrelated and complementary
- core functions articulate the work required to effectively address public health nutrition problems or issues, and consequently provide a framework for identifying and conceptualising workforce development needs
- current public health nutrition work practices do not accurately align with these core functions (Hughes 2004b). They are therefore aspirational, outlining the practices required for effective public health nutrition action, and are a pointer to practice improvement.

There are three overarching function categories for the public health nutrition practice outlined in this listing of core functions — research and analysis, building capacity and intervention management. The functions are covered in the following chapters of this section, as outlined below.

1. Monitor, assess and communicate population nutritional health needs and issues

Chapter 12 on the monitoring of the food and nutrition situation of populations by Rutishauser, Webb and Marks, provides a detailed overview of this core function. Workforce research in Australia has demonstrated that monitoring and surveillance of nutrition is currently neither a common practice

Table Ten core functions for public health nutrition practice (practice functions)

Research and Analysis	1	Monitor, assess and communicate population nutritional health needs and issues.	
	2	Develop and communicate intelligence* about determinants of nutrition problems, policy impacts, intervention effectiveness and prioritisation through research and evaluation.	
Building Capacity	3	Develop the various tiers of the public health nutrition workforce and its collaborators through education, disseminating intelligence* and ensuring organisational support.	
	4	Build community capacity and social capital to engage in, identify and build solutions to nutrition problems and issues.	
	5	Build organisational capacity and systems to facilitate and coordinate effective public health nutrition action.	
Intervention Management	6	Plan, develop, implement and evaluate interventions that address the determinants of priority public health nutrition issues and problems and promote equity.	
	7	Enhance and sustain population knowledge and awareness of healthy eating so that dietary choices are informed choices.	
	8	Advocate for food- and nutrition-related policy and government support to protect and promote health.	
	9	Promote, develop and support healthy growth and development throughout all life stages.	
	10	Promote equitable access to safe and healthy food so that healthy choices are easy choices .	

* Intelligence refers to information and knowledge from various sources used to inform decisions relating to problem resolution in public health nutrition practice.

Source: adapted from Hughes 2003a; Hughes 2003b; Hughes 2004

function (Hughes 2004b), nor a function expected of the workforce by many employers (Hughes 2004a). This reflects the reality that monitoring and surveillance requires considerable resourcing, systems and an advanced competency mix that is often outside the reach of individual practitioners. Nonetheless, practitioners need to be able to access, interpret, use and critique intelligence gained by monitoring and surveillance systems in their daily practice. Similar issues are addressed within the context of physical activity in chapter 13, prepared by Timperio and colleagues.

2. *Develop and communicate intelligence about determinants of nutrition problems, policy impacts, intervention effectiveness and prioritisation through research and evaluation*

Closely related to the first core function because of its analytical emphasis, this function articulates the importance of research and evaluation in public health nutrition practice. Chapter 14, on research skills by McNaughton, Ball and Crawford, outlines the key principles relating to population health research. While workforce research in Australia suggests that there is a small proportion of the current workforce engaged in research and evaluation as a regular feature of their practice (Hughes 2004b), the need for evidence of practice effectiveness and intelligence-based intervention planning indicates that this aspect of practice needs considerable strengthening.

3. *Develop the various tiers of the public health nutrition workforce and its collaborators through education, disseminating intelligence and ensuring organisational support*

Empowering other health and community members via nutrition upskilling and training is an important capacity building function of public health nutrition practice. It is acknowledged that public health nutrition work involves many disciplines at many levels, and that an inclusive, capacity building approach is required to best achieve health gains. Public health nutrition specialists therefore need to employ many of the skills, such as leadership, partnership development and communication, in this aspect of practice, as outlined in chapter 15, on professional practice, by Yeatman and Begley.

4. *Build community capacity and social capital to engage in, identify and build solutions to nutrition problems and issues*

Community development is widely accepted as an important component of building capacity for organised efforts to address public health problems, but appears yet to become established in current workforce practices (Hughes 2004b). Community development involves engaging and empowering community stakeholders in identifying, prioritising and deciding on strategies to address agreed problems. It is an often neglected aspect of public health nutrition intervention planning and as a result is likely to be a significant determinant of intervention success or failure. This core function is discussed briefly by Yeatman and Begley in chapter 15.

5. *Build organisational capacity and systems to facilitate and coordinate effective public health nutrition action*

One of the most potent barriers to effectively practising public health nutrition among practitioners is the organisational structure of the workplace. Research in Australia has consistently identified workforce disorganisation as a major capacity impediment (Hughes 2006). This means that practitioners are not organisationally supported to work in a way consistent with public health nutrition (that is, implementing core functions) but instead are limited to clinical, low-reach and restricted strategy-type service provision. The reality of practice indicates that the leadership, communication and emotional intelligence competencies, outlined by Yeatman and Begley in chapter 15, are needed to support organisational capacity building. Recent workforce capacity gains in some areas of Australia indicate that public health nutritionists often need to drive this organisational change agenda rather than waiting for someone else to do it.

6. *Plan, develop, implement and evaluate interventions that address the determinants of priority public health nutrition issues and problems and promote equity*

Intervention management (the design, planning, implementation and evaluation of public health interventions) is the most common employer function expectation, and one of the most common aspects of practice that the Australian workforce report doing (Hughes 2004a; Hughes 2004b). This research, however, suggests that a considerable proportion of the designated workforce's project activity is inconsistent with recognised public health nutrition workforce functions and priorities. Strategy utilisation and practices involving food supply changes, policy processes and health service reorientation are used infrequently, suggesting a limited strategic approach to addressing public health nutrition issues in this workforce. Chapter 16, on project management, by Caraher, Cowburn and Coveney, provides the practice basis for good intervention management. As practitioners, we need to ensure our intervention activity addresses community needs rather than our individual interests. This can be challenging because much of the need in public health nutrition requires difficult and time-consuming work, considerable ongoing competency development, with little short-term reward. Needs-based practice also forces us to work on issues often outside what many of us consider 'sexy'.

7. *Enhance and sustain population knowledge and awareness of healthy eating so that dietary choices are informed choices*

Nutrition education and communication is the most frequently reported aspect of public health nutrition practice in Australia; however, much of this effort relies on limited reach and person-to-person communication. Few reported regularly participating in state or national media campaigns, and mass media use and social marketing were rarely used in interventions. This suggests limited-reach approaches dominate and limit the capacity of the workforce to successfully perform this function (Hughes 2004b). Chapter 17, on promotion and communication, by Worsley, demonstrates that there is much more to this function in the public health nutrition practice context than the person-to-person communication so ingrained in traditional dietetic training. Use of the various media will increasingly become a practice tool for nutrition promotion and advocacy, and is a competency development challenge for the majority of the workforce.

8. *Advocate for food- and nutrition-related policy and government support to protect and promote health*

Chapter 18, on policy and politics, by Lawrence, outlines the complexity and importance of a strong public health nutrition footprint in the policy-making process. Workforce practice research suggests, however, that the current workforce is largely disengaged from the political process and unprepared for this type of work (Hughes 2003b). This reinforces the aspirational nature of the listed core functions for public health nutrition, and points to the practices and competencies we need to develop in this profession.

9. *Promote, develop and support healthy growth and development throughout all life stages*

Nutrition and physical activity are key determinants of healthy growth and development, and are a key focus of the competency needs of the public health nutrition practitioner (Hughes 2006). The chapters in section 2, Populations, provide an analysis of the key issues in healthy growth and development throughout the critical life stages of maternity and infancy, childhood and adolescence, and older adults.

10. *Promote equitable access to safe and healthy food so that healthy choices are easy choices*

The health-advancing objectives of public health nutrition are contingent on a safe, healthy and sustainable food supply. As a result, it is not surprising that there is an increasing interest by practitioners on food-supply strategies as an environmental change approach to healthy eating. This is based on the simple premise that improving accessibility to healthy food (lowering prices, point-of-sale promotions, etc.) will make healthy choices easy. In section 3, Priorities, McMichael's chapter on the global developments with the food system and ecological sustainability illustrates that the importance of the food supply goes well beyond this interventionist perspective, and underpins all of what we do in public health nutrition.

Conclusion

The core functions proposed are future-oriented and provide direction for workforce development in public health nutrition. The current state of public health nutrition practice suggests that we as a group of practitioners and soon-to-be practitioners have significant continuing development needs, and that there is a significant need for a reorientation of the way we do business. In a relatively new and emerging profession, this is not unexpected, but it does challenge us to reflect on our practice and strive to be more effective in our work. This is what makes public health nutrition as an area of practice the most dynamic, challenging and interesting areas of nutrition work. I hope readers have the passion and capacity to take up this challenge for the sake of the public health. The chapters that follow in this section can help us focus on the functions and competencies we need to develop to be more effective in practice.

REFERENCES

Barcelona (draft) Declaration on the Formation of the World Public Health Nutrition Association, The, 2006 (in press), Inaugural Planning Meeting, 30 September, Barcelona.

Hughes, R. 2003a, 'Competency development needs of the Australian public health nutrition workforce' in *Public Health Nutrition*, vol. 6, pp. 839–47.

—— 2003b, 'Public health nutrition workforce composition, core functions, competencies and capacity: Perspectives of advanced level practitioners in Australia' in *Public Health Nutrition*, vol. 6, no. 6, pp. 607–13.

—— 2004a, 'Employers' expectations of core functions and competencies for the public health nutrition workforce' in *Nutrition and Dietetics*, vol. 61, pp. 105–11.

—— 2004b, 'Work practices of the community and public health nutrition workforce in Australia' in *Nutrition and Dietetics*, vol. 61, pp. 38–45.

—— 2006, 'A competency framework for public health nutrition workforce development', Australian Public Health Nutrition Academic Collaboration, Griffith University, Gold Coast, cited at <http://www.aphnac.com>.

12

Monitoring the food and nutrition situation of populations

INGRID RUTISHAUSER
KAREN WEBB
GEOFFREY MARKS

The aim of collecting information about the food and nutrition situation ultimately should be to make improvements. Ritualistic collection of information is a waste of effort, resources, and an opportunity missed. There are several important uses for food and nutrition information, including:

- assessment of individuals for diagnosis, education, and management of nutrition-related conditions or risk factors
- food- and nutrition-related research and evaluation on groups and populations to investigate causes, determinants and mechanisms of diet-related disease, develop evidence-based nutrition policies and population dietary guidance, plan and evaluate the effects of interventions to reduce diet-related disease and its determinants
- monitoring and surveillance of selected indicators of the food and nutrition situation of populations and important sub-groups to assess differences and trends, track progress on achievement of policy goals, garner support for investment and action, fine-tune policies, develop and target programmes, and identify emerging problems that require a public health response.

[273]

In this chapter, we deal with the third of these purposes — monitoring and surveillance of the food and nutrition situation in populations. The terms 'monitoring' and 'surveillance' often are used interchangeably, and their definitions have in common 'the routine collection of information to watch over a situation' to guide policy, investment, and programme responses. We use the term 'monitoring' in preference to surveillance in this chapter to mean a system of routine data collection, analysis and reporting, to keep track of aspects of the food and nutrition situation of a population and important sub-groups, on the assumption that the information will be useful for a variety of purposes, particularly those outlined above.

Purposes for food and nutrition information relating to populations

The need for monitoring the food and nutrition situation at the national level has long been recognised, but the scope of monitoring efforts varies widely across countries. Many developed and developing countries have had a national nutrition survey programme for decades to monitor the nutrition situations of their populations, and more recently for use in formulating and harmonising relevant food regulations. Most countries have also produced food balance sheets for many years to assess food supply trends and nutrient adequacy. In the past two to three decades, behavioural risk factor monitoring has become commonplace in some countries to track progress towards health policy goals, such as national dietary guidelines and chronic disease risk factor reduction programmes. Monitoring at the sub-national level is also well developed in many countries, providing information at the state and even local community levels.

It is clear that there are a variety of important needs for data that can be met from a food and nutrition monitoring system, and several important user groups who are key stakeholders in such a system, including national, state and local governments as policymakers and regulators, health agencies charged with service provision and accountability for quality, the food-related industries, non-government and consumer organisations with responsibility for protection of vulnerable population groups, and research and academic institutions. Some uses of the data for each of these groups are shown in Table 12.1.

It is recognised that data from a food and nutrition monitoring system can enable user groups to answer important policy questions in relation to their constituencies and responsibilities. Some examples of policy questions answerable by data from a monitoring system include:

Table 12.1 Potential users and uses of data from a food and nutrition monitoring system

Stakeholder	Uses
National government	*Food*: Development, monitoring and enforcement of food regulations and standards (food safety risk assessment, food composition database maintenance and labelling requirements), development of fortification and health claims policy and other food regulation policy issues, contribution to international food standards (Codex), provision of ministerial advice, monitoring trends in self-sufficiency and adequacy of food supply to meet population needs. *Nutrition*: Development of national food and nutrition guidelines, nutrient reference values, nutrition goals and targets, nutrition policies, strategies and programs (e.g. Eat Well Australian and National Aboriginal and Torres Strait Islander Nutrition Strategy and Action Plan), health promotion, provision of nutrition services, ministerial advice. *Nutrition-related health status*: Development of health strategies (e.g. for chronic disease prevention and addressing inequalities between population sub-groups), meeting international reporting obligations (OECD/WHO/FAO).
Regional public health agencies and primary care providers	Development of nutrition education, health promotion programmes. Enforcement of food standards. Development of regional and specific settings, food and nutrition health policies and strategies. Guidance for service planning, resource allocation and a basis for client advice.
Food industry ('paddock to plate')	Guiding primary produce research and development, and marketing and distribution strategies. Food product development, labelling and marketing. Research, development and innovation.
Non-government and consumer organisations	Basis for nutrition and health-promotion policies and programmes, and provision of advice to the general public.
Research and academic institutions	Identifying relevant directions for applied research, including methods research for health and nutrition monitoring and for health professional training.

Source: Adapted from Ministry of Health, NZ, 2003

- Is a nutritionally adequate food supply available and accessible to all segments of the population?
- Is there equitable food access within countries or regions?
- Is the composition of foods in the food supply changing, and are the changes associated with increased or decreased risk of nutrition-related ill health?
- What are the implications of technological and regulatory changes on the composition of the food supply, for population health and for the nation's food industry?
- Are the risks of exposure to bioactive compounds in food acceptable at current levels of consumption?
- Is the composition of the overall diet changing, and is this associated with increased or decreased risk of morbidity, chronic disease and mortality?
- Are food habits and nutrient intake of the population changing in line with dietary targets and guidelines and nutrient reference values?
- What are the current trends in eating patterns that may affect food industry growth and innovation?
- Is the nutritional status of the population changing, and is this associated with increasing or decreasing risk of morbidity, chronic disease and mortality?
- Is nutritional status different for particular population sub-groups, and what environmental, socioeconomic and personal factors are associated with these differences?
- Is the use of nutritional supplements changing, and what are the implications for nutrient intake, nutritional status and the health of the population?

Costs and disadvantages associated with inadequate information

Conversely, the lack of a national food and nutrition monitoring system incurs significant costs and disadvantages. Among them, there is a reduced ability to appropriately develop, target and monitor the outcomes of costly and labour-intensive public health nutrition interventions. Health authorities, nationally and internationally, are promoting evidence-based policies and practice, yet countries without monitoring systems are making policy in an evidence-free environment, reliant on no or outdated, one-off or serendipitous data collected for other purposes to signal whether things are moving in the right direction. A related risk is the late detection of new, or accelerating, nutrition problems in the community, and the lack of trend information about the possible causes. For example, are changes in obesity levels linked to changes in certain diet patterns or exercise or both? Is there an emerging problem with, for instance, vitamin D, iodine or folate?

In the absence of a food and nutrition monitoring system, food regulatory decisions may be made without a rational basis. Effective risk assessment for food additives, fortification with vitamins and minerals, chemical residues, novel foods and so on cannot be carried out without current data on food and nutrient intake. This is because risk analysis depends on accurate dietary exposure assessments, which are only possible if there is current knowledge of food intake and composition, particularly of foods that have emerged recently in the marketplace. From industry's standpoint, there is a concern that the introduction of new technologies, initiatives or innovations may be inhibited because, in the absence of current data about food and nutrient intake, risk assessments must err on the side of caution.

In summary, risks arising from the absence of data from a food and nutrition monitoring system include:

- the 'invisibility' of some food and nutrition problems
- an inability to develop policy and programme responses leading to policy or programme inertia
- an inability to determine clear priorities for resource allocation
- ineffective/inappropriate food regulation
- lack of credibility/targeting of public health messages
- an inability to properly assess existing policy initiatives and programmes
- an inability to reliably determine trends over time
- the atrophy of organisational and user capacity to support regular data collection, analysis and use
- evidence-free decision-making.

Priorities and principles for monitoring

Because the resources required for supporting an ongoing system of data collection, analysis and reporting are substantial, the information collected usually needs to be kept to a minimum, including that most widely useful to users/stakeholders. The types of information about food and nutrition that are most commonly identified as core elements of a monitoring system can be classified into four domains, including:

- the food supply: information on the availability of foodstuffs and the composition of foods available
- food distribution and access: information on household and individual expenditure on food, types of food purchased, prices paid and quantities bought, food security
- food habits and dietary intake: selected food behaviours and detailed information on food and nutrient intake
- nutritional status: physical and biochemical measures related to food and nutrient intake.

These are shown in Figure 12.1. Information such as population socio-demographic characteristics, other health-related behaviours, and health status are also considered to be essential data from health monitoring systems that link to and underpin the interpretation of food and nutrition data. A wide range of data within each of the core domains could be collected and used; considerations in setting priorities, and basic principles for monitoring these aspects of food and nutrition are considered in the next section.

Priority setting
Nutrition is multidimensional in that different aspects of diet are important for a range of health outcomes of interest. Thus, the most relevant food and nutrition data for monitoring will differ according to purpose and audience, as described in Table 12.1. The question of what to monitor is fundamental to developing a food and nutrition monitoring system. Further, the resources to support a monitoring system are generally limited, and so establishing priorities among the range of food and nutrition issues in a population typically requires setting priorities among the competing users and uses of the data. Similarly, the most appropriate measures for use in monitoring will vary, depending on the purpose of collecting the information, and may be a dietary, anthropometric, biochemical or another type of measure.

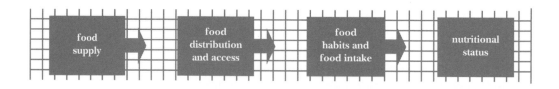

Figure 12.1 Framework for a national food and nutrition monitoring system

Monitoring systems can be developed around a set of individual priorities, such as the monitoring of chronic disease risk factors, or addressing a more comprehensive agenda. An example of the former is the STEPwise approach to chronic disease risk factor surveillance (STEPS) developed by the World Health Organization. The core of the system is information collected by questionnaire, with other components such as simple physical measurements and blood samples included if resources permit (see <www.who.int/steps/en>). Two approaches that are useful for developing more comprehensive monitoring systems are the development of a framework based on policy and programme objectives, and categorisation of food and nutrition issues based on the evidence for an adverse impact on health.

To illustrate the first of these, a core agenda for monitoring in Australia can be developed through considering national nutrition policies and guidelines; for example, Eat Well Australia and the Australian Dietary Guidelines. Australian governments endorsed Eat Well Australia in 2001 as the national public health nutrition strategy to provide guidance to government agencies and other organisations for activities to further improve the nutritional health of the population (Strategic Intergovernmental Nutrition Alliance 2001). The Australian Dietary Guidelines are developed under the auspices of the National Health and Medical Research Council, and form the basis for dietary advice to Australians. The food and nutrition issues identified in these are listed in Table 12.2. The documents also specify particularly vulnerable groups in the population that would potentially need to be monitored for specific issues. Further development of the agenda would require consultation with key stakeholders to include, for instance, the additional data required to meet regulatory needs.

An example of the second approach to priority-setting is the US national monitoring system, where priority is assigned to monitoring food components for which there is sound evidence regarding adverse health consequences. The decision-making process is summarised in Figure 12.2, which shows that information on the intake of specified food components is combined with other evidence to determine whether it is a current public health issue, a potential public health issue, or not a current public health issue. This approach has the advantage of not only determining priority for monitoring, but also identifying issues where evidence is lacking and more research or information is needed before a judgement can be made. An agenda developed on this basis would not meet the data requirements of all key stakeholders, and further consultation would be needed.

Considering that food and nutrition monitoring is intended to describe the nutrition situation over the long term, care should be taken to retain comparability

Table 12.2 Food and nutrition issues identified from Australian national policy documents and guidelines

Food supply, distribution & access
- food supply/access
- food security

Food habits & food intake

Infants:
- breastfeeding
- introduction of solid

General population:
- diversity/five food groups
- vegetables & legumes, fruit, breads & cereals
- alcoholic beverages & water
- energy, fat & saturated fat, added sugars
- folate, iron, calcium, sodium
- supplement intake (folate, iron, calcium)

Nutritional status
- birthweight
- overweight and obesity
- folate, iron, calcium

and also the flexibility for introducing new components and re-analysis of the situation to address new questions and challenges; for example, in response to:

- changing patterns of consumption of dietary supplements
- changes to the food supply – fortification, growth in consumption of functional foods, introduction of genetically modified foods, other regulatory changes
- changes in nutritional sciences – recognition of new food factors that may have important health impacts such as glucosinolates and flavonoids.

Indicator development

In order to provide relevant information for important policy decisions, the priorities identified for national, regional or local monitoring need to be translated into a limited number of clearly defined measures. This process is generally more complex than making a state-of-the-art measurement in a clinical or research context. For effective monitoring, relatively simple procedures must be able to provide a reliable assessment in a specific individual at a given point in time, as well as to provide consistent data for representative samples of a

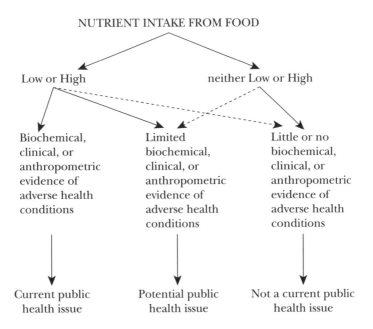

NUTRIENT INTAKE FROM FOOD

Low or High   neither Low or High

| Biochemical, clinical, or anthropometric evidence of adverse health conditions | Limited biochemical, clinical, or anthropometric evidence of adverse health conditions | Little or no biochemical, clinical, or anthropometric evidence of adverse health conditions |

| Current public health issue | Potential public health issue | Not a current public health issue |

Note. Whenever nutrient intake data were available from surveys, they were used and evaluated by established criteria. When survey data were not available, Total Diet Study data were used and evaluated by established criteria. Dashed lines indicate less likely outcomes.

Figure 12.2 Decision-making process used to categorise food components by monitoring priority status

Source: Life Sciences Research Office 1995

population or population sub-groups at more than one point in time. Measures that provide this kind of information are often referred to as indicators. Indicators are measurable statistical constructs for monitoring progress towards a goal, and may be defined in terms of a proportion or as a mean or median. Mathers and Schofield (1997) define indicators as:

Public health indicators are summary statistics, which facilitate concise, comprehensive and balanced judgments about the condition of a major aspect of health, a determinant of health, or progress towards a healthier society.

A discussion paper on the development of indicators (Australian Institute of Health Welfare 1999) proposed a number of criteria to guide the definition and development of national public health indicators that can also be used to guide the development of food and nutrition indicators. The criteria suggested that indicators should be:

- national in scope, or applicable to regional or local population issues of national significance
- as aggregated as possible, that is, summarise as much as is consistent with the level of monitoring or surveillance required
- 'normative' — subject to the interpretation that if the indicator changes in the right direction, while other things remain equal, people will be better off
- based on evidence of a clear link between the indicator and improvement in outcome
- reliable and valid — its values must be meaningful in relation to public health
- scientifically credible and ethical
- consistent and comparable with indicators used in other jurisdictions, as far as possible
- easy to understand
- described in a standard manner
- have an explicit operational definition in terms of measurable constructs
- capable of being monitored to provide statistically verifiable time series, and preferably applicable to a broad range of age groups and populations; responsive to measurable change; and able to be monitored with relative ease at suitable intervals.

Some examples of indicators that have been used in the US National Nutrition Monitoring and Related Research Program (Life Sciences Research Office 1995) to report on food and nutrition issues of importance to the health of Americans, which cover many of the components of food and nutrition monitoring illustrated in Figure 12.1, are:

- annual per capita consumption of non-alcoholic beverages
- percentage of total food expenditures away from home
- prevalence of breastfeeding among mothers aged 15 to 44 years
- precent distribution of servings of fruit and vegetables
- percentage with total fat intake: 30, greater than 30, and 40 and greater than 40 per cent of energy intake
- prevalence of physical activity among adults and percentage meeting Healthy People 2000 Objective for vigorous physical activity
- prevalence of reported family food sufficiency problems
- prevalence of low birthweight among low-income, high-risk females

- prevalence of shortness and thinness in children and adolescents
- percentage of adults who are overweight
- percentage of adults who have hypertension
- percentage with desirable, borderline and high serum total cholesterol levels.

Indicators suitable for national monitoring, while basically simple measures, often undergo a lengthy process of development, which involves discussions about a number of issues, including the following, before consensus is reached and they become part of an ongoing monitoring programme:

- definition of the construct to be measured by the indicator (for example, in relation to nutrition policies, guidelines, recommendations)
- availability of appropriate data
- consultations with relevant stakeholders
- how data are to be derived and presented
- limitations and appropriate interpretation of the indicator.

One of the dilemmas for those engaged in the process of indicator development is that indicators, in order to be useful, should be robust enough to be able to provide medium- to long-term trend data while remaining responsive to changes within the policy environment within which they operate. The various stages and considerations involved in the process of indicator development are illustrated by a case study of the process and considerations involved in the development of recommendations for indicators for monitoring breastfeeding in Australia (Webb et al. 2001).

Data requirements
While both the process and the specific considerations related to the development of indicators for food and nutrition monitoring differ for different types of food and nutrition information, an issue common to all is data quality. In the context of monitoring, it is important that the data obtained for monitoring purposes are:

- as representative as possible of the target group
- not merely reproducible but also valid in relation to the construct being measured
- not influenced by the method of administration, that is, by face-to-face or telephone interview or with the type of equipment used, provided that both conform with the requirements for standard methods

- consistent, that is, able to provide the same information over time
- obtained by clearly defined standard methods.

In order to be representative, the measurement methods should be acceptable to the target group so that response rates are high. Individuals should be both able and willing to respond, and this in turn requires that the respondents clearly understand the question(s) posed or tasks involved, and that the demands made on them are not so great as to discourage their participation.

It goes without saying that data that do not provide a reliable reflection of the construct to be assessed and are not reproducible have no place in food and nutrition monitoring. It is simply not true that any data are better than none. Unreliable or inappropriate data are worse than no data at all, because they have the potential to mislead, and thus to lead to the development of inappropriate policy and/or misallocation of limited resources. This does not mean that the data for monitoring need to be perfect, only that they must be reliable. Agreement with more detailed information does not need to be absolute, but it should be possible to demonstrate that the indicator used for monitoring is clearly associated with the reference or preferred measurement for the parameter of interest, so that the indicator increases when the reference measurement increases and vice versa.

Consistency over time requires not only that the indicator be reproducible when remeasured at a time close to the original measurement, but also that it continues to reflect the same construct in the same way over time. For example, a survey question about vegetable intake administered at a time when dietary guidelines and other public education resources include potatoes as a vegetable is unlikely to provide data that are comparable with the data that would be obtained for the same question at another time when potatoes were no longer generally considered as a vegetable, that is, when the construct for what is a vegetable has changed.

Clearly defined standard methods are important in relation to the method of data collection and also in relation to the way in which the data are subsequently recorded, analysed and reported. One example where this has been done is for the measurement of weight and height and the derivation of body mass index (Australian Institute for Health and Welfare 1999). A similar process needs to be undertaken for a wider range of public health nutrition measures, and the recommendations routinely implemented. Until such time, data that at first sight appear to be comparable may in fact have been obtained and derived in different ways that compromise their comparability and their ability to accurately reflect trends over time.

Measurement of system components

This section briefly describes the main approaches to data collection and the types of data collected for each of the main components of the food and nutrition system (Figure 12.1). It does not provide details of the various measurement methods because this information can readily be found in standard texts on nutrition assessment. Instead, this section focuses on the practical considerations relevant to different types of data, and guidance on evaluation and appropriate interpretation of the data.

Food supply

Some of the longest time-series data available for food and nutrition monitoring are those on national food supplies. In Australia, the *Apparent Consumption of Foodstuffs and Nutrients* series was begun in the mid-1930s and published annually until 2000. Similarly, standardised international food supply data, known as food balance sheets, have been compiled and published by FAO since 1949 for a large number of countries. Different terms have been used to describe such data, but all aim to provide information on the amount of food available for consumption within a country over a specified period of time, and are calculated from data on the annual production, changes in stocks, imports and exports of foodstuffs, and, where available, non-food uses; for example, for animal feed, estimates of home production, and losses in the supply chain. Detailed descriptions of the methods used to collect and compile the data compiled by FAO are available at <http://www.fao.org/> and in the publications produced by individual countries.

Practical considerations

Food balance sheets are compiled from a wide range of data sources, which can differ markedly in terms of coverage, accuracy, consistency over time, and availability from year to year. The main challenge is the maintenance of consistent data collection over the longer term. It is inevitable that, with time, the methods, scope and frequency of data collection will change, and not unlikely that at least some of these changes will lead to 'apparent' changes in the food supply. It is therefore crucial that all methodological changes are documented and, when possible, their impact assessed. Because of these complexities, published food supply data are *always* accompanied by explanatory or technical notes. It is essential that this technical information, often in appendices rather than 'up front', is read carefully before using the data. It is also important to review the technical data for the *whole* time period of interest, and not simply in the most recent publication. Unless this is done, the reasons for apparent changes cannot be distinguished reliably from real changes.

Interpretation

Food supply data can be used to monitor shifts between and within major commodity groups as a guide to the direction of changes in dietary patterns. In Australia, for example, commodity data have clearly demonstrated the gradual shift from butter to margarine, the changing role of sugar in the food supply, the increased contribution of poultry to the meat supply, and, since 1988–89, the marked increase in the availability of aerated and carbonated beverages. An important point about use of the data in this way is that it depends only on consistent methodology for the commodity of interest.

In contrast, using the data to assess nutrient availability requires reliable data for the whole of the food supply. This is clearly a more difficult requirement to meet, and the resulting estimates are subject to greater error. The standard approach used by FAO is to convert the weights of processed foods to the equivalent primary commodity weights for the purpose of nutrient estimation. This works well for macronutrients, but does not allow for the varying micronutrient losses associated with different types of processing, both commercial and domestic. Some attempt to take these into account can be made by incorporating predicted loss factors for the most common processing operations. National estimates of the micronutrient supply are primarily useful for identifying the nutrients most likely to be in short supply, and whether the supply is increasing or decreasing in the short term.

An alternative approach for estimating nutrients in the food supply, which may be more appropriate to countries where much of the food consumed is processed or manufactured, are total diet studies or market basket surveys, which were originally developed to estimate the level of contaminants in the food supply (Ockhuizen et al. 1991). The procedures used to determine the relative amounts and types of foods to be analysed in such studies are documented in detail in the periodic published reports of such studies. The advantages of this approach over using estimates of average intake/per person/per day are that estimates of micronutrient availability are based on direct chemical analysis, and that estimates can be derived for 'typical' diets consumed by different age-sex groups in the population.

The most practical way to allow for relatively minor changes in food supply data collection methodology is by using three-year averages for assessing trends rather than year-to-year data. FAO have adopted this process as standard for reporting purposes. Major changes in methodology, which are likely to have an ongoing and systematic effect, are best accommodated by showing a clear break in the data set and, where possible, recalculating earlier data using the revised methodology and reporting both sets of data.

Food distribution

National food supply data provide no information on how food is distributed within the population, and therefore no guidance on where and to which population sub-groups nutrition interventions are best targeted. The most obvious approach for obtaining the information needed is to collect data on the food intake of different population sub-groups. This approach has not been widely used on a regular basis because it is expensive, requires dedicated staff and resources, and may be difficult to obtain for the whole population. Instead, regularly conducted surveys of household expenditure have, in many countries, become a standard source of information on differences in food patterns and nutrient availability by locality and household characteristics such as size, composition, education and income level (Trichopoulou 1992).

Practical considerations

The common feature of household expenditure/budget surveys is that they collect data on the amount of money spent on food by households. In nearly all cases, the initial purpose of the surveys was to provide data for economic rather than nutritional analysis. Some, however, also collect data on the quantities of food entering the household, both from purchases and from other sources such as gifts and home production (Slater 1991), and thus enable estimates of both food and nutrient availability to be derived from the data. In general, household expenditure surveys, even those that collect information on food quantities, have not been widely used for nutritional analysis, mainly because foods purchased and consumed outside the home are generally not included, data on waste and other losses are not collected, and the broad level of classification of the food items recorded limits the estimation of nutrient availability.

In Europe, the DAFNE (Data Food Networking) initiative was specifically undertaken to standardise data collection and processing, and to explore options for using retail prices for the conversion of expenditure data to quantities (Friel et al. 2001) in order to increase the value and use of household expenditure data for nutrition monitoring and policymaking (Trichopoulou 1992; Lagiou et al. 2001). In Australia, the data available from the Australian Bureau of Statistics (ABS) Household Expenditure Surveys, conducted first in 1975–76 and five-yearly since 1988–89, have also been under-utilised for nutrition monitoring. During this time, expenditure on food and non-alcoholic beverages has remained relatively stable at 18 to 20 per cent of total household expenditure in both low- and high-income households, but the actual amount of money spent on food by households in the lowest income quintile expressed as a proportion of that spent by households in the highest income quintile has decreased markedly, from around 75 per cent in 1984 to 34 per cent in 1998–99 (ABS 1986 and 2003). Changes of this magnitude are clearly worthy of further exploration in terms of expenditure differences between commodities, even if they cannot readily be expressed in quantitative or nutrient terms. This is particularly relevant in view of increasing food insecurity in some population groups within affluent societies, and observations that food insecurity, however defined, is more prevalent in households with lower income and education level, and those from socioeconomically disadvantaged areas.

Interpretation
Instruments developed to assess the level of food insecurity, such as that developed by the US Department of Agriculture <http://www.ers.usda.gov/briefing/foodsecurity/> and for the 1997 New Zealand National Nutrition Survey (Quigley & Watts 1997), provide estimates of the prevalence of different levels of selected aspects of food insecurity for individuals from different types of households, but do not allow comparison with information about diet quality unless the food security data are obtained in the context of a nutrition survey in which the food intake of respondents is also assessed.

When food security modules are used in regularly conducted population health surveys, it would be useful to collect similar socio-demographic data as that collected in national household expenditure surveys to enable classification of respondent households by at least some of the same characteristics. Data from the two sources cross-classified by household type could then be used to identify food purchasing patterns associated with different levels of food insecurity, and in this way contribute to the development of relevant public health policy and interventions for those in greatest need.

Food habits
National nutrition policies, such as dietary guidelines and food selection guides, are generally concerned with promoting food habits or food behaviours that will lead to improved overall diet quality, and, in turn, better nutritional status. Because the term 'habit' implies a constancy of behaviour, food habits of individuals and populations can best be described by methods that seek information about usual food behaviours, such as survey questions about frequency, quantity and types of foods usually consumed, on average, over a period of time, such

as the past year. By contrast, detailed information about total food and nutrient intake of individuals is best assessed from a snapshot of recent or current food consumption (see national nutrition surveys later in this chapter).

Short questions about food habits often seek to assess the types, frequency or quantities of foods or food groups consumed, as these relate to dietary guidelines or food selection guide recommendations. Other specific types of food-related behaviours, such as use of nutritional supplements and breast-feeding practices, can also be measured by one or more short questions, as can some factors thought to be substantial influences on food habits for vulnerable population groups (for example, food security, barriers to change).

Practical considerations
Federal and state/regional/provincial level health surveys often seek to monitor how the populations of their jurisdictions are 'travelling' with regard to current recommended health behaviours, including food habits, physical activity, smoking, alcohol consumption and safe sexual practices. Data from these surveys is often used for accountability with regard to the relevance and effectiveness of the health services and programmes they provide. In such a multidimensional health survey, which covers many health behaviours and issues, survey space to assess food habits is usually limited to a few short questions; existing tools to measure usual intake of selected foods, such as food-frequency questionnaires, are generally too lengthy to include.

The use of short questions about food habits is appealing to health surveyors, as they can be readily incorporated into most health surveys, and are inexpensive and uncomplicated to administer. They can provide both qualitative and quantitative information on intake over varying periods of time, be used to report on key indicators of food intake and key influences, be included in local as well as national surveys, and can be administered via the telephone, mail surveys or face-to-face interviews. It is therefore not surprising that short questions about food habits and other health behaviours are now a regular feature in population health surveys in many countries of the world, such as that used in the Center for Disease Control Behavioural Risk Factor Surveillance System in the United States and adapted for use in many developing countries. In Australia, the Australian Bureau of Statistics 2001 and 2005 National Health Surveys (NHS) included some questions that were also included in the 1995 National Nutrition Survey (NNS). A technical document describing the development and testing of the dietary indicators module for 2001 NHS (ABS 2003) provides information on contextual differences that are relevant to the interpretation of differences between 1995 and 2001 (Table 12.3).

Because of the space limit in most surveys, it is important that short questions are of direct relevance to issues of significance in public health nutrition, and that they can be interpreted in relation to defined policies. For example, questions about fruit and vegetable consumption are indicative of aspects of diet, directly relevant to the dietary guidelines of most countries, and responses can be interpreted in relation to recommended frequencies and quantities. By contrast, questions about breakfast consumption or number of meals and snacks usually consumed per day are not directly relevant to most national guidelines, and therefore responses cannot be interpreted in relation to a recommendation, or as indicative of diet quality.

In order to assess change in food habits over time and between population groups, it is crucial that short survey questions and response categories be standardised to ensure comparability over time and between surveys of different population groups. Significant variation in the types and wording of short questions and response categories in health surveys has, to date, rendered the data obtained from many short questions useless for monitoring changes in food habits in Australia and elsewhere. Efforts to standardise survey questions with

Table 12.3 Comparison of data for some dietary indicators from the 1995 NNS and the 2001 and 2004/5 National Health Surveys

Dietary indicator	Percentage of persons older than 12 years		
	1995 NNS	2001 NHS	2004/5 NHS
Type of milk usually consumed			
Not stated/unknown	1.9	0.2	0.9
Whole	50.9	48.7	45.4
Low/reduced fat	31.9	29.9	30.8
Skim	11.8	12.4	13.2
Other type of milk	0.6	4.1	4.6
None	4.0	4.9	5.1
Usual daily serves of vegetables			
Not stated/unknown	0.6	0.0	0.0
1 serve or less	27.2	22.5	20.5
2–3 serves	54.4	47.8	46.7
4 or more serves	17.8	29.7	32.8
Usual daily serves of fruit			
Not stated/unknown	0.6	0.0	0.0
1 serve or less	48.1	47.3	46.1
2 or more serves	51.4	52.7	53.9

supportive documentation about their origins and any modifications made over time are essential for monitoring purposes.

The ability of short questions to measure usual food habits is a key consideration. Ideally, the results obtained from the short question are compared with information about the same food habit from another data source known to give valid information. In practice, information is usually only available or obtainable from other self-reported data, which itself may have limitations and measurement error. Nevertheless, such attempts to document the comparative validity of short questions with another measure of dietary intake are helpful in evaluating the usefulness of the data obtained.

The use of short questions as indicators of diet quality are also of interest because changes in population food habits are often recommended to effect change in nutrient intake. For example, national dietary guidelines often recommend the use of reduced-fat dairy products as a means of reducing saturated fat intake. In this instance, it is important to know whether short questions about type of milk or other dairy products usually consumed (which contribute substantially to saturated fat intake) can differentiate between respondents with higher and lower intake of saturated fat. Occasionally, the validity of short questions has been assessed in relation to biomarkers; for example, fruit and vegetable intake in relation to blood folate and carotenoid levels (Coyne et al. 2005). Overall, relatively little work has been devoted to the assessment of the performance of short questions about food habits, including their ability to detect change over time (Marks et al. 2001). At least two studies in which the authors have been involved have shown selected short questions to have acceptable validity for classifying people as higher and lower consumers of particular foods or food groups, and reflect at least some differences in intakes of selected nutrients found in those foods (Riley et al. 2001; Rutishauser et al. 2001).

Data from short questions are particularly useful in 'triangulation' with other sources of information about changes in the food and nutrition situation; for example, changes in reported number of serves of fruit and vegetables, compared with food balance sheet information about the long-term supply of fruit and vegetables available, and more detailed data about changes in types and portion sizes of fruit and vegetables consumed, and the nutrient contribution they make to the total diet.

Interpretation
Because of the limited nature of the information obtainable from short questions, there are also clear limitations to the interpretation of data. Validation

studies to date have shown that, on average, quantitative estimates of foods consumed (when expressed in standard serves) differ from the number of serves as measured by short questions. Thus, using short questions to identify the percentage of individuals who meet specific recommendations, for example, greater than four serves of vegetables, is likely to result in misclassification error. Preferable ways of expressing and interpreting the data are to report the mean or median number of serves consumed, mean or median frequency of consumption or mean body mass index (BMI), and the distribution of responses in several categories from lowest to highest (either the response categories) or grouped response categories. These methods of summarising the data from short questions are less susceptible to misinterpretation and attaching a precision to the estimates that is not warranted. They also have the advantage of capturing more detail about which groups are making what changes over time.

Detailed dietary assessment (food and nutrient intake)

Routinely collected detailed information about the food and nutrient intake of the population and major sub-groups is essential for regulators to model the likely effects of changes in the food supply, to assess the extent of nutrient adequacy, and to provide a sound basis for nutrition policy and programmes. However, because surveys to obtain this kind of data involve the allocation of considerable resources, they have in the past tended to be conducted at often irregular intervals rather than routinely. Internationally, this situation is changing, with the National Center for Health Statistics in the United States having moved to a continuous dietary survey programme since 2002, and the Food Standards Agency in United Kingdom proposing to do so. Annual ongoing data collection will make it much more likely that real trends in dietary change can be assessed, and that responses to changing circumstances can be more timely.

More detailed information than can be obtained by means of the semi-quantitative food frequency questionnaires widely used in epidemiological studies is needed for quantitative assessment of food and nutrient intake. In such studies' information on habitual intake is essential in order to allow correlation with risk factor and/or disease status in the same individuals. In the context of food and nutrition monitoring, however, population subgroups rather than individuals are the units of interest, and what is needed is reliable data on the mean/median and the usual distribution of intake in groups. This does not require information on the *habitual* intake of individuals, but reliable information about actual foods and portion sizes from representative samples of the groups of interest. Samples need to be large enough to minimise sampling error, and the method must be acceptable to a wide range of respondents and be able to elicit an accurate quantitative response from those willing to participate. A standardised 24-hour recall procedure is generally regarded as the method most likely to meet these criteria. This method is used in the US NHANES surveys, and was recommended as the European Food Consumption Method (EFCOSUM)) for monitoring food consumption in nationally representative samples of all ages (Biro et al. 2002).

Practical considerations
Objective evidence from validation studies using doubly labelled water (DLW) as the reference method for energy intake clearly demonstrates that intake from self-reports such as 24-hour recalls often underestimates energy expenditure by as much as 20 per cent on average (Black et al. 1993), and that the extent of underestimation varies with gender and body mass index (Briefel et al. 1997). For this reason, the 24-hour recall method has been further refined, based on a structure that provides respondents with multiple recall strategies and memory cues to help them to remember the foods eaten the previous day (Ingwersen et al. 2004). In a study that compared energy intake by the Automated Multiple Pass Method (AMPM) with total energy expenditure obtained by DLW, no significant difference was found between the methods, nor were there any significant differences by gender or BMI category, suggesting that the AMPM is likely to be more effective than earlier 24-hour recall procedures (Cleveland et al. 2004). In surveys where it is not possible to measure energy expenditure by DLW, standard questions should be used to classify individuals according to their physical activity level to enable evaluation of the level of underreporting in the 24-hour recall data (Black 2000).

A single day's intake from each individual limits the value of the data for estimation of nutrient adequacy. This is because the one-day intake distribution invariably has a greater spread than the longer-term average intake distribution for the same individuals, because it includes day-to-day variation within individuals. Data for a second day of intake, or at least a sub-sample, and preferably for the whole group, is needed to remove the effect of within-person variation and obtain a better approximation of the usual distribution of intakes between individuals (Carriquiry 1999; Carriquiry 2003). Up-to-date food composition data, and comprehensive recipe and portion size information are also essential for accurate estimation of nutrient intake.

Interpretation
The data from one-off surveys conducted at intervals of five to ten years are difficult to compare without special studies to take into account methodological differences between them such as different age and geographical coverage,

nutrient databases and dietary methods. Guenther and Perloff (1990) have reviewed the effects of procedural differences on food and nutrient estimates from the 1977 and 1987 US Nationwide Food Consumption Surveys, and Cook and colleagues (2001) have described the process used to derive comparable data to assess time trends from two Australian surveys conducted more than ten years apart.

Assessing the adequacy of nutrient intake of populations and subgroups involves comparison with nutrient reference values published and updated from time to time by FAO and WHO, and by individual countries. Until the 1991 report on Dietary Reference Values for Food Energy and Nutrients in the United Kingdom, the published values have usually been a level of requirement designed to exceed the needs of virtually all (approximately 97 per cent) members of the population. Thus, they have been primarily useful for planning food supplies rather than evaluating intake, since they are not estimates of average requirements. The problems arising from the use of the same reference values both for planning diets and for assessing the prevalence of nutrient inadequacy have long been recognised (Beaton 1994), but detailed guidelines for the use of reference values were not published until 2000 (Institute of Medicine 2000). The effect of adjusting 24-hour intakes for day-to-day variation and under-reporting, and of using different nutrient reference values, is illustrated by Mackerras and Rutishauser (2005).

Nutritional status

The measures described above all provide clues to the nutritional status of the population, but are *not* measures of nutritional status. Assessment of nutritional status requires anthropometric (body measurements, in particular body weight and height), biochemical (for instance, blood lipids, urinary sodium and red cell folate), and physiological (such as, blood pressure) data on individuals.

Anthropometry

Anthropometric assessment is widely used for monitoring, not only because it is simple, inexpensive and non-invasive, but also because it provides exceedingly valuable information. Body weight and height are the fundamental measures of nutritional status — body weight because it is an overall measure of the individual's current nutritional status, and height because it reflects growth and development to date. In adults, height also provides the basis for assessing weight status as BMI.

Practical considerations

The apparent simplicity of weight and height measurements has, not infrequently, led to non-standard measurement techniques, use of inappropriate equipment, and inconsistent reporting of the data. Unless consistent approaches are used, comparisons with reference standards or assessment of trends over time will not be reliable. International recommendations for reference data for all ages, together with guidelines for their use and interpretation, were published by WHO in 1995 (De Onis & Habicht 1996). Standards for the reporting and analysis of data are also important, but may vary according to the use of the data.

Interpretation

Assessment of the prevalence of both under- and overweight is based on the availability and use of appropriate reference cut-offs. While classification categories for adult BMI (thin less than 18.50, normal 18.50 to 24.99, overweight 25.00 to 29.99, obese greater than 30.00) are well established (WHO 1995), there has been no universally accepted standard definition for child overweight and obesity. Adult value cut-offs are inappropriate because in childhood BMI changes with age. Cole et al. (2000) have proposed a new definition based on BMI centiles, developed from pooled international data, and constructed to pass through the adult overweight and obesity cut-off point of 25 and 30 at eighteen years. Agreement on, and use of, a standard set of reference values for anthropometric assessment, even if not ideal, enables more informative comparisons not only between population subgroups, but also over time, and in turn lead to more appropriate public health nutrition policy.

Biomedical assessments

In contrast to anthropometry, a large number of measurements (for example, biochemical measures of nutrient or metabolite levels in blood, urine and tissues, and physiological measures such as blood pressure) are used for the assessment of nutritional status in clinical practice. In the context of population-level monitoring, only some of these measures are practicable in terms of respondent acceptability and technical feasibility under survey conditions and/or resources. Most importantly, they must have a predictable relation to nutritional status. Thus, while it might be desirable to monitor the population's status for a wide range of nutrients, in practical terms little is to be gained from expenditure of limited resources and the goodwill of respondents on measurements for which there are no indications of excess or inadequate nutrient status from other sources of information.

Practical considerations

The first consideration is to identify which measurements will provide the most valuable information for addressing existing nutrition problems and/or confirming concerns about emerging problems that have been suggested by other data. Priorities for biochemical, clinical and anthropometric monitoring can be determined in different ways, as discussed previously, and depend on the availability of resources and on the existence of other information about the nutrition situation in the population. The focus should always be on measures for which there is clear evidence that changes of practical significance are possible and that such changes are associated with improved health status.

The technical considerations associated with the measures chosen for monitoring are measurement specific and beyond the scope of this chapter, except to reiterate that, irrespective of the measurement, it is always important to identify and document factors *other* than nutrition or the diet that may influence the relevant indicators, for example, smoking status, supplement use, medications and/or conditions that interfere with the measurement in question (see Gibson 2005 for detailed information about tests for assessing nutritional status.)

Interpretation

As for other measures of food and nutrition status, the interpretation of biomedical measurements is based on reference data and cut-off values based on the relationship between the measurement and various aspects of impaired nutritional status. Different approaches for deriving reference values for such measurements have been described by Habicht (1982). Not infrequently, the reference values used for classification simply represent the distribution of values found in an ostensibly healthy population. In this case, the cut-offs are statistically rather than biologically based, and classify individuals with values that fall in the lower and upper 2.5 per cent of the population distribution (that is, outside the 95 per cent confidence interval) as having unusually low or high values. Use of any cut-off value potentially misclassifies some individuals, and an understanding of the source and meaning of the cut-off is always needed for appropriate interpretation. (A discussion of sensitivity and specificity and the influence of prevalence on the predictive value of measures can be found in Gibson 2005.)

Consistency in the methods used to obtain biomedical data also needs to be taken into account. Over time, improved methods, new instrumentation and changes in measurement protocols designed to enhance data quality can affect the values obtained and introduce systematic differences that may be interpreted (erroneously) as secular trends, unless, as indicated earlier for food supply data, the changes are clearly documented and, where possible, their impact assessed.

The need for a system to support the collection and use of information about food and nutrition of populations

The term 'monitoring' has been used in this chapter to mean a system of routine data collection, analysis and reporting, to keep track of aspects of the food and nutrition situation of a population and important subgroups. In practice, the data may be collated from sources that are collected for other purposes (for example, from growth monitoring clinics; from food production statistics), or they may be collected in surveys specifically conducted for the purpose of monitoring, or some combination of the two. The essence of monitoring is that it is an ongoing activity, with routine reporting. The following are two examples of monitoring systems.

United States

Regular nutrition surveys have been conducted in the United States for more than three decades, and consolidated in 1990 through a congressional mandate to publish a report at least every five years on the dietary, nutritional and related health status of Americans, and the nutritional quality of the food they consume. The US Department of Agriculture (USDA) and the US Department of Health and Human Services (DHSS) jointly implement and coordinate the activities of the system. The central activity is a continuing survey programme conducted at the national level (National Health and Nutrition Examination Survey). However, the system includes a range of other components and data sources such as the Pediatric Nutrition Surveillance System and the Pregnancy Surveillance System, which monitor the nutritional status of low-income infants, children and women in federally funded maternal and child health programmes. Both the USDA and DHSS have technical groups that support the development and implementation of the system. An interagency board is responsible for planning, coordination and communication among agencies engaged in nutrition monitoring. Interpretation, data analysis and preparation of regular reports is carried out under contract by a scientific body such as the National Academy of Sciences.

New Zealand

Monitoring was introduced in New Zealand in response to the 1995 National Plan of Action for Nutrition (NPAN) and the need to monitor food, nutrition targets and weight targets, as well as a need for up-to-date knowledge about food and nutrient intake and nutritional status of the population at a time of rapid change in the food supply. The core of the system is a coordinated national survey programme, with a nutrition survey of adults and of children planned every ten years, commencing with the 1997 National Nutrition Survey (which was conducted on a sub-sample of participants in the previous NZ Health Survey), and the 2002 national Children's Survey, which was a stand-alone survey. The Public Health Directorate within the NZ Ministry of Health is responsible for planning and coordination, while the development and conduct of the surveys are contracted out. Further plans to develop the system include identifying secondary sources that may be used for monitoring food supply at national and household level, and to develop a reporting schedule and networks to improve dissemination of food and nutrition monitoring data.

While much of the discussion so far has focused on monitoring by governments at the national level, other successful models have been effectively implemented at state and local levels by government and non-government organisations to address specific issues. For example, Helen Keller International began nutrition monitoring in Bangladesh in 1990 to assess the health impact of severe floods in the country. They continue to report on health and programme issues more than a decade later. Similarly, nutrition monitoring was commenced in Indonesia at the time of the economic crisis in 1997, with regular reports published for the next five years (see <www.hki.org/research/ nutrition_surveillance.html>). In this case, a non-government organisation is involved with monitoring food security and malnutrition at both national (Bangladesh) and regional levels (Indonesia), with the mandate and resources coming from outside the national governments, and with support from international agencies.

The scope, agenda and methods used for food and nutrition monitoring systems have changed over time. Recent trends in the evolution of systems include the following:

- a shift in stakeholders and agendas — the initial priorities of most monitoring systems were based on public health concerns such as malnutrition; increasingly, food industry and the requirements for food regulation are shaping the priorities
- a shift from household to individual-based surveys — in response to the desire for more detailed information on the status of individual household members as they represent particular population subgroups
- introduction of continuing surveys, whereby data collection is an ongoing

activity, but with smaller sample sizes than in fixed cross-sectional surveys — a response to budget pressures, with experience showing that it is frequently easier to get political and administrative support for the smaller recurrent budgets

- harmonisation of methods across countries/regions in response to demands for comparable data — the prime example being EFCOSUM, a European project to develop methods for European food consumption surveys that provide internationally comparable data on a set of policy-relevant nutritional indicators; similar initiatives have been discussed elsewhere, but are not yet well developed
- international guidelines and models for priority issues — such as the WHO STEPwise approach for monitoring chronic disease risk factors, and the FAO recommendations for measurement and assessment of food deprivation and undernutrition.

The best model for a monitoring system in a particular situation depends very much on the specific priorities, the purpose of the system, and the resources available. Up until the late 1980s, much of the effort in nutrition monitoring focused on improving data quality and other technical aspects of monitoring, to the exclusion of broader organisational issues. Many developments failed to have any impact and were not sustainable because they ignored the needs of users. More recent, and successful, approaches have focused much more on the information users and uses. International experience across a range of circumstances has shown that the following conditions promote effective monitoring systems as they:

- have a person or unit responsible for coordinating the activities
- have a political and organisational mandate
- have a clear monitoring agenda and links with information users (that is, there is a demand for the information)
- include appropriate and timely analysis, interpretation, presentation and dissemination of information
- include mechanisms for evaluation and feedback regarding the information's usefulness for policy-setting and decision-making
- are practical and cost-effective.

Conclusion

This chapter has described the need for and considerations in selecting, using and interpreting methods for monitoring the nutritional status of populations.

A key premise of the chapter is that the ultimate purpose of monitoring is to improve the food and nutrition situation of populations by informing policy and programme development, monitoring progress towards national nutrition goals and guidelines, and identifying emerging nutrition problems that require action. International experience in nutrition monitoring has shown that conditions for successful systems include a clear mandate for continuity, adequate resources, effective, coordination, and relevance to food and nutrition policy and programmes, and to data users.

REFERENCES

Australian Bureau of Statistics (ABS) 1986 and 2000, *Household Expenditure Survey, Australia: Summary of results*, cat. 6530.0, ABS, Canberra.

— 2003, *Measuring Dietary Habits in the 2001 National Health Survey, Australia*, cat. 4814.0.0.5.001, ABS, Canberra.

Australian Institute of Health and Welfare (AIHW) 1998, 'Data standards for indicators of body fatness in Australian Adults' in *National Health Data Dictionary* (version 7), AIHW, Canberra.

— 1999, *Development of national public health indicators,* discussion paper, Health Division Working Paper No. 1, AIHW, Canberra.

Beaton, G.H. 1994, 'Criteria of an adequate diet' in Shils, R.E., Olsen, J.A. and Shike M. (eds) 1994, *Modern Nutrition in Health and Disease* (8th edn), Lea and Febiger, Philadelphia, pp. 1491–1505.

Biro, G., Hulshof, K.F.A.M., Ovesen, L. and Amopim Cruz, J.A. for the EFCOSUM Group 2002, 'Selection of methodology to assess food intake' in *European Journal of Clinical Nutrition,* vol. 56, pp. S25–32.

Black, A.E. 2000, 'The sensitivity and specificity of the Goldberg cut-off for EI:BMR for identifying diet reports of poor validity' in *European Journal of Clinical Nutrition*, vol. 54, pp. 395–404.

Black, A.E., Prentice, A.M., Goldberg, G.R., Jebb, S.A., Bingham, S.A., Livingstone, B.E. and Edward, A. 1993, 'Measurements of total energy expenditure provide insights into the validity of dietary measurements of energy intake' in *Journal of the American Dietetic Association*, vol. 93, pp. 572–79.

Briefel, R.R., Sempos, C.T., McDowell, M.A., Chien, S., and Alaimo, K. 1997, 'Dietary methods research in the third National Health and Nutrition Examination Survey: Underreporting of energy intake' in *American Journal of Clinical Nutrition*, vol. 65, pp. S1203–09.

Carriquiry, A.A. 1999, 'Assessing the prevalence of nutrient inadequacy' in *Public Health Nutrition*, vol. 2, pp. 23–33.

——. 2003, 'Estimation of usual intake distributions of nutrients and foods' in *Journal of Nutrition*, vol. 133, pp. S601–08.

Cleveland, L., Rhodes, D., Sebastian, R., Kuczynski, K., Clemens, J., Moshfegh, A. 2004, 'Validation of national 24-hour recall and physical activity methodology' [abstract], XIVth International Congress of Dietetics, Chicago.

Cole, T.J., Bellizzi, M.C., Flegal, K.M. and Dietz, W.H. 2000, 'Establishing a standard definition of child overweight and obesity worldwide: International survey' in *British Medical Journal*, vol. 320, pp. 1240–43.

Cook, T., Rutishauser, I.H.E. and Allsopp, R. 2001, *The Bridging Study: Comparing results from the 1983, 1985, and 1995; Australian national nutrition surveys*, National Food and Nutrition Monitoring and Surveillance Project, Commonwealth Department of Health and Aged Care, Canberra.

Coyne, T., Ibiebele, T.I. and McNaughton, S., Rutishauser, I.H.E., O'Dea, K., Hodge, A.M., McClintock, C., Findlay, M.G. and Lee, AZ. 2005, 'Evaluation of brief dietary questions to estimate vegetable and fruit consumption: Using serum carotenoids and red-cell folate' in *Public Health Nutrition*, vol. 8, pp. 298–308.

De Onis, M. and Habicht, J-P. 1996, 'Anthropometric reference data for international use: Recommendations from World Health Organization Expert Committee HOE' in *American Journal of Clinical Nutrition*, vol. 64, pp. 650–58.

Friel, S., Nelson, M., McCormack, K., Kelleher, C. and Thriskos, P., 2001, 'Methodological issues using household budget survey expenditure data for individual food availability estimation: Irish experience in the DAFNE pan-European project' in *Public Health Nutrition*, vol. 4, pp. 1143–48.

Gibson, R.S. 2005, *Principles of Nutritional Assessment* (2nd edn), Oxford University Press, New York.

Guenther, P.M. and Perloff, B.P. 1990, 'Effects of procedural differences between 1977 and 1987 in the Nationwide Food Consumption Survey estimates of food and nutrient intakes: Results of the USDA 1988 bridging study', NFCS Report No. 87-M-1, Accession No. PB92–178193, USDA, Beltsville, p. 48.

Habicht, J-P., Meyers, L.D. and Brownie, C. 1982, 'Indicators for counting the improperly nourished' in *American Journal of Clinical Nutrition*, vol. 35, pp. 1241–54.

Ingwersen, L., Cleveland, L., Heendeniya, K. and Moshfegh, A. 2004, 'How to ask people what they eat: Improved 24-hr intake method aids recall of foods eaten' (abstract) in *Journal of Nutrition Education*, vol. 36, p. S30.

Institute of Medicine (IOM) 2000, *Dietary Reference Intakes: Applications in dietary assessment*, National Academy Press, Washington D.C.

Lagiou, P., Trichopoulou, A. and the DAFNE contributers 2001, *Public Health Nutrition*, 4: pp. 1135–42.

Life Sciences Research Office 1995, *Executive Summary: Third Report on Nutrition Monitoring in the United States*, prepared for the Interagency Board for Nutrition Monitoring and Related Research, US Government Printing Office, Washington D.C., p. ES–24.

Mackerras, D.M. and Rutishauser I.H.E. 2005, '24-Hour national dietary survey data: How do we interpret them most effectively?' in *Public Health Nutrition*, vol. 8, pp. 657–65.

Marks, G.C., Webb, K., Rutishauser, I.H.E. and Riley, M. 2001, *Monitoring food habits in the Australian population using short questions*, National Food and Nutrition Monitoring and Surveillance Project, Commonwealth Department of Health and Aged Care, Canberra.

Mathers, C. and Schofield, D.J. 1997, 'Development of national public health indicators', paper presented to the National Public Health Information Working Group meeting, December.

Ministry of Health (NZ) 2003, 'Food and Nutrition Monitoring in New Zealand' in *Public Health Intelligence Occasional Bulletin*, no. 19, Wellington, cited at <http://www.moh.govt.nz>.

Ockhuizen, T., Vaessen, H.A.M.G., de Vos R.H. 1991, 'The validity of total diet studies for assessing nutrient intake' in MacDonalds, I. (ed.) 1991 *Monitoring Dietary Intakes*, Springer Verlag, Berlin, pp. 9–18.

Quigley, R. and Watts, C. 1997, *Food Comes First: Methodologies for the National Nutrition Survey of New Zealand*, Public Health Report Number 2, Ministry of Health, Wellington.

Riley, M., Rutishauser, I.H.E. and Webb, K. 2001, *Comparison of Short Questions with Weighed Dietary Records*, National Food and Nutrition Monitoring and Surveillance Project, Commonwealth Department of Health and Aged Care, Canberra.

Rutishauser, I.H.E., Webb, K., Abraham, B. and Allsopp, R. 2001, *Evaluation of Short Dietary Questions from the 1995 National Nutrition Survey*, National Food and Nutrition Monitoring and Surveillance Project, Commonwealth Department of Health and Aged Care, Canberra.

Slater, J.M. (ed.) 1991, *Fifty Years of the National Food Survey 1940–1990*, proceedings of a symposium held in December 1990, Her Majesty's Stationery Office, London.

Strategic Intergovernmental Nutrition Alliance 2001, *Eat Well Australia: An agenda for action in public health nutrition 2000–2010*, Commonwealth Department of Health and Aged Care, Canberra.

Trichopoulou, A. (ed.) 1992, 'Methodology and public health aspects of dietary surveillance in Europe: The use of household budget surveys' in *European Journal of Clinical Nutrition*, vol. 46, pp. S1–153.

Webb, K., Marks, G.C., Lund-Adams, M., Rutishauser, I.H.E. and Abraham, B. 2001, *Towards a National System for Monitoring Breastfeeding in Australia*, National Food and Nutrition Monitoring and Surveillance Project, Commonwealth Department of Health and Aged Care, Canberra.

World Health Organization (WHO) 1995, *Physical Status: The use and interpretation of anthropometry*, report of a WHO Expert Committee, Technical Report Series No. 854, WHO, Geneva.

13

Physical activity

Anna Timperio
Clare Hume
Julie Saunders
Jo Salmon

The purpose of this chapter is to describe the importance of physical activity within the context of public health nutrition, and introduce key concepts and methods of assessing physical activity in populations. The chapter also examines physical activity within a behavioural epidemiology framework. Behavioural epidemiology combines methods, applications and theory of epidemiology and behavioural science (Raymond 1989), and thus describes the distribution of behaviour and provides a promising method of investigating why a behaviour is performed and how that behaviour may be influenced. The behavioural epidemiology of physical activity is examined throughout the life course, with a focus on youth, adults and older adults.

Physical activity and public health nutrition

The discipline of public health nutrition has continually evolved in response to emerging population needs. Most recently, it has broadened its focus to include physical activity in response to the significant and increasing threat to population health posed by cardiovascular disease (CVD), obesity, type 2 diabetes and osteoporosis − non-communicable diseases that share their origins in both poor nutrition and inadequate physical activity (Sjöström et al. 1999). It is recognised that these threats to population health are unlikely to be resolved by focusing on nutrition alone.

Defining physical activity

Physical activity is commonly defined as 'bodily movement that is produced by the contraction of skeletal muscle and that substantially increases energy expenditure' (US Department of Health and Human Services 1996). It is a complex behaviour that can be planned or unplanned (incidental). Among adults, physical activity typically occurs within one of four domains (circumstance or purpose): household, leisure-time, occupational and transport. The distinction between these domains is important for the assessment of physical activity, as well as for understanding the various influences on different types of physical activity. Adult physical activity is rarely a stable behaviour, differing from 'day to day, season to season, and year to year' (Sallis & Owen 1999). Among children, physical activity usually consists of active play, organised and non-organised sports, school physical education (PE), transport-related activity (for example, walking and cycling), chores, and other incidental activities, and, unlike adults, is characterised as spontaneous, sporadic and intermittent (Pangrazi et al. 1997).

In general, there are four dimensions of physical activity among adults and children: frequency, intensity, duration and type (Sallis & Owen 1999). Different combinations of these dimensions constitute a dose of physical activity and may have different relationships with health outcomes (for example, vigorous-intensity activity is beneficial for cardiovascular fitness; strength training assists functional health; weight-bearing, high-impact physical activity benefits bone health).

Public health benefits of physical activity

Regular physical activity contributes to healthy growth among children, and good health and the prevention of disease among people of all ages. The act of being physically active affects multiple systems within the body, including the musculoskeletal, cardiovascular, respiratory and endocrine systems (US Department of Health and Human Services 1996). Thus, regular physical activity has a broad range of benefits for physical and mental health at all stages of the lifespan. Among adults, there is consistent epidemiological evidence that physical activity reduces the risk of all-cause mortality, coronary heart disease, CVD, hypertension, colon cancer and type 2 diabetes (US Department of Health and Human Services 1996). There is also evidence that physical activity helps to control body weight, improve musculoskeletal health, achieve and maintain peak bone mass, relieve symptoms of depression and anxiety, improve mood and enhance psychological wellbeing and physical functioning (US Department of Health and Human Services 1996). The benefits of physical activity among older adults are similar. Further, age-related deterioration of the cardiovascular system can be reversed by physical activity, and the combination of balance exercises and regular resistance training contribute to preventing frailty and falls, and lead to improved functional status and independent living (Taylor et al. 2004). Among children, although there are limited studies, there is some evidence of links between physical inactivity and risk factors for CVD, overweight/obesity and type 2 diabetes, and positive associations between physical activity and psychosocial outcomes and bone health (Biddle et al. 2004).

Recommendations

Recommendations for physical activity among children and adults provide a benchmark for population monitoring, and inform public health policy and programmes. The recommended dose and intensity of physical activity for youth is reasonably consistent across countries. The United States, United Kingdom, and Australia recommend that youth should participate in at least 60 minutes of moderate- to vigorous-intensity physical activity every day (Strong et al. 2005; UK Department of Health 2004; Australian Government Department of Health and Ageing 1994). In addition to physical activity recommendations for youth, many countries have also developed guidelines for sedentary behaviour that endorse no more than two hours per day using electronic entertainment media (that is, television viewing, computer games and Internet use). The Canadian guidelines, however, are less prescriptive, recommending all youth increase their physical activity by 30 minutes per day and reduce their electronic entertainment media use by 30 minutes per day (Health Canada 2002).

Current public health recommendations for physical activity among adults consistently endorse the accumulation of at least 30 minutes of moderate-intensity physical activity on five to seven days per week (UK Department of Health 2004; Commonwealth Department of Health and Aged Care 1999; US Department of Health and Human Services 1996). Each 30-minute session may consist of a single bout of activity or an accumulation of three or more eight- to ten-minute bouts of activity. Moderate-intensity activity is usually defined as a brisk walking pace, equivalent to approximately 3 METs (multiple units of resting metabolic rate), which confers approximately 800 kjoul/calorie of physical activity energy expenditure per week. In addition to following these general population guidelines, most recommendations for older adults also endorse regular participation in physical activities that contribute to functional living capabilities, such as muscle strength, coordination, balance and flexibility (US Department of Health and Human Services 1996; UK Department of Health 2004).

Assessment

There are numerous tools currently available for the assessment of physical activity. Some assess physical activity 'behaviour', while others are measures of energy expenditure (a consequence of physical activity). In general, six key criteria are used to evaluate measurement tools:

1. reliability
2. validity
3. sensitivity to change
4. non-reactivity (do not cause the respondent to change their behaviour)
5. acceptability to respondent (low burden)
6. acceptable cost (Sallis & Owen 1999).

No available method meets each criterion; few methods are able to provide information about all the dimensions of physical activity and the domains in which it occurs; few methods of physical activity assessment are appropriate for use across all age groups. Selection of the most appropriate assessment tool depends on the purpose (for example, population monitoring) and outcome of interest (for example, population health relating to metabolic diseases).

Assessment for individuals versus populations

Physical activity is usually assessed using questionnaires or diaries, interviews, observation, or direct measurement using objective tools. Each method of assessment has varying levels of accuracy (error) and practicality, and thus some are more suitable for assessment in individuals or small samples, while others are more suited to assessment of populations. Assessment of physical activity in individuals requires accurate measures that are sufficiently sensitive to detect differences over time. Intervention research also requires measures that are sensitive to change. For population-based research, less accurate tools that are practical and acceptable to large groups of people, such as self-report instruments, are commonly used to provide information about levels of activity in relative terms (Kriska & Casperson 1997). Objective instruments, such as pedometers and accelerometers, can also be used in populations.

Self-report measures

Self-report instruments require the respondent to recollect their past physical activity behaviour, and can be classified as global, recall or quantitative history instruments, based on the level of detail they request and resultant burden to respondents (Matthews 2002). Recall surveys are most commonly used in population-based studies and can be self- or interviewer-administered (face-to-face or telephone). Interviewer-administered instruments generally tend to have greater validity than self-administered instruments (Matthews 2002).

Recall surveys are inexpensive, easy to administer and process with large groups, unobtrusive and non-reactive, with low to medium subject burden — five to fifteen questions (Matthews 2002). They allow the assessment of physical activity dose through questions about frequency, duration and intensity of recent physical activity. Thus, many recall surveys are able to be used to assess compliance with physical activity recommendations. Recall surveys also vary in the amount of contextual information captured. Some assess just one or two domains (for instance, Active Australia Survey), while others assess physical activity across multiple domains (for example, the International Physical Activity Questionnaire). In addition, some require respondents to recall specific types of activities, such as organised sport or strength training, while more cognitively challenging surveys request respondents to recall and sum many different types of physical activity performed at the same intensity in one response (for example, all moderate-intensity activity).

Self-report surveys are associated with several limitations (see Table 13.1). Cognitively, the act of recalling physical activity, particularly broad categories of physical activity, can be a challenging task (Matthews 2002). Recall capabilities and memory may hinder an individual's ability to accurately recall their physical activity, particularly over long timeframes. Similarly, ambiguous or new terms (such as moderate-intensity activity) and poor comprehension of the specific information to be reported (for example, recall of activity performed in bouts of at least ten minutes) may also affect accuracy, with the potential for wide variation between individuals (Sallis & Saelens 2000). Social desirability biases may also contribute to over-reporting. Several studies have found that vigorous-intensity physical activity is recalled with greater accuracy than less intense physical activity (Matthews 2002; Sallis & Saelens 2000), potentially because vigorous-intensity activity is more likely to be planned.

Limitations of self-report instruments vary for different life stages. For example, the validity of self-report responses is of concern among children under the age of ten years, who typically lack the cognitive ability to accurately recall their activity (Sallis & Owen 1999). Proxy-report instruments administered to parents and/or teachers can be used instead; however, parents and teachers may not be aware of all activities undertaken while the child was not in their care (Sirard & Pate 2001). In addition, the sporadic and spontaneous nature of children's activity is difficult to recall, and may be more readily captured using objective measures.

Table 13.1 Limitations of self-report measures of physical activity, pedometers and accelerometers

Type	General	Children & youth	Older adults
Self-report	• social desirability bias • cognitively challenging • may be affected by memory • unplanned physical activity not a 'memorable' event • poor understanding of terms (e.g., moderate-intensity)	• not suitable for children under ten years • sporadic/spontaneous physical activity difficult to recall	• recall can be challenging • may require large font • should include age-appropriate activities and activities related to functional living
Pedometers	• only captures walking • no behavioural information • no contextual information (e.g. information about domain) • accuracy may be affected among abdominally obese • may influence physical activity	• some common activities performed by children (e.g. climbing, cycling and swimming) do not involve walking • compliance	• unable to detect shuffled steps
Accelerometers	• no behavioural information • no contextual information • some models not waterproof • underestimation of physical activity for activities where the torso remains relatively static (e.g. strength training)	• cycling, a popular activity for children, is underestimated • compliance	• little validation undertaken specifically among elderly

There may also be challenges in assessing physical activity among older adults, particularly those with cognitive impairments or poor vision or hearing (Harada et al. 2001). Several instruments have been designed specifically for older adults, which are presented in large font and include age-appropriate activities (Harada et al. 2001). Consistent with physical activity recommendations for this life stage, instruments designed for older adults should assess factors relating to functional living (for instance, participation in strengthening exercises, flexibility, balance, household activities and light-intensity activities).

Pedometers and accelerometers

New technologies have been developed to overcome the limitations associated with using self-report instruments in population studies. Although not yet widely used for population-based studies, pedometers and accelerometers have distinct advantages over self-report measures. Both are small, lightweight devices, usually worn at the hip. The pedometer detects and counts steps, and is thus used as an objective measure of walking behaviour. It is particularly useful for capturing incidental walking (for instance, while doing chores at home), which is usually difficult to recall and quantify. Accelerometers quantify intensity and amount (frequency and duration) of physical activity, resulting in a measure of movement counts/minute, with higher counts/minute indicating greater intensity of activity. They allow unrestricted movement, collect data in real time over long periods, and are able to be used in all age groups. Recent models are also waterproof.

Pedometers have been shown to be reliable and valid (Tudor-Locke & Myers 2001), and accelerometers have been shown to provide valid estimates of heart rate and energy expenditure among children (Trost et al. 1998) and adults (Melanson & Freedson 1995). However, neither instrument can collect behavioural information on the type of activities undertaken or the contexts in which they occurred, and some activities may be underestimated if the accelerometer is worn on the hip and the torso remains relatively static during the activity (for example, cycling, strength training). Although pedometers and accelerometers can be used with most age groups, their accuracy may be lower in certain population groups, such as the elderly (the pedometer is unable to detect shuffled steps) and those with abdominal obesity (if positioning is not vertical) (Tudor-Locke & Myers 2001).

Prevalence and trends

Physical activity prevalence among youth

As identified in the previous section, children's physical activity can be challenging to assess at the individual and the population level. Many countries have only recently established or updated their physical activity recommendations for youth; therefore, few have reported compliance with current recommendations in the population.

Most of the available data on population prevalence of youth physical activity are based on adult recommendations. The 2003 US Youth Risk Behavior Survey found that 63 per cent of adolescents (9th to 12th grade) had exercised or participated in vigorous-intensity physical activity for more than twenty minutes, three or more days per week, and one-quarter had participated in moderate-intensity physical activity for more than 30 minutes, five or more days per week (Centers for Disease Control and Prevention 2004). More than one-third of youth surveyed failed to meet adult physical activity recommendations for health. In contrast, just nineteen per cent of Finnish youth and young adults (15 to 24 years) were physically active four to six times per week for at least 30 minutes each time during their leisure-time (Helakorpi et al. 2005). Also based on adult physical activity recommendations, in 1996, 20 to 25 per cent of Australian youth failed to participate in 30 minutes moderate-intensity physical activity, five or more days per week (Booth 2000).

One of the few nations to have reported the prevalence of youth meeting the 60-minute per day recommendation is the United Kingdom. In 2002, it was found that 30 per cent of boys and 40 per cent of girls in the United Kingdom failed to meet physical activity recommendations for children (Department of Health 2003). In Scotland, 27 per cent of boys and 40 per cent of girls were not active enough to meet the youth physical activity guidelines (Physical Activity Taskforce 2003).

It is difficult to compare these population estimates across countries, as different methods of assessment have been used and prevalence estimates have also been based on different recommendations (mainly adult). One of the challenges of monitoring children's physical activity is the assessment of this complex, multifaceted health behaviour. Methodological studies to develop internationally acceptable youth physical activity instruments suitable for population monitoring are required.

Physical activity prevalence among adults

Data on the proportion of the population meeting physical activity recommendations are more readily available for adults than they are for children. In

Australia, there have been three population surveys (1997, 1999, 2000) of adults aged 18 to 75 years (Bauman et al. 2002). From 1997 to 2000, the proportion of Australians who were sufficiently active for health benefits decreased from 62 to 57 per cent. Physical activity rates were higher in Finland in 2005, with 60 and 68 per cent of men and women, respectively, physically active at least twice a week (Helakorpi et al. 2005). However, this is a lower threshold (two physical activity sessions/week) than those employed in the Australian prevalence estimates. In contrast, the 2003 Health Survey for England found that only 37 per cent of men and 24 per cent of women were sufficiently active for health benefits (Stamatakis 2005), with the proportion meeting recommendations declining with age from 41 per cent of 16 to 24 year olds to 5 per cent of those aged 75 years and over.

Consistent use of survey instruments and interpretation of physical activity recommendations is essential for population monitoring. To illustrate, in 2000 the US Behavioral Risk Factor Surveillance System found 26 per cent of adults met physical activity recommendations; however, in 2001 the proportion who met the recommendations increased to 45 per cent after a modified version of the physical activity survey was used that included moderate-intensity activities (Centers for Disease Control and Prevention 2003).

In summary, in many countries it is estimated that approximately half (or fewer) of adults are meeting physical activity recommendations for health. These figures suggest that there is an urgent need for the development of effective population strategies to promote physical activity, particularly if countries are to meet physical activity goals and targets.

Physical activity prevalence among older adults

As with adults, older adults' physical activity estimates vary according to the definition applied and to the instrument used. In 2003, 48 per cent of older men and 44 per cent of older women (65 to 84 years) in Finland walked for at least 30 minutes every day of the week; and 15 per cent of older men and women engaged in exercise (other than walking) every day of the week (Sulander et al. 2004). A smaller proportion of older adults (those over 50 years) met the physical activity recommendations in Switzerland, with approximately 9 per cent engaged in moderate-intensity physical activity, and 18 per cent participating in vigorous-intensity activity (Meyer et al. 2005). However, half of those aged 65 to 79 years and 80 years or over reported they were habitually active. In 2004, fewer men in the United States aged 70 years or more were physically inactive (approximately 30 per cent) compared with women in the same age group (approximately 40 per cent) (Centers for Disease Control and Prevention

2005). These estimates represent a significant decline in US population levels of inactivity from 1996 to 2004 (approximately a five per cent absolute decline for men and women).

Although many countries have developed physical activity recommendations for older adults, few have reported the prevalence of participation in specific domains or participation in activities that contribute to functional living. Future population surveys should assess what proportions of older adults engage in strength, balance or coordination activities.

Influences on physical activity

To increase the proportion of the population who are physically active, it is important to understand why many individuals do not participate in sufficient levels of physical activity. As the influences on participation are extremely diverse, conceptual theories or models are often applied as a means of summarising and understanding those factors most likely to be important (Sallis & Owen 1999).

Using theory to understand physical activity

Several behavioural theories have been applied to explain physical activity. Early theoretical models of health behaviours, such as the Health Belief Model and the Theory of Planned Behaviour, posit that health behaviour is primarily influenced by psychological factors such as attitudes and intentions; however, these models are often criticised for their failure to consider the broader contexts in which health behaviours occur (Sallis & Owen 1999).

Social-ecological theories are gaining in popularity as they incorporate broader contextual influences on behaviour (Sallis & Owen 1999). Ecological models, for example, acknowledge the connections between people and the environments in which they live (Stokols 1996; Sallis & Owen 2002), with behaviours influenced by interactions between individuals, their social systems, and their physical and policy environments (Stokols 1996). Influences on physical activity, particularly contextual influences in the social and physical environment, are likely to differ across life stages. Parental support, for example, is likely to be an important influence on physical activity during childhood and perhaps during adolescence, but is less likely to be influential during young adulthood.

The following sections explore individual, social and environmental influences on physical activity across the lifespan.

Individual-level influences on physical activity

Individual-level influences incorporated in ecological models can be broadly grouped as demographic, biological, cognitive/psychological and behavioural (Sallis et al. 2000; Trost et al. 2002). Age and gender are important demographic influences on physical activity throughout the lifespan; younger people are more active than older people, and males are generally more active than females (Sallis et al. 2000; Trost et al. 2002). Individual socioeconomic status (SES, usually indicated by parent's education levels, own education level, occupation or income) has been positively associated with physical activity in all age groups, particularly among adults (Trost et al. 2002; US Department of Health and Human Services 1996). Conversely, body mass index and physical activity has been negatively associated among all age groups (Sallis et al. 2000; Trost et al. 2002; Di Francesco et al. 2005).

Among cognitive or psychological factors, self-efficacy, or one's confidence in their ability to be physically active in various circumstances (Sallis & Owen 1999), is one of the most consistent predictors of physical activity among adults (Trost et al. 2002) and older adults (Booth et al. 2000), although studies of children and youth have produced mixed results (Sallis et al. 2000). Adults and older adults who perceive that there are benefits from physical activity tend to be more active than those who do not (Trost et al. 2002; Burton et al. 1999), while in all age groups, individuals who perceive barriers to physical activity, particularly having a lack of time for exercise among adults, are less likely to be active than those perceiving fewer barriers (Booth et al. 1997; Sallis et al. 2000; Trost et al. 2002).

Intention to be active is positively associated with physical activity during childhood and adolescence (Sallis et al. 2000) and during adulthood (Trost et al. 2002), but has not been examined among older adults. Adults who enjoy physical activity tend to be more active than those who do not (Trost et al. 2002), but there is no consistent relationship among children or youth (Sallis et al. 2000). However, perceived physical competence is positively associated with physical activity during adolescence (Sallis et al. 2000). Fear of injury is often inversely associated with physical activity among older adults (Ewing Garber & Blissmer 2002), but has not been comprehensively examined among youth or young adults. Among behavioural attributes, previous participation in physical activity is consistently positively associated with current physical activity among children and adolescents (Sallis et al. 2000), and a history of physical activity during adulthood, but not childhood, is consistently related to physical activity among adults (Trost et al. 2002).

Social influences on physical activity

An individual's social environment generally consists of influences from proximal sources such as family members and peers or friends, as well as distal sources such as neighbourhood relations and the neighbourhood social environment.

Social support is one of the most consistent factors associated with physical activity. Adolescents, adults and older adults who receive support for physical activity from significant others, including family members, friends and peers, tend to be more likely to be physically active than those who do not receive support (Sallis et al. 2000; Ewing Garber & Blissmer 2002; Trost et al. 2002). Receiving support for physical activity from a physician is also a positive influence on physical activity among adults (Trost et al. 2002) and older adults (Ewing Garber & Blissmer 2002). There is mixed evidence of the influence of modelling on physical activity among children, adolescents and adults (Sallis et al. 2000; Trost et al. 2002). However, the frequency others are observed being active in the neighbourhood has been positively associated with physical activity among adults (Trost et al. 2002).

Though not commonly studied, the sociability of local neighbourhoods also appears to be important. For example, emerging research suggests that having social opportunities in the neighbourhood is positively associated with youth physical activity (Carver et al. 2005). Another study has found that adults who live in a friendly neighbourhood are more physically active than those living in less friendly areas (Lindstrom et al. 2001). Further, social isolation appears to be inversely associated with participation in physical activity among adults and older adults (Ewing Garber & Blissmer 2002; Trost et al. 2002).

Environmental influences on physical activity

The concept of a 'behaviour setting' has often been used to study the influence of the environment on physical activity (Sallis & Owen 2002). Current physical activity guidelines encourage the accumulation of physical activity throughout the day. Thus, physical activity is encouraged in all settings within the contexts of people's everyday lives. This section focuses on the home and neighbourhood environments, as these behaviour settings are broadly applicable to people of all ages, and only limited research has examined correlates of physical activity within other settings.

Within the home environment, both youth (Trost et al. 1999) and adults (Trost et al. 2002) who have access to physical activity equipment at home tend to be more physically active than those without such equipment. It is not known, however, whether physical activity equipment within the home is supportive of physical activity among older adults.

The physical environment within the neighbourhood is a growing area of physical activity research, and emerging studies suggest that it may be an important influence on physical activity (Sallis et al. 2005). Among children and adolescents, a small number of studies have found that access to facilities and opportunities to exercise are positively associated with physical activity, but there is mixed evidence about whether seasonality and residing in an urban or rural location are related to physical activity in these age groups (Sallis et al. 2000). Among adults, several studies have shown that living in an urban location is a negative influence on physical activity (Trost et al. 2002). Weak associations have also been found between physical activity and weather, and safety among adults (Humpel et al. 2002). Although neighbourhood safety is often assumed to influence physical activity, the evidence among studies of children is mixed (Sallis et al. 2000). This may be because 'safety' is a complex concept comprising environmental hazards (for instance, traffic), incivilities (such as litter and graffiti) and aspects of social safety such as bullying or being approached by strangers. Each dimension is likely to have different relationships with physical activity and should be examined separately. It is also possible that perceptions about elements of safety may differ from reality. Recently, however, studies have shown that features of neighbourhoods that assist safe negotiation of traffic, such as lights and crossings, may support walking or cycling among children (Timperio et al. 2004a; Timperio et al. 2006).

Among adults, aesthetic attributes, convenience of walking facilities (for example, footpaths, trails) and accessibility of destinations (like shops, parks) have been associated with walking (Owen et al. 2004), while aesthetics, opportunities to be active, and access to facilities have been associated with overall physical activity (Humpel et al. 2002). There is also consistent evidence from transportation studies that aspects of urban form, such as population density, mixed land use and highly connected streets, are supportive of utilitarian walking and cycling among adults (Saelens et al. 2003).

Few studies have examined environmental influences on physical activity specifically among older adults. Emerging research suggests that living in a rural area (Lim & Taylor 2005) and living within walking distance of a park, store, or bicycle or walking trail (King et al. 2003) may be important. Booth and colleagues (2000) also found that older adults were more likely to be active if they found footpaths to be safe for walking and perceived good access to local facilities. Emerging approaches to examining influences on physical activity within a social-ecological framework are presented in Box 13.1.

Box 13.1 Emerging methodologies in physical activity research

The connections between people and the environments in which they live is a central tenet of ecological models (Stokols 1996; Sallis & Owen 2002). These models are based on interactions between individuals and the multiple contexts in which they live (for example, family, school or workplace, neighbourhood environments); however, few studies have examined such interactions in relation to physical activity. Multi-level analyses provide an ideal method of examining these interactions (Duncan et al. 2004). These kinds of analyses take into account the level at which data is nested. For example, individual-level data comprises factors related only to individuals (such as level of education, self-efficacy), while area-level data comprises characteristics of an area that is shared by all those living in that area or who interact with that setting (for instance, the school environment or the neighbourhood environment). Multi-level models take into account the shared variance associated with area-level data.

In their multi-level study van Lenthe and colleagues (2005) studied participants from 78 neighbourhoods. They found inequities in leisure-time physical activities according to socioeconomic disadvantage within these neighbourhoods; and that neighbourhood characteristics (for example neighbourhood design) contributed to these inequities. Multi-level studies provide a more appropriate technique for analysing data that is shared at a group level. They also provide rich data to help researchers understand how people and their environments interact to influence behaviour. Thus, such studies may have important implications for the promotion of physical activity as they aid in understanding where the majority of efforts should be directed (for example it may be that individual influences on physical activity are stronger than environmental influences).

Promotion of physical activity

The evidence presented in this chapter shows a clear need to promote physical activity across populations to improve public health. However, little is known about how best to influence physical activity. Physical activity promotion should be based on the best evidence available, employ a comprehensive range of strategies, have sound theoretical underpinnings, and be appropriately evaluated to enable the effectiveness of initiatives to be measured and potentially improved. Tailoring interventions to the target group is crucial, given that the determinants of physical activity vary across the lifespan and also between certain population groups. Physical activity interventions can occur at a number of levels; some are tailored to specific individuals, others to particular target groups, communities or populations. The types of strategies employed, and the degree of behaviour change that can be expected, differ according to the level, intensity and effectiveness of the intervention. Many interventions use a settings-based approach, whereby a range of strategies are employed within a particular setting (for example, schools, primary care settings, worksites). These settings comprise captive audiences, where physical activity messages or programmes can be delivered efficiently (Sallis & Owen 1999). In this section, selected interventions trialled within common settings will be described.

Children and adolescents

Many interventions to increase young people's participation in physical activity have been trialled within the school setting, though a number have been delivered in other settings (Timperio et al. 2004b; Salmon & King 2005).

School settings

Within the school setting, Bauman and colleagues (2002) suggest that limiting options for sedentary behaviours, improving links between schools and communities, emphasising participation and skill development rather than competition, curriculum changes and pre- and in-service training for primary teachers may be promising strategies for increasing physical activity among youth. Timperio and colleagues (2004b) stress the importance of comprehensive, whole-of-school approaches, suggesting that approaches that were inclusive of curriculum, policy and environmental strategies were more effective than curriculum-only strategies.

Specific initiatives that have had some success in increasing physical activity among youth within the school setting include policy and environmental strategies such as the introduction of playground markings and PE classes with better trained specialist teachers and greater emphasis on being active for a greater proportion of class time (Matson-Koffman et al. 2005).

Other settings

Other settings in which physical activity interventions for children or adolescents have been trialled include family, primary care, community and transport (Timperio et al. 2004b; Salmon & King 2005). Those interventions that implement strategies both in schools and in families appear to hold most promise (Salmon & King 2005). Specific intervention strategies that have achieved moderate success include mother/daughter exercise classes and the promotion of dancing among adolescent girls, after-school programmes with regular family contact, counselling by primary care providers (potentially coupled with screening and goal setting) and comprehensive strategies to support active transport to school, such as mapping of safe routes, education, walking buses or cycle trains, competitions and promotions (Salmon & King 2005). Few interventions have sought to change aspects of the environment in an effort to increase physical activity among children.

Adults

To date, interventions targeting adults have led to short- to mid-term increases in physical activity, and there is very limited evidence of their long-term effectiveness (Hillsdon et al. 2005).

Workplace settings

Although there are few examples of the long-term effectiveness of workplace interventions, the available evidence suggests that comprehensive worksite approaches that include education, employee and peer support, incentives and access to exercise facilities are most successful in increasing physical activity (Matson-Koffman et al. 2005). However, some simple workplace interventions, such as environmental adaptations to stairwells (Kerr et al. 2004) and individual physical activity counselling (Proper et al. 2003), have achieved moderate short-term success.

Primary care settings

There is mixed evidence of the effectiveness of efforts of primary care practitioners to intervene to increase their patient's physical activity (Salmon & King 2005). However, some randomised controlled trials have shown that the provision of professional advice and guidance by primary care practitioners, coupled with continued support, can encourage adults to be more physically active (Hillsdon et al. 2005).

Community settings

Within the community setting, mass media is generally perceived as a cost-effective means of reaching large numbers of people. While mass media can increase awareness, particularly for those who are at earlier stages of exercise adoption, mass media alone is unlikely to change behaviour. A range of strategies are needed to support messages promoted by mass media, including environmental and policy approaches (Bauman et al. 2002). Examples of policy and environmental strategies that have been shown to be successful include prompts to increase stair use, and increased access to places and opportunities for physical activity (Matson-Koffman et al. 2005). Intersectoral collaboration, including involvement from health, local government, education and transport sectors, is required to implement the range of strategies needed to support community wide interventions to increase physical activity.

Older adults
Key considerations for planning interventions for older adults include the need for pre-activity screening and the need to determine whether the target group has any special needs or limitations, such as lack of mobility, transport options or social support.

Community vs home settings
Reviews of physical activity interventions suggest that, among older adults, participation rates are higher in home-based compared to group-based interventions (Taylor et al. 2004). Furthermore, interventions that employ strategies relying solely on community facilities have been shown to be less effective than those that also include home-based strategies and those that are home-based only, regardless of whether the home-based intervention is supervised (Taylor et al. 2004).

Primary care settings
Among older people, interventions in primary care settings, particularly those that maintained contact for a long period and individually tailored programmes, have been moderately successful in increasing physical activity (Cyarto et al. 2004). Taylor and colleagues (2004) suggest that reinforcing physical activity by providing advice to exercise more may make older adults more receptive to other efforts to increase physical activity within the community setting (for example, public walking promotion signs). Salmon and King (2005) also highlight the importance of the role of the general practitioner as an advocate for physical activity.

Conclusions

Physical inactivity is a significant public health issue. While the nutrition and physical activity disciplines have traditionally worked separately, there is a need to view nutrition and physical activity from a holistic perspective and to recognise that progress toward resolving many public health issues requires combined efforts (Sjöström et al. 1999). Considering physical activity in the context of public health nutrition is critical, given that poor nutrition and inadequate levels of physical activity both contribute to the development of many increasingly prevalent non-communicable diseases. However, the benefits of physical activity to health and wellbeing also extend beyond the prevention of obesity, diabetes and CVD, to include healthy growth and development, as well as functional and psychological health. Thus, it is important to work towards improved levels of physical activity among all age groups. The data described in this chapter suggest that many children, adolescents, adults and older adults are insufficiently active for health benefits. A significant proportion of the population do not meet public health recommendations to accrue one hour per day of physical activity among youth and 30 minutes of physical activity on most days among adults and older adults. However, few studies have examined whether older adults are meeting recommendations to engage in activities to improve or maintain functional living.

A large body of literature has examined potential influences on physical activity behaviour among youth and adults, but less has focused on older adults. Consistent with ecological models, correlates of physical activity are varied, and include individual, social and environmental influences. However, to date, most studies have been cross-sectional observation studies, thus it is not possible to infer causal relationships. In recent years, there has been a strong research focus on understanding how the built or physical environment influences physical activity; most of this research has focused on adults. However, the most salient features of the environment that may support or hinder the physical activity of youth and older adults may differ to those that are important among adults. Furthermore, as children lack complete autonomy, their parent's perceptions of the local environment in relation to risk and the child's level of maturity may be more important than objectively determined features of the environment.

Despite recent interest in the environment as an influence on physical activity, few studies to date have considered individual, social and environmental influences simultaneously, and even less have examined interactions between individuals and the social and physical environmental contexts in which they exist. Although multi-level studies are emerging (see Box 13.1), a strong evidence base is needed to guide the development of more effective interventions to increase physical activity that consider the complexities between the multiple contexts within which people live. Studying physical activity from a lifecourse perspective is also important, as different factors are likely to be influential at certain life stages. In particular, few studies have examined influences on physical activity during key life transitions, such as the transition from childhood to adolescence, adolescence to young adulthood, school to work, and work to retirement (Salmon & King 2005).

Although some stand-alone physical activity promotion strategies have achieved short-term success, comprehensive interventions are more likely to lead to longer-term behaviour change. Thorough evaluation of all physical activity interventions (regardless of the setting through which it is delivered and the simplicity or complexity of its strategies) is needed to provide data to guide the modification of existing programmes and enhance the development of new interventions. Many intervention studies have included short follow-up periods, are based on small sample sizes, and are evaluated using self-report measures (Timperio et al. 2004b). However, self-report measures may not be sensitive enough to detect changes in physical activity, particularly over short periods.

Recommendation

Physical activity is a complex behaviour and thus is difficult to assess. Better measurement tools are required to assess physical activity among children and older adults, and monitoring needs to be consistent with current recommendations for different age groups. In particular, it is important to assess whether older adults participate in activities that enhance functional health. The use of objective tools may be more accurate than self-report; however, without concurrent self-report data collection, little contextual information can be obtained. Contextual information is important, as it can be used to select targets and foci for physical activity interventions and guide the allocation of resources.

There is a specific need to develop strategies designed to target population groups who are least active, such as adolescent girls. Further, physical activity interventions should be guided by appropriate theoretical models. Emerging research supports the use of social-ecological theories, and there is considerable scope to trial more extensive environmental and policy interventions that focus on multiple levels of influence.

Research to practice

The opportunity exists to trial innovative physical activity programmes in real-life settings. While existing physical activity interventions provide some guide to the selection of promotion strategies, many novel strategies have yet to be trialled. Given the wide range of influences on physical activity, effective interventions are likely to be those that engage people across multiple contexts, targeting individual factors as well as the social and physical environments. Such interventions are likely to involve multiple settings, disciplines and sectors (for example, schools, healthcare providers, facility management, recreation, urban and transport planners, local and regional government, etc.). Thus, stronger links between health-promotion agencies and government departments who are better equipped and resourced to translate research to practice need to be established to ensure that multidisciplinary approaches can be enacted. Furthermore, interventions shown to be effective in controlled research conditions may not be feasible for implementation in the community without collaboration with other sectors that can provide the necessary structures to support the strategies at a population level.

Finally, public health practitioners who implement programmes or interventions that include a focus on physical activity need to consider evaluation from the outset, regardless of the size of the intervention. Evaluation is needed to build an evidence-base regarding the types of strategies that are likely to be successful, and to discourage others from repeating strategies of limited efficacy.

Acknowledgements

Anna Timperio and Jo Salmon are supported by Public Health Research Fellowships from the Victorian Health Promotion Foundation (VicHealth).

REFERENCES

Australian Government Department of Health and Ageing 2004, *Australia's Physical Activity Recommendations for Children and Young People*, Department of Health and Ageing, Canberra.

Bauman, A., Bellew, B., Vita, P., Brown, W. and Owen, N. 2002, *Getting Australia active: Towards Better Practice for the Promotion of Physical Activity*, National Public Health Partnership, Melbourne.

Biddle, S.J., Gorely, T. and Stensel, D.J. 2004, 'Health-enhancing physical activity and sedentary behaviour in children and adolescents' in *Journal of Sports Science*, vol. 22, no. 8, pp. 679–701.

Booth M. 2000, 'What proportion of Australian children are sufficiently active?' in *Medical Journal of Australia*, vol. 173, pp. S6–7.

Booth, M.L., Bauman, A., Owen, N. and Gore, C.J. 1997, 'Physical activity preferences, preferred sources of assistance, and perceived barriers to increased activity among physically inactive Australians' in *Preventive Medicine*, vol. 26, no. 1, pp. 131–37.

Booth, M.L., Owen, N., Bauman, A., Clavisi, O. and Leslie, E. 2000, 'Social-cognitive and perceived environment influences associated with physical activity in older Australians' in *Preventive Medicine*, vol. 31, no. 1, pp. 15–22.

Burton, L.C., Shapiro, S. and German, P.S. 1999, 'Determinants of physical activity initiation and maintenance among community-dwelling older persons' in *Preventive Medicine*, vol. 29, no. 5, pp. 422–30.

Carver, A., Salmon, J., Campbell, K., Baur, L., Garnett, S. and Crawford, D. 2005, 'How do perceptions of local neighborhood relate to adolescents' walking and cycling?' in *American Journal of Health Promotion*, vol. 20, no. 2, pp. 139–47.

Centers for Disease Control and Prevention (US) 2003, 'Prevalence of physical activity, including lifestyle activities among adults: United States, 2000–2001' in *Morbidity and Mortality Weekly Report*, vol. 52, no. 32, pp. 764–69.

—— 2004, 'Surveillance summaries: Youth risk behavior surveillance' in *Morbidity and Mortality Weekly Report*, vol. 53, no. SS–2, pp. 21–25.

—— 2005, 'Trends in leisure-time physical inactivity by age, sex, and race/ethnicity: United States, 1994–2004' in *Morbidity and Mortality Weekly Report*, vol. 54, no. 39, pp. 991–94.

Commonwealth Department of Health and Aged Care 1999, *National Physical Activity Guidelines for Australians*, Commonwealth Department of Health and Aged Care, Canberra.

Cyarto, E.V., Moorhead, G.E. and Brown, W.J. 2004, 'Updating the evidence relating to physical activity intervention studies in older people' in *Journal of Science and Medicine in Sport*, vol. 7, no. 1, pp. 30–38.

Davison, K.K. and Birch, L.L. 2001, 'Childhood overweight: A contextual model and recommendations for future research' in *Obesity Research*, vol. 2, no. 3, pp. 159–71.

Department of Health (UK) 2003, *Health survey for England 2002: The health of children and young people*, Her Majesty's Stationery Office, London.

—— 2004, *At least five a week: Evidence of the impact of physical activity and its relationship to health; a report from the Chief Medical Officer*, Her Majesty's Stationery Office, London.

Di Francesco, V., Zamboni, M., Zoico, E., Bortolani, A., Maggi, S., Bissoli, L., Zivelonghi, A., Guariento, S. and Bosello, O. 2005, 'Relationships between leisure-time physical activity, obesity and disability in elderly men' in *Aging Clinical and Experimental Research*, vol. 17, no. 3, pp. 201–06.

Duncan, S.C., Duncan, T.E., Strycker, L.A. and Chaumeton, N.R. 2004, 'A multilevel approach to youth physical activity research' in *Exercise and Sport Sciences Reviews*, vol. 32, no. 3, pp. 95–99.

Ewing Garber, C. and Blissmer, B.J. 2002, 'The challenges of exercise in older adults' in Burbank, P.M. and Riebe, D. (eds) 2002, *Promoting Exercise and Behaviour Change in Older Adults: Interventions with the Transtheoretical Model*, Springer Publishing Company, New York, pp. 29–56.

Harada, N.D., Chiu, V., King, A.C. and Stewart, A.L. 2001, 'An evaluation of self-report physical activity instruments for older adults' in *Medicine and Science in Sports and Exercise*, vol. 33, no. 6, pp. 962–70.

Health Canada, The College of Family Physicians of Canada, Canadian Paediatric Society, Canadian Society for Exercise Physiology 2002, *Physical activity recommendations for children*, Minister of Public Works and Government Services Canada, Ottawa.

Helakorpi, S., Patja, K., Prättälä, R. and Uutela, A. 2005, *Health Behaviour and Health Among the Finnish Adult Population*, Publications of the National Public Health Institute, Helsinki.

Hillsdon, M., Foster, C. and Thorogood, M. 2005, 'Interventions for promoting physical activity' in *The Cochrane DataBase of Systematic Reviews*, John Wiley & Sons Ltd.

Humpel, N., Owen, N. and Leslie, E. 2002, 'Environmental factors associated with adults' participation in physical activity: A review' in *American Journal of Preventive Medicine*, vol. 22, no. 3, pp. 188–99.

Jamner, M.S., Spruijt-Metz, D., Bassin, S. and Cooper, D.M. 2004, 'A controlled evaluation of a school-based intervention to promote physical activity among sedentary adolescent females: Project FAB' in *Journal of Adolescent Health*, vol. 34, no. 4, pp. 279–89.

Kerr, N.A., Yore, M.M., Ham, S.A. and Dietz, W.H. 2004, 'Increasing stair use in a worksite through environmental changes' in *American Journal of Health Promotion*, vol. 18, no. 4, pp. 312–15.

King, W.C., Brach, J.S., Belle, S., Killingsworth, R., Fenton, M. and Kriska, A.M. 2003, 'The relationship between convenience of destinations and walking levels in older women' in *American Journal of Health Promotion*, vol. 18, no. 1, pp. 74–82.

Kriska, A.M. and Casperson, C.J. 1997, 'Introduction to a collection of physical activity questionnaires' in *Medicine and Science in Sports and Exercise*, vol. 29, no. 6, pp. S5–9.

Lim, K. and Taylor, L. 2005, 'Factors associated with physical activity among older people: A population-based study' in *Preventive Medicine*, vol. 40, no. 1, pp. 33–40.

Lindstrom, M., Hanson, B.S. and Ostergren, P.O. 2001, 'Socioeconomic differences in leisure-time physical activity: The role of social participation and social capital in shaping health related behaviour' in *Social Science in Medicine*, vol. 52, no. 3, pp. 441–51.

Matson-Koffman, D.M., Brownstein, J.N., Neiner, J.A. and Greaney, M.L. 2005, 'A site-specific literature review of policy and environmental interventions that promote physical activity and nutrition for cardiovascular health: What works?' in *American Journal of Health Promotion*, vol. 19, no. 3, pp. 167–93.

Matthews, C.E. 2002, 'Use of self-report instruments to assess physical activity' in Welk W.J. (ed.) 2002, *Physical Activity Assessments for Health-related Research*, Human Kinetics, Champaign, pp. 107–23.

Melanson, E.L. and Freedson, P.S. 1995, 'Validity of the Computer Science and Applications, Inc (CSA) activity monitor' in *Medicine and Science in Sports and Exercise*, vol. 27, no. 6, pp. 934–40.

Meyer, K., Rezny, L., Breuer, C., Lamprecht, M. and Stamm, H.P. 2005, 'Physical activity of adults aged 50 years and older in Switzerland' in *Sozial und Praventivmedizen*, vol. 50, no. 4, pp. 218–29.

Owen, N., Humpel, N., Leslie, E., Bauman, A. and Sallis, J.F. 2004, 'Understanding environmental influences on walking: Review and research agenda' in *American Journal of Preventive Medicine*, vol. 27, no. 1, pp. 67–76.

Pangrazi, P., Corbin, C. and Welk, G. 1997, 'Physical activity for children and youth' in *CAHPERD Journal*, summer, pp. 4–7.

Pate, R.R., Trost, S.G., Felton, G.M., Ward, D.S., Dowda, M. and Saunders, R. 1997, 'Correlates of physical activity behavior in rural youth' in *Research Quarterly for Exercise and Sport*, vol. 68, no. 3, pp. 241–48.

Physical Activity Taskforce 2003, *Let's Make Scotland More Active: A strategy for physical activity*, Scottish Executive, Edinburgh.

Proper, K.I., Hildebrandt, V.H., Van der Beek, A.J., Twisk, J.W. and Van Mechelen, W. 2003, 'Effect of individual counselling on physical activity, fitness and health: A randomised controlled trial in a workplace setting' in *American Journal of Preventive Medicine*, vol. 24, no. 3, pp. 218–26.

Ransdell, L.B., Taylor, A., Oakland, D., Schmidt, J., Moyer-Mileur, L. and Shultz, B. 2003, 'Daughters and mothers exercising together: Effects of home- and community-based programs' in *Medicine and Science in Sports and Exercise*, vol. 35, no. 2, pp. 286–96.

Raymond, J.S. 1989, 'Behavioral epidemiology: The science of health promotion' in *Health Promotion*', vol. 4, no. 4, pp. 281–86.

Saelens, B.E., Sallis, J.F. and Frank, L.D. 2003, 'Environmental correlates of walking and cycling: Findings from the transportation, urban design, and planning literatures' in *Annals of Behavioral Medicine*, vol. 25, no. 2, pp. 80–91.

Sallis, J.F. and Owen, N. 1999, *Physical Activity and Behavioural Medicine*, Sage Publications, Thousand Oaks, p. 72.

—— 2002, 'Ecological models of health behaviour' in Glanz, K., Rimer, B.K. and Marcus Lewis, F. (eds), *Health Behavior and Health Education: Theory, Research and Practice*, Jossey-Bass, San Fransisco, pp. 462–84.

Sallis, J.F. and Saelens, B.E. 2000, 'Assessment of physical activity by self-report: Status, limitations and future directions' in *Research Quarterly for Exercise and Sport*, vol. 71, no. 2, pp. 1–14.

Sallis, J.F., Linton, L. and Kraft, K. 2005, 'The first Active Living Research Conference: Growth of a transdisciplinary field' in *American Journal of Preventive Medicine*, vol. 28, no 2S2, pp. 93–5.

Sallis, J.F., Prochaska, J.J. and Taylor, W.C. 2000, 'A review of correlates of physical activity of children and adolescents' in *Medicine and Science in Sports and Exercise*, vol. 32, no. 5, pp. 963–75.

Salmon, J. and King, A.C. 2005, 'Population approaches to increasing physical activity among children and adults' in Crawford, D. and Jeffery, R.W. (eds) 2005 *Obesity Prevention and Public Health*, Oxford University Press, Oxford, pp. 129–52.

Sirard, J.R. and Pate, R.R. 2001, 'Physical activity assessment in children and adolescents' in *Sports Medicine*, vol. 31, no. 6, pp. 439–54.

Sjöström, M., Yngve, A., Poortvliet, E., Warm, D. and Ekelund, U. 1999, 'Diet and physical activity: Interactions for health; public health nutrition in the European perspective' in *Public Health Nutrition*, vol. 2, no. 3a, pp. 453–59.

Stamatakis, E. 2005, 'Physical activity' in Sposton, K. and Primatesta, P. (eds), *Health Survey for England 2003, volume 2: Risk factors for cardiovascular disease*, Her Majesty's Stationery Office, London.

Stokols, D. 1996, 'Translating social ecological theory into guidelines for community health promotion' in *American Journal of Health Promotion*, vol. 10, no. 4, pp. 282–98.

Strong, W.B., Malina, R.M., Blimkie, C.J.R., Daniels, S.R., Dishman, R.K., Gutin, B., Hergenroeder, A.C., Must, A., Nixon, P.A., Pivarnik, J.M., Rowland, T., Trost, S. and Trudeau, F. 2005, 'Evidence based physical activity for school-age youth' in *Journal of Pediatrics*, vol. 146, no. 6, pp. 723–27.

Sulander, T., Helakorpi, S., Nissinen, A. and Uutela, A. 2004, *Health Behaviour and Health Among Finnish Elderly, Spring 2003, with trends 1993–2003*, Publications of the KTL-National Public Health Institute, Helsinki.

Taylor, A.H., Cable, N.T., Faulkner, G., Hillsdon, M., Narici, M. and Van Der Bij, A.K. 2004, 'Physical activity and older adults: A review of health benefits and the effectiveness of interventions' in *Journal of Sports Sciences*, vol. 22, no. 8, pp. 703–25.

Timperio, A., Crawford, D., Ball, K., Giles-Corti, B., Roberts, R., Simmons, D., Baur, L. and Salmon, J. 2006, 'Personal, and family, social and physical environment correlates of active commuting to school among children' in *American Journal of Preventive Medicine*, vol. 30, no. 1, pp. 45–51.

Timperio, A., Crawford, D., Telford, A. and Salmon, J. 2004a, 'Perceptions about the local neighborhood and walking and cycling among children' in *Preventive Medicine*, vol. 38, no. 1, pp. 39–47.

Timperio, A., Salmon, J. and Ball, K. 2004b, 'Evidence-based strategies to promote physical activity among children, adolescents and young adults: Review and update' in *Journal of Science and Medicine in Sport*, vol. 7, no. 1, pp. S20–29.

Trost, S.G., Owen, N., Bauman, A.E., Sallis, J.F. and Brown, W. 2002, 'Correlates of adults' participation in physical activity: Review and update' in *Medicine and Science in Sports and Exercise*, vol. 34, no. 12, pp. 1996–2001.

Trost, S.G., Pate, R.R., Ward, D.S., Saunders, R. and Riner, W. 1999, 'Correlates of objectively measured physical activity in preadolescent youth' in *American Journal of Preventive Medicine*, vol. 17, no. 2, pp. 120–26.

Trost, S.G., Ward, D.S., Moorehead, S.M., Watson, P.D., Riner, W. and Burke, J.R. 1998, 'Validity of the computer science and applications (CSA) activity monitor in children' in *Medicine and Science in Sports and Exercise*, vol. 30, no. 4, pp. 629–33.

Tudor-Locke, C.E. and Myers, A.M. 2001, 'Methodological considerations for researchers and practitioners using pedometers to measure physical (ambulatory) activity' in *Research Quarterly for Exercise and Sport*, vol. 72, no. 1, pp. 1–12.

US Department of Health and Human Services 1996, *Physical Activity and Health: A report of the Surgeon General*, Department of Health and Human Services, Centers for Disease Control and Prevention, National Center for Chronic Disease Prevention and Health Promotion, Atlanta, p. 21.

van Lenthe, F.J., Brug, J. and Mackenbach, J.P. 2005, 'Neighbourhood inequalities in physical inactivity: The role of neighbourhood attractiveness, proximity to local facilities and safety in the Netherlands' in *Social Science in Medicine*, vol. 60, no. 4, pp. 763–75.

14

Research skills

Sarah McNaughton
Kylie Ball
David Crawford

Public health nutrition is concerned with the nutritional health of populations, encompassing a focus from the local community level, through to national and global levels. In taking a population health perspective, public health nutrition research draws heavily on the principles and methods of epidemiology. Epidemiology is defined as 'the study of the distribution and determinants of health-related states or events in specific populations, and the application of this study to control of health problems' (Last 1998). In other words, epidemiologists are interested in understanding who develops ill-health, and why.

'Nutritional epidemiology' focuses specifically on the relationship between diet and disease, by combining nutritional knowledge with epidemiological methods developed to investigate the determinants of health and disease in populations. Nutritional epidemiology is also concerned with monitoring the nutritional status of populations; and with the development of interventions aimed at promoting healthy eating patterns among populations.

'Social epidemiology' and 'behavioural epidemiology' are also highly relevant to our work as public health nutritionists. Social epidemiology is concerned particularly with investigating social determinants of population health. Behavioural epidemiology is concerned with the distribution and determinants of behaviours that influence health. Research questions of interest to public health nutrition researchers are often best considered by a combination of these disciplinary approaches. For example, an understanding of the relationships between diet and disease may be facilitated through the application of behavioural and nutritional epidemiological methods to define and assess dietary behaviours in populations; and principles of social epidemiology may enhance nutritional epidemiologists' insights into the social and contextual influences on eating behaviours in different population groups.

A sound understanding of epidemiological concepts is an important prerequisite to understanding and conducting public health nutrition research. The first part of this chapter outlines key epidemiological concepts as they apply to nutrition. In particular, we focus on definitions of outcome and exposure; measures of disease frequency; and methods of comparing disease occurrence. Examples of public health nutrition research issues are provided to illustrate these concepts. The second part of the chapter is concerned with the practical aspects of public health nutrition research. It examines the issues in defining the research question, reviewing the literature, selecting the study design, selecting measurement tools, and dealing with data.

Key epidemiological concepts

Epidemiology is concerned with the distribution of disease states, which are termed 'outcomes' or effects; and the relationships between exposures and outcomes. Outcomes in nutritional epidemiological studies are the health- or disease-related states or events of interest. They may include chronic diseases or conditions, such as cancer, cardiovascular disease, arthritis, malnutrition or depression; or more acute conditions, such as food poisoning or migraines. Exposure refers to whether or not an individual, or group of individuals, have encountered a risk (or protective) factor.

Insights into the aetiology (potential causes) of disease are obtained by comparing disease rates (outcomes) in groups of individuals exposed and unexposed to a hypothesised risk factor. Disease rates may also be compared between people with different levels of exposure to a risk factor. For instance, a nutritional epidemiologist may investigate whether high saturated-fat consumption (exposure) is associated with increased risk of coronary heart disease (the outcome), by comparing rates of coronary heart disease among an exposed group – people with high intakes of saturated fat – against those in an unexposed group – people with low saturated-fat intake. In order to make such comparisons, sound and unbiased methods of quantifying disease occurrence and of comparing disease occurrence among exposed and unexposed groups are required.

Measures of disease occurrence

Quantifying disease occurrence in epidemiological studies involves considering the correct numbers of individuals who are at risk, or potentially susceptible to the disease under study. For example, estimates of risk of prostate cancer should exclude women from calculations. Measures of the frequency of disease occurrence are often based on rates, which reflect the number of cases or events per population at risk. Two commonly used measures of disease frequency are the incidence and prevalence rates. There is some debate about the most appropriate definitions of these terms; the descriptions provided below are based on those provided in *A Dictionary of Epidemiology* (Last 1998).

'Incidence' refers to the number of new cases of a disease/health state that occur in a population during a specified time period. Calculating an incidence rate involves dividing the number of new cases by the corresponding number of people in the population at risk, expressed, for instance, as cases per 100 000 people. This is usually expressed per time unit (that is, per year). Incidence rates are commonly calculated (assuming the size of the population is stable) as:

$$\frac{\textit{Number of new cases of a disease in a specified time period}}{\textit{Population at risk} \times \textit{length of time during which cases were determined}}$$

As an example, the incidence of breast cancer among women in Australia rose from 100.5 cases per 100 000 population in 1991 to 117.2 cases per 100 000 population in 2001 (Australian Institute of Health and Welfare and Australasian Association of Cancer Registries 2001).

'Prevalence' refers to the number of cases (new and old) in a defined population at a specified point or period in time. The prevalence rate is generally calculated as:

$$\frac{\textit{Number of cases of a disease at a specified time}}{\textit{Population at risk at the specified time}}$$

For instance, the prevalence of obesity among Australian adults in 2001 was 16 per cent among women, and 17 per cent among men (Australian Bureau of Statistics 2002).

Two indicators of population health/disease occurrence that are often routinely available and used by epidemiologists are mortality and morbidity measures.

'Mortality' refers to the incidence of death from a disease in a population. Being an incident rate, it is calculated relative to the population at risk, as:

$$\frac{\textit{Number of deaths in a specified period}}{\textit{Average total population during that period}}$$

For instance, the death rate in Turkey in 2005 was 5.96 deaths/1000 population (see http://www.indexmundi.com/turkey/death_rate.html).

'Morbidity' refers to a state of ill-health produced by a disease or condition. Morbidity rates can be indicated by either the prevalence or the incidence of a disease. Morbidity may be assessed using such indicators as hospital admissions, notifications (such as communicable diseases), or disease registers that exist in many countries.

Crude and adjusted rates

Crude incidence, prevalence, morbidity and mortality rates are based on the at-risk population as a whole, without subdivision or adjustment for the composition of the populations. One limitation of such an approach is that these rates do not account for the fact that disease and mortality risk often vary across population subgroups; for instance, the incidence and prevalence of arthritis are much higher among the elderly than among young adults or children. Ignoring these disproportionate risks can result in misleading conclusions. Two communities, for example, may have highly divergent prevalences of arthritis that are primarily attributable to the different age structures of the populations within them – a community in which many elderly people reside is likely to have a higher prevalence of arthritis than a new estate full of young families. For these reasons, rates are sometimes provided for specific age and sex groups. Alternatively, standardised rates, rather than crude rates, may be presented. Standardised rates 'adjust' the crude rate to enable consistent comparisons across populations with divergent sociodemographic characteristics. As such, age-standardised mortality rates reflect the number of deaths that a population would expect if it had a given age structure, hence eliminating the influence of different population age distributions on rates being compared (Beaglehole et al. 1993).

Methods of comparing disease occurrence

Investigating disease incidence, prevalence, morbidity or mortality rates provides interesting descriptive information about the health of populations and the magnitude of diseases. However, public health nutrition researchers are often more interested in the underlying aetiology (potential causes) of these diseases or conditions, and particularly the aetiological role of nutrition-related factors. For example, we might be curious about links between fish consumption and risk of depression; or between high-carbohydrate diets and risk of obesity. Alternatively, we might question whether cardiovascular disease rates have decreased in the past two decades, or after the introduction of a community based nutrition programme. Public health nutritionists interested in monitoring the nutritional status of populations might wish to examine how intake of micronutrients has altered over time, or in response to a policy change (take, for example, the fortification of breakfast cereals with folate).

The investigation of these research questions involves the comparison of disease rates, typically those of an exposed and an unexposed group. A number of measures are used to summarise comparisons of disease rates between populations, and describe the strength of associations between exposures and outcomes; the most common being odds ratio and relative risk.

Odds ratio is closely related to relative risk, and is defined as the odds of disease in exposed persons divided by the odds of disease in unexposed persons. A rate of one in 100, for instance, corresponds to odds of 99 to one against. See Box 14.1 for an example of the use of the odds ratio.

Relative risk (also termed risk ratio) refers to the ratio of the disease rate in exposed persons to that in people unexposed to a risk factor. See boxes 14.2 and 14.3 for examples of the use of the relative risk.

Study design

There are number of different study designs that can be employed in public health nutrition research. Each has strengths and weaknesses that need to be considered when planning a study or when evaluating the literature. Study designs fall into two main categories: observational studies, where the researcher does not attempt to intervene; and experimental studies, where the researcher purposefully manipulates exposure to examine the effect of doing so (for example, manipulating the amount of calcium in the diet to examine the effect on bone density). Figure 14.1 presents a schema of the commonly used epidemiological studies.

Observational studies
Cross-sectional surveys are descriptive studies, and involve the measurement of exposures and outcomes at a given time. Examples include the descriptions of diet or health outcomes in relation to other factors, such as age, socioeconomic status, education level and geographical regions (Food Standards

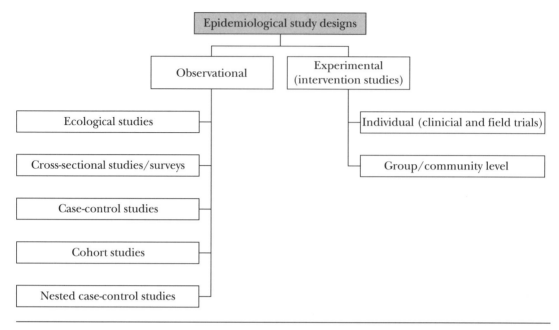

Figure 14.1 Types of epidemiological study designs

Source: Rothman & Greenland 1998

Agency 2004), and prevalence studies of obesity or other health conditions such as diabetes or hypertension (Cameron et al. 2003).

Surveys are often used to describe the associations between exposure and disease; however, they are limited in their ability to determine causality (that is, whether the exposure produces the disease or outcome). They are useful in providing information on the amount and distribution of disease and exposures, which can provide vital information for health planning and resource allocation and may be useful for hypothesis-generating.

Ecological studies

Ecological studies are cross-sectional studies that investigate exposures and health outcomes at the group level rather than at the individual level. They include cross-country comparisons and analysis of trends over time within a population. As with cross-sectional studies, these studies are useful for generating hypotheses, but they are unable to determine causality. For example, ecological studies may investigate how the density of fast-food outlets in different neighbourhoods relates to obesity prevalence in those neighbourhoods; or how changes in average working hours over a decade within a country are associated with increases in national rates of fast-food consumption.

Case-control studies

In a case-control study, individuals with disease (cases) are identified, and are compared with individuals who do not have disease (controls). The exposure of the two groups to the factors of interest is compared (see Box 14.1).

BOX 14.1
CASE-CONTROL STUDIES

In a population-based case-control study, the fruit and vegetable intake of subjects with pancreatic cancer were compared with healthy subjects (Chan et al. 2005). Comparing the highest and lowest levels of intake, the odds ratio (and 95 per cent confidence interval) was 0.45 (0.32 to 0.62) for total vegetable intake and 0.72 (0.54 to 0.98) for total fruit intake, indicating that higher total vegetable and fruit intake was associated with a reduced risk of pancreatic cancer.

Case-control studies are useful for rare diseases, such as specific cancers, which would require very large cohort studies in order to obtain a sufficient number of people with the disease. They are relatively quick to complete, as there is no waiting to see who develops the disease of interest. Subsequently, they are less costly due to their shorter duration and the smaller sample sizes used.

There are also a number of weaknesses of case-control studies (Rothman & Greenland 1998). Selection bias can affect case-control studies if an inappropriate sample of controls is used. For example, many studies have used hospital-based controls rather than population- or community-based controls. Also, case-control studies are subject to recall bias (such as, when those with a disease/outcome remember risk factors differently than those without the disease/outcome) in a number of ways. Exposures are generally measured through recall, and the presence of disease may affect the reporting. The recall of past dietary intake has been shown to be influenced by recent dietary intake, and recent diet may have been altered by the development of disease (Margetts & Nelson 1997). Use of biological indicators of diet (also known as biomarkers) is limited due to potential alterations in physiology and metabolism due to the presence of disease (Sempos et al. 1999). With respect to the temporal relationship required for causality, the measurement of exposure occurs after the onset of disease (Potischman & Weed 1999). Finally, in most case-control study designs, only one disease can be studied at a time.

Cohort studies

A cohort study involves identifying a group or cohort of disease-free people who are followed over time (Beaglehole et al. 1993). Information is collected at baseline on the exposures of interest, and subjects who subsequently develop disease are identified. The rates of disease in those who were exposed are compared to those who were not exposed (see Box 14.2).

Box 14.2
Cohort studies

Example 1: In the European Prospective Investigation into Cancer (EPIC), plasma vitamin C was measured in subjects at baseline, with mortality from all causes over a four-year period identified (Khaw et al. 2001). Comparing the mortality rates of subjects with high and low plasma vitamin C subjects, the relative risk (and 95 per cent confidence interval) for all-cause mortality was 0.48 (0.33 to 0.70) for men and 0.50 (0.32 to 0.81) for women, indicating that higher plasma vitamin C was associated with a lower risk of death.

Example 2: Shunk and Birch (2004) conducted a longitudinal cohort study in which 153 five-year-old girls were followed up until age nine with assessment of weight, height and a range of psychological factors relating to eating behaviour every two years. Girls who were at risk of overweight at age five (defined as a BMI greater than 85th percentile) showed significantly higher levels of dietary restraint, disinhibited eating, weight concerns and body dissatisfaction by age nine than girls who were normal weight at age five.

Advantages of cohort studies include its prospective nature, that is, the measures of exposure are determined before the onset of disease (Freudenheim 1999) and the ability to investigate multiple health outcomes simultaneously.

Cohort studies also have a number of weaknesses. They are also susceptible to selection bias, as subjects lost during follow up may be different in important characteristics from those subjects who continue to participate (Margetts & Nelson 1997). Cohort studies are expensive to conduct, as the time required for completion is usually long depending on the health outcome, and large samples are generally required for sufficient statistical power.

Nested case-control studies

Nested case-control studies are a cross between a cohort study and a case-control study in that a case-control study is 'nested' within a cohort study

(Sempos et al. 1999). As with a cohort study, a group of disease-free individuals is identified and exposure is measured, and the cohort is followed up to identify those who develop disease. Over a set period of time, subjects that developed disease are compared with a random sample of disease-free subjects selected from the cohort. These studies benefit from the advantages of a cohort study and overcome part of the practical disadvantages relating to cost normally associated with cohort studies.

Experimental studies

In an intervention study or a randomised controlled trial (RCT), subjects are randomly assigned either to an intervention or control group, and then followed to identify the development of disease (Beaglehole et al. 1993). After a defined period of time, the treatment group and the control group are compared (see Box 14.3). In intervention studies that are double blind, both the subject and researcher do not know which treatment the subject has received.

Box 14.3
INTERVENTION STUDIES

Example 1: The Lyon Diet Heart Study (De Lorgeril et al. 1999) randomised subjects with a previous history of myocardial infarction to either a treatment group, who were asked to consume a Mediterranean-style diet, or a control group, who were asked to consume a prudent diet for two years. The rates of cardiac death and non-fatal heart attacks were compared between the two groups. The relative risk (and 95 per cent confidence interval) was 0.27 (0.12 to 0.59), demonstrating that the Mediterranean-style diet was protective against subsequent coronary events.

Example 2: The TACOS (Trying Alternative Cafeteria Options in Schools) study was a two-year group randomised school-based environmental intervention (French et al. 2004). Twenty schools in the United States were randomised to an intervention group involving increasing the availability of lower-fat food choices available in the cafeteria and peer-led promotion of the lower-fat food options, or to a control group. During the second year of the intervention, the intervention schools had a significantly higher mean percentage of sales of lower-fat foods (33.6 per cent versus 22.1 per cent), suggesting that environmental interventions can increase the purchase of lower-fat food choices among adolescents.

There are particular advantages of intervention studies. First, they provide direct evidence of cause and effect, as only the exposure under consideration has been altered. Second, the randomisation process minimises biases that may occur through allocation of subjects to the intervention or control group, and minimises confounding, as known and unknown covariates are assumed to be evenly distributed across the treatment and control groups (Margetts & Nelson 1997; Freudenheim 1999). However, intervention studies are generally expensive to conduct, partly due to the long follow-up periods required to detect the effect of treatments, particularly for chronic diseases, and generally only one or two exposures can be assessed at any time (Sempos et al. 1999). More recent dietary interventions, though, have been based on an overall dietary pattern rather than individual constituents in the diet (Appel et al. 1997; De Lorgeril et al. 1999).

Within the field of nutrition, there are a number of particular considerations for intervention studies. Blinding of subjects may not be possible as the subjects' diet may be altered significantly; for example, when the intervention involves alterations to the macronutrients intake (Freudenheim 1999). When the intervention involves changes to micronutrient intake, supplements and placebo tablets that are identical in appearance can be used so that subjects are blinded to their treatment status. However, often only single nutrients are investigated, and usually a single dose or level of intake is tested (Sempos et al. 1999).

Levels of evidence

All types of public health recommendations or guidelines require systematic evaluation of the available evidence. The concept of evidence-based practice in a public health nutrition context was introduced in chapters 1 and 2 of this book. In this chapter, we adopt the view that the level of evidence that supports a public health recommendation is determined by the hierarchy of studies, which is based on the strength of the evidence that each provides (Figure 14.2). Case-control studies provide the weakest evidence of a relationship compared with other study designs (Beaglehole et al. 1993). Methodologically sound cohort and nested case-control studies provide good evidence, and sound intervention studies are considered to provide the best evidence.

In recent years, there has been increasing debate about the value of observational studies versus intervention studies (Lawlor et al. 2004). This has arisen due to the contradictory findings of a number of observational studies and RCTs. For example, observational studies suggested that betacarotene was

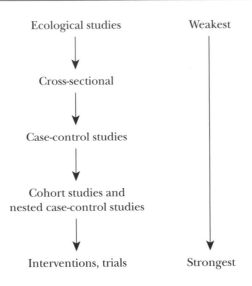

Figure 14.2 Levels of evidence

protective against lung cancer, however when supplemental betacarotene was used in randomised controlled trials, no protective effect was seen, and in fact, betacarotene supplementation resulted in an increased incidence of lung cancer (Duffield-Lillico & Begg 2004). A variety of reasons for the contradictory findings have been put forward, including biological or mechanistic possibilities. Much of the criticism of cohort studies relates to the issue of confounding and, in particular, residual confounding. Residual confounding refers to confounding that has not been accounted for due to either unmeasured or unknown confounders, or poorly measured confounders. In observational studies, confounding can be accounted for at the design stage through matching of subjects on important confounders, although there is usually a limit to the number of factors that a subject can be matched for due to practical consider-ations (Rothman & Greenland 1998). Confounding may also be dealt with at the analysis phase through multivariate statistical analysis. This requires adequate consideration and identification of all relevant confounders through the devel-opment of conceptual models and the use of appropriate measurement tools in the design phase of the study.

Despite their strengths, it has been suggested that RCTs will not be the best method of assessing causality for all research questions. This is particularly relevant for many public health nutrition issues, as often there are few or no intervention studies or RCTs on which to base recommendations. Therefore, a broader approach to evaluation of the evidence is required. For example, the World Cancer Research Fund (WCRF) is currently assessing the evidence between diet and cancer in order to update its recommendations (World Cancer Research Fund 1997). The WCRF is using 'a portfolio approach to the evidence, where all available evidence, including all types of epidemiological studies, are considered along with experimental studies using animal and *in vitro* models, particularly for the understanding of biological mechanisms contributing to understanding of causality (Heggie et al. 2003).

Key practical considerations

Clarifying the research question

The first question any public health nutrition researcher must ask themselves is, 'What (specifically) is it that I am trying to understand?' Before embarking on any study, the question and study aims need to be clearly defined and articled. It is the research question that defines the size and scope of the review of the literature, drives the selection of the overall study design, determines the means of gathering the data, the sampling methods, and determination of the sample size, the measures to be used, and the approach to statistical analysis. While the need to clarify the research question may seem obvious, with so many important questions to address in public health nutrition, and so many potentially potent influences on population nutrition, defining your question can be a difficult task.

For public health nutritionists, it is important to be clear whether one is interested in examining or influencing the overall diet, patterns of food intake, consumption of specific foods, particular dietary habits, nutrient intake, or the intake of non-nutritive substances contained in foods. It is also necessary to be clear as to whether the aim is to examine the influence of one or more of these factors on some aspect of health (where the nutrition-related factor is an exposure), or whether the aim is to examine the influence of other factors on some aspect of diet/nutrition (where this is the outcome). For example, in a nutritional epidemiology study, a researcher might be interested in answering the following question: 'What is the role of fast-food consumption on obesity risk?' In a study that takes a social or behavioural epidemiology approach, the researcher is more likely to be interested answering the question, 'What influences the intake of fast foods?' The two questions are both important, but are vastly different, and different methodological approaches are required to address them.

In research focused on understanding the influences on nutrition-related behaviours, it is important to recognise that the range of potential influences on nutrition-related behaviours is huge, ranging from personal factors such as knowledge, beliefs, attitudes and personal values, social factors such as peer and family support, environmental factors such as the availability and cost of foods, policy factors, and cultural factors. It may not be appropriate or feasible to assess all of these potential influences in any one study, so how does a researcher decide what to include and what to ignore? This is where theoretical models of health behaviour can help. A theoretically based approach is essential since it defines the boundaries of research and provides a framework to build upon previous work. Theoretical models are also useful since they help identify key factors influencing behaviours, and can lead to the development of more effective interventions. A detailed discussion of theoretical models is beyond the scope of this chapter, however interested readers should refer to the review by Baranowski and his colleagues (1999) for more information.

Regardless of the research question, once it has been defined, the researcher should carefully consider whether they need to design and implement a study to address the question, or whether there is existing data that would allow them to address the question. There is a wealth of data that has been and continues to be collected that may be relevant to the question you wish to address. Research that is based on secondary analysis of existing data is completely acceptable and can potentially save time, effort and money.

Critical review of the literature

A critical review of the literature aims to identify all relevant research on a specific topic, assess the studies in terms of their quality, and systematically summarise the findings. When starting a critical review, it is important to determine the objective of the review (that is, clarify the research question, as described above). There may be an abundance of studies for consideration, and if the research question is not clearly defined, then it will be impossible to restrict the scope of the review. This will lead to defining set criteria for selecting and excluding studies from the review (Box 14.4).

Identifying studies is a major task of the review. The most common approach is the use of electronic bibliographic databases, such as MEDLINE and EMBASE. Depending on the issues being investigated, they may also be other relevant discipline or topic-specific databases. However, the use of these databases is unlikely to identify all relevant studies, and other strategies should be used to ensure that the search is comprehensive, such as cross-checking of reference lists of already identified studies and other reviews. These approaches will identify published studies. However, it may also be necessary to identify the 'grey literature' – unpublished and ongoing studies – through direct contact with researchers in the field and via professional networks.

[339]

BOX 14.4
SELECTING STUDIES FOR THE CRITICAL REVIEW

Defining criteria for the selection and exclusion of studies to be evaluated in a critical review will depend upon the specific nature of research question, but may include aspects of the following:

- the overall study design
- the method of exposure measurement
- the method of health outcome measurement
- the population group studied (for example, men, women, adults, children)
- the settings for the study (for instance, school-based interventions, community interventions, workplace)
- other aspects of the study design (such as, the length of interventions or follow-up).

Once all the relevant studies have been identified, it is necessary to consider each of the studies and to assess them in terms of the internal validity and the external validity of the study. External validity refers to the *generalisability* of the study or how applicable the results of the study are to other groups of people (Beaglehole et al. 1993). Internal validity refers to the degree to which the results of an observation are correct for the particular group of people being studied (Beaglehole et al. 1993).

The three main issues to consider when evaluating the internal validity of individual studies are the possible effects of bias, confounding and chance. With respect to bias, the primary concerns are selection bias (relating to the way in which the subjects in the study have been selected), and information bias (relating to measurement issues). The presence and likely effect of confounding, and the use of strategies to avoid, minimise or account for potential confounders must also be evaluated. The third issue to address is whether the association that has been observed could be explained by chance. This is usually assessed through the statistical analysis through formal significance tests and determination of confidence intervals. For a discussion of these issues, see Rothman & Greenland (1998).

While these three issues must be considered for each type of study design, the specific questions for each will vary. There are many tools available in the literature that can be used to evaluate studies; for example, see Greenhalgh (1997), Greenhalgh and Taylor (1997) and Public Health Resource Unit (UK) National Health Service (2005). Similarly, Margetts and colleagues (1995) have developed a scoring system specifically for case-control and cohort studies involving diet. Assessment of study quality may be used to exclude poorly conducted studies, it may be used to explain inconsistent results between the studies, or it may be used in quantitative summaries to weight individual studies. After each study has been considered separately, it is necessary to summarise the findings of all relevant research either qualitatively or quantitatively (see Box 14.5).

One approach to summarising the findings of a critical review is a meta-analysis, which is a formal statistical process for quantitatively summarising the findings of multiple studies; however, this is not appropriate in all situations. For a detailed discussion of the issues involved in conducting and interpreting a meta-analysis, see Rothman & Greenland (1998).

The Cochrane Collaboration (http://www.cochrane.org) is aimed at promoting evidence-based health care via the conduct of systematic reviews of intervention studies. With respect to nutrition, reviews have primarily been conducted in areas relating to clinical nutrition. However, there are an increasing number of reviews in areas relevant to public health nutrition such as interventions for obesity (Summerbell et al. 2005).

BOX 14.5
SUMMARISING THE FINDINGS OF THE CRITICAL REVIEW

The body of research should be considered in the context of:
- the hierarchy of epidemiological studies and levels of evidence
- the consistency of results across study designs, methods and study populations and to determine possible explanations for inconsistencies in research findings
- the strength or size of the effect (for example, even if the study results are statistically significant, it is also important to assess the practical significance or public health significance of the findings).

Measurement issues

When selecting measurement tools or methods, it is important to consider the following questions:

- What type of information do you require? That is, what is your objective or what question are you trying to answer?
- Who are your subjects/participants? (Different methods will often be required for children versus adults, and you will need to consider the respondent burden of each method.)
- What are your limitations in terms of time, budget and personnel?

Nutrition-related factors and diet

Different types of measurement tools are required to assess the wider range of nutrition-related factors or aspects of diet that may be of interest in any research study (see Table 14.1). In addition, depending on the specific aspect of diet or nutrition you are interested in, there are a range of further considerations. For example, consider betacarotene; in order to choose the appropriate assessment tool, the following will need to be considered. Are you interested in:

- betacarotene intake or the amount of betacarotene available in the body
- intake of foods rich in betacarotene
- absolute levels of betacarotene intake or classifying subjects as high and low consumers
- group intake or individual intake
- changes in intake

A detailed description of each of the available assessment methods is beyond the scope of this chapter, but may be found in Margetts and Nelson (1997).

Measurement of health outcomes

There are a number of ways of gathering information on health outcomes. For example:

- self-report by the subjects, such as, subjects may be asked, 'Have you ever been told by a doctor that you have diabetes?'
- observation or direct measurement, for instance, blood pressure, oral glucose tolerance tests, clinical examinations and biopsies
- access to medical records, disease-specific registries (like cancer registries) and death registries – these can provide information on all-cause mortality and cause-specific mortality if the specific cause of death is available via the use of the International Classification of Disease (ICD) codes.

Assessment of other variables

In any research study, other information will be required on the subjects in order to consider the impact of bias and confounding, interpret the findings, and to allow comparisons with previous research. The following are examples of the methods available and the types information that can be collected.

- Self-report: Information on other health behaviours such as smoking, alcohol consumption and socio-demographic information such as age, sex, education level and socioeconomic status.

Table 14.1 Examples of the broad range of nutrition-related factors and possible measurement tools

	Examples	Measurement tools
Cultural factors	• cultural norms and beliefs regarding food and eating	• qualitative methods • questionnaires
Environmental factors	• availability, accessibility and cost of foods	• questionnaires • objective audits
Social factors	• family and peer support and sabotage of healthy eating	• qualitative methods • questionnaires
Psychological factors	• nutrition knowledge • nutrition-related attitudes and beliefs • food security	• qualitative methods • questionnaires
Eating and food-related behaviours	• cooking skills • use of low-fat products • food purchasing behaviours	• questionnaires • qualitative methods
Food intake and food patterns	• intake of specific foods • intake of food groups • dietary variety	• food frequency questionnaire • food records • food recalls • diet history • household food surveys • short dietary questions
Nutrient intake	• macronutrients • micronutrients • phytochemicals and non-nutrients	• food frequency questionnaire • food records • 24-hour recalls • diet history • household food surveys • biomarkers, e.g. urinary sodium, urinary nitrogen
Nutritional status	• waist circumference • body fat • plasma folate	• anthropometry • body composition methods • biomarkers

- Observation or direct measures, for example, anthropometric measures such as height and weight.
- Access to medical records: information on current and previous health conditions or other health-related information such as birth weight.

Reliability and validity

Reliability, also known as reproducibility, refers to the ability of a method to produce the same answer when used on different occasions under similar circumstances (Armstrong et al. 1992). To assess reliability, the measurement is repeated in the same subjects after an appropriate length of time. The time interval will vary depending on the assessment tool; however, it must be long enough to avoid subjects remembering their answers, and short enough to minimise real changes.

Validity refers to the ability of a method to measure what it claims to measure (Beaglehole et al. 1993). There are a number of types of validity, including face validity, content validity, criterion validity and predictive validity (Abramson & Abramson 1999). Criterion validity is how well the measure compares to a better measure of the same variable, and is the type of validity most commonly referred to. The aim is to compare your test method with the truth; however, as the 'truth' can often not be measured, it is compared to a 'gold standard' method, that is, a more accurate (but not perfect) reference method.

There is an extensive body of literature concerning the reliability and validity of dietary assessment measures. For further detailed discussion of the issues relating to dietary assessment, see Willett (1998) and Margetts and Nelson (1997). For a broader discussion of reliability and validity in health research, see Streiner and Noman (1991) and Abramson & Abramson (1999).

Questionnaire design

Questionnaires are widely used in health research to collect information on a range of factors. Some examples include:

- dietary questionnaires, such as food frequency questionnaires (Willett 1998), or food behaviour questionnaires like the Three Factor Eating Questionnaire (Stunkard & Messick 1985)
- health questionnaires, such as the SF36 General Health Questionnaire (http://www.sf-36.org/)
- questionnaires used to collect socio-demographic information, health behaviour information (for example, smoking behaviour, alcohol consumption, physical activity) or other information of interest (such as family history).

Before embarking on the development of a new questionnaire, consider whether there is an existing questionnaire available. Developing a questionnaire and conducting reliability and validation studies is expensive and time-consuming. However, it will be important to consider the objective of the original tool and its intended study population, and to investigate whether it has been evaluated with respect to reproducibility and validity. This will determine whether the tool is appropriate for use in the new situation.

In addition, for any questionnaire that is examining nutrition-related factors, the questions will need to be considered in terms of whether they are appropriate with respect to:

- the study population (such as children versus adolescents versus adults)
- the food supply (for instance, the types of foods available and commonly eaten change over time)
- the culture (as in different foods contribute to the diet).

If a new questionnaire needs to be developed, there are a range of other issues that will need to be considered:

- will the questionnaire be self-administered (paper-based or web-based) or interviewer-administered (via face-to-face or telephone interviews)
- are closed or open questions appropriate
- what types of responses are required — consider the use of Likert scales, tick boxes, visual analogue scales
- are there sufficient response categories
- how will responses be coded
- how will data entry be conducted (for example automated or manual data entry)?

Unwieldy questionnaires will contribute to respondent burden, non-completion and subject drop-outs, and will affect the quality of information collected. Therefore, it is necessary to consider the use of appropriate language, the length of the questionnaire, the format and layout. Further detailed discussion on the development and use of questionnaires can be found in Armstrong and colleagues (1992).

In summary, questionnaires are means of communication between the researcher and his/her subjects. It is important that they are well designed, thoroughly pilot tested, and, wherever possible, their validity and reliability established. Poorly designed questionnaires will yield poor data.

Pilot studies

Pilot studies aim to test the practical aspects of the research study and to identify and resolve problems in the study design and measurement tools or methods before substantial resources are invested in the main study. Small numbers of subjects, who are similar to the actual study population (but not part of the study population) are recruited. If major changes are required to the study protocol or questionnaires, it may be necessary to conduct further pilot testing. Aspects of the research study that may require consideration during piloting include:

- testing questionnaires for comprehension, readability and time taken to complete
- testing the feasibility of an intervention
- feasibility of other measurements, for example, biomarkers (can the samples be transported to the laboratory under appropriate storage conditions and within required time frames for analysis?).

Qualitative methods

Qualitative research is designed to obtain rich, detailed, descriptive insights into a phenomenon, typically through examining the meanings and interpretations of data derived from observation, interviews, or verbal communication between people (Holloway & Wheeler 1995). Qualitative data is typically verbal or textual, rather than numerical or quantitative, and often involves smaller sample sizes than those required in quantitative studies. Qualitative studies are particularly useful for understanding beliefs, perceptions, attitudes and cultural factors affecting health and health-related behaviours (Abramson & Abramson 1999). Qualitative research can be useful in generating hypotheses (for instance, the reasons that some individuals have less healthy diets than others), or assessing the feasibility of instruments (such as investigating individual's understanding and perceived response burden of dietary questions) or interventions (as in assessing the difficulty of adhering to a dietary regimen or adopting certain nutrition-related behaviours). Further details of qualitative methods and analyses can be found in Holloway and Wheeler (1995) and Strauss and Corbin (1990).

Working with data

Data entry and storage

In most epidemiological studies, large amounts of information (or data) will be collected, and therefore it will be necessary to give adequate consideration to the issues of data entry and storage in the planning and design of the project with advice from experts in computerised databases and data management.

Subjects will usually be given a unique identifier or numerical code, which will appear on all data recording forms pertaining to that individual. Subject details such as name and contact details are generally kept separately to meet confidentiality requirements, and are available only to authorised research personnel.

Researchers will be faced with the choice of using manual data entry or an automated process such as optical recognition scanning. Use of an automated process can be more efficient with respect to time required for data entry and a reduction in the number of data entry errors. In some circumstances, it may be possible to use computerised software for direct entry while conducting an interview.

Quality control of data entry is important at a number of stages along the data entry process. Development of coding manuals will be required and staff will require adequate training, as consistency between staff is vital. This is particularly important for dietary intake data, as coders may be required to make decisions on the coding of food products and portion sizes. Automated data validation procedures (also known as logical checks), where values outside specified ranges are flagged or identified during data entry. These processes can also be used after the data has been entered with flagged entries requiring cross-checking with the original data. Double data entry can be used where all data is entered twice and computerised cross-checking of data verifies the records. An alternative approach is to randomly select a proportion of records (for example, ten per cent) and have them recoded and cross-checked.

Data files must be adequately stored, with sufficient backups and archiving to prevent loss of data, and data files should be stored securely to avoid unauthorised access through the use of appropriate security measures such as password-protected computer access.

Data analysis

Before data can be used in any analysis, it important that the data is checked thoroughly for errors and inconsistencies, which is known as data cleaning. Although many data errors will have been picked up during coding though use of double data entry, data validation or logical checks, it is still important to perform additional data cleaning. It is important to check individual variables, for example, by checking the ranges of variables, but also cross-tabulations by other variables (such as age and sex), which can often highlight implausible values.

Initial steps in data analysis often involve the recoding of data into new variables (for example, age in years converted to five-year age categories) or the calculation of new variables (such as calculation of body mass index based on height and weight data). It is preferable to retain original variables rather than overwriting variables as this allows any errors made in recoding or calculations to be rectified at a later date or development of new recoding categories as necessary. It is equally important to document all manipulations of the data carefully, as this information will be needed by other users and for reporting of the data.

Analysis of the data should commence by examining each variable separately (univariate analysis) and then progress to investigate how one variable varies according to a second variable (bivariate analysis). It will be important to consider the types of variables you have, that is, whether they are quantitative (continuous/discrete), or categorical (nominal/ ordinal), as this will determine many aspects of the analysis (Bland 1997). Final steps in the analysis involve multivariate models where advice from a statistician is crucial. Although advice will have been sought during the planning stages, with major issues already resolved, additional assistance with the specific techniques and interpretation may be required during analysis, particularly for more complex study designs and hypotheses. Although statistical analysis programmes are becoming increasingly easier to use, this can lead to use of inappropriate models and statistical tests being applied.

Planning for how you will deal with the data (information) you collect in your research, and how you will make sense of it, is essential to the conduct of any public health nutrition project. This is a key step that needs to be undertaken early in the development of your project, and wherever possible the input of an experienced data analyst and statistician should be sought.

Conclusion

Research in public health nutrition draws on ideas and principles from a range of fields including nutritional, social and behavioural epidemiology. A detailed understanding of the research question is essential as this will determine many aspects of the design and conduct of the research, such as selecting the appropriate study design, the target population and measurement tools for your needs, through to analysis and interpretation of the data. Understanding the basic principles of epidemiology is necessary for conducting your own research, projects, evaluating and interpreting the existing research, and in order to put your own work into the wider public health nutrition context.

REFERENCES

Abramson, J.H. and Abramson, Z.H. 1999, *Survey Methods in Community Medicine* (5th edition), Churchill Livingstone, London.

Appel, L.J., Moore, T.J., Obarzanek, E., Vollmer, W.M., Svetkey, L.P., Sacks, M., Bray, G.A., Vogt, T.M., Cutler, J.A., Windhauser, M.M., Lin, P.H. and Karanja, N. 1997, 'A clinical trial of the effects of dietary patterns on blood pressure: DASH Collaborative Research Group' in *New England Journal of Medicine*, vol. 336, no. 16, pp. 117–24.

Armstrong, B.K., White, E. and Saracci, R. 1992, *Principles of exposure measurement in epidemiology*, Oxford University Press, New York.

Australian Bureau of Statistics (ABS) 2002, *2001 National Health Survey: Users' guide*, ABS, Canberra.

Australian Institute of Health and Welfare (AIHW) and Australasian Association of Cancer Registries 2001, *Cancer Survival in Australia 2001: Part 1–National summary statistics*, AIHW, Canberra.

Baranowski, T., Weber Cullen, K. and Baranowski, J. 1999, 'Psychosocial correlates of dietary intake: Advancing dietary intervention' in *Annual Review of Nutrition*, vol. 19, pp. 17–40.

Beaglehole, R., Bonita, R. and Kjellstrom, T. 1993, *Basic Epidemiology*, World Health Organization, Geneva.

Bland, M. 1997, *An Introduction to Medical Statistics* (2nd edition), Oxford Univeristy Press, Oxford.

Cameron, A.J., Welborn, T.A., Zimmet, P.Z., Dunstan, D.W., Owen, N., Salmon, J., Dalton, M., Jolley, D. and Shaw, J.E. 2003, 'Overweight and obesity in Australia: The 1999–2000 Australian Diabetes, Obesity and Lifestyle Study (AusDiab)' in *Medical Journal of Australia*, vol. 178, no. 9, pp. 427–32.

Chan, J.M., Wang, F. and Holly, E.A. 2005, 'Vegatable and fruit intake and pancreatic cancer in a population-based case-control study in the San Francisco Bay Area' in *Cancer Epidemiology, Biomarkers and Prevention*, vol. 14, no. 9, pp. 2093–7.

De Lorgeril, M., Salen, P., Martin, J.L., Monjaud, I., Delaye, J. and Mamelle, N. 1999, 'Mediterranean diet, traditional risk factors, and the rate of cardiovascular complications after myocardial infarction: Final report of the Lyon Diet Heart Study' in *Circulation*, vol. 99, no. 6, pp. 779–85.

Duffield-Lillico, A.J. and Begg, C.B. 2004, 'Reflections on the landmark studies of b-carotene supplementation' in *Journal of the National Cancer Institute*, vol. 96, no. 2, pp. 1729–31.

Food Standards Agency 2004, *National Diet & Nutrition Survey: Adults aged 19 to 64 years; Volume 5; Summary Report*, Her Majesty's Stationery Office, Norwich.

French, S.A., Story, M., Fulkerson, J.A. and Hannan, P. 2004, 'An environmental intervention to promote lower-fat food choices in secondary schools: Outcomes of the TACOS study' in *American Journal of Public Health*, vol. 94, no. 9, pp. 1507–12.

Freudenheim, J.L. 1999, 'Study design and hypothesis testing: Issues in the evaluation of evidence from research in nutritional epidemiology' in *American Journal of Clinical Nutrition*, vol. 99, pp. S1315–21.

Greenhalgh, T. 1997, 'How to read a paper: Assessing the methodological quality of published papers' in *British Medical Journal*, vol. 315, pp. 305–08.

Greenhalgh, T. and Taylor, R. 1997, 'How to read a paper: Papers that go beyond numbers (qualitative research)' in *British Medical Journal*, vol. 315, pp. 740–43.

Heggie, S.J., Wiseman, M.J., Cannon, G.J., Mile, L.M., Thompson, R.L., Stone, E.M., Butrum, R.R. and Kroke, A. 2003, 'Defining the state of knowledge with respect to food, nutrition, physical activity and the prevention of cancer' in *Journal of Nutrition*, vol. 133, pp. S3837–42.

Holloway, I. and Wheeler, S. 1995, 'Ethical issues in qualitative nursing research' in *Nursing Ethics*, vol. 2, no. 3, pp. 223–32.

Khaw, K.T., Bingham, S., Welch, A., Luben, R., Wareham, N., Oakes, S. and Day, N. 2001, 'Relation between plasma ascorbic acid and mortality in men and women in EPIC-Norfolk prospective study: A prospective population study' in *Lancet*, vol. 357, pp. 657–63.

Last, J.M. (ed.) 1998, *A Dictionary of Epidemiology* (2nd edition), Oxford Medical Publications, Oxford University Press, New York.

Lawlor, D.A., Davey-Smith, G.D., Bruckdorfer, K.R., Kundu, D. and Ebrahim, S. 2004, 'Those confounded vitamins: What can we learn from the differences between observational versus randomised trial evidence?' in *Lancet*, vol. 363, pp. 1724–27.

Margetts, B.M. and Nelson, M. (eds) 1997, *Design Concepts in Nutritional Epidemiology* (2nd edition), Oxford University Press, New York.

Margetts, B.M., Thompson, R.L., Key, T., Duffy, S., Nelson, M., Bingham, S. and Wiseman, M. 1995, 'Development of a scoring system to judge the scientific quality of information from case-control and cohort studies of nutrition and disease' in *Nutrition and Cancer*, vol. 24, no. 3, pp. 231–39.

Potischman, N. and Weed, D.L. 1999, 'Causal criteria in nutritional epidemiology' in *American Journal of Clinical Nutrition*, vol. 99, pp. S1309–14.

Public Health Resource Unit (UK) 2005, 'Critical Appraisal Tools', National Health Service, cited at <http://www.phru.nhs.uk/casp/critical_appraisal_tools.htm> on 25 January 2006.

Rothman, K.J. and Greenland, S. 1998, *Modern Epidemiology*, Lippincott-Raven, Philadelphia.

Sempos, C.T., Liu, K. and Ernst, N.D. 1999, 'Food and nutrient exposures: What to consider when evaluating epidemiologic evidence' in *American Journal of Clinical Nutrition*, vol. 69, pp. S1330–38.

Shunk, J.A. and Birch, L.L. 2004, 'Girls at risk for overweight at age 5 are at risk for dietary restraint, disinhibited overeating, weight concerns, and greater weight gain from 5 to 9 years' in *Journal of the American Dietetic Association*, vol. 104, pp. 1120–26.

Strauss, A. and Corbin, J. 1990, *Basics of Qualitative Research: Grounded theory procedures and Techniques*, Sage Publications, Newbury Park, CA.

Streiner, D.L. and Norman, G.R. 1991, *Health Measurement Scales: A practical guide to their development and use*, Oxford University Press, New York.

Stunkard, A.J. and Messick, S. 1985, 'The three-factor eating questionnaire to measure dietary restraint, disinhibition and hunger' in *Journal of Psychosometric Research*, vol. 29, no. 1, pp. 71–83.

Summerbell, C.D., Waters, E., Edmunds, L.D., Kelly, S., Brown, T. and Campbell, K.J. 2005, 'Interventions for preventing obesity in children' in *The Cochrane Database of Systematic Reviews*, July 20, no. 3, CD001871.

Willett, W. (ed.) 1998, *Nutritional Epidemiology*, Oxford University Press, New York.

World Cancer Research Fund 1997, *Food, Nutrition and the Prevention of Cancer: A global perspective*, American Institute for Cancer Research, Washington.

15

Professional practice

HEATHER YEATMAN
ANDREA BEGLEY

The practice of public health nutrition includes a variety of services and activities that provide an environment in which populations can be healthy (Johnson et al. 2001). The ability to deliver effective and targeted services and activities to address current health concerns requires public health nutritionists to not only have the knowledge content but also the insight and skills to address the organisational and public expectations of the position.

Research on the nature and basics of practice is essential to guide future practice and hence to improve public health nutrition outcomes. Recent research on public health nutrition competencies has identified a range of key expectations of practitioners and employers (Hughes 2003; Hughes 2004a). Hughes (2004a) demonstrated that the scope of public health nutrition practice is a fluid concept, changing as a result of advances in knowledge, technological developments, and organisational and team dynamics. It is also needs to be responsive to broader social and policy issues that may impact on public health nutrition outcomes.

A range of practice skills have been identified through international consensus and examination of job description position statements. These skills include human resource management, continuing professional development, submission writing, quality management, consultation and negotiation skills, interpersonal communication skills, ability to work in a multidisciplinary manner, being independent and self-directed and cultural competency (Hughes 2003; Hughes 2004b).

This chapter outlines the range of issues under six areas that need to be considered by the public health nutrition practitioner, reflecting and developing their own professional practice, including working to maximise organisational support:

1. Leadership: identified as an essential attribute to ensure nutrition is on the agenda of key decision-makers to influence policies and programmes within the community or in organisations, as well as to challenge established ideas and practice.
2. Working in partnerships: with others can be formal or informal, advocacy or technically based, long or short term, focused on outcomes or on achieving an intermediate goal, such as building capacity within a community.
3. Professional ethics and conduct: particularly pertinent to public health nutrition, as there are many situations where conflicts of interest (perceived or otherwise) can function to undermine the achievement of public health nutrition outcomes. In addition, as public health nutritionists often work in professionally sole situations, diligence must be given to maintain a current and comprehensive public health nutrition knowledge and skill base, to ensure that professional advice is soundly based.
4. Personal communication skills: critical, due to the often controversial nature of the field, the eloquence and influence of other stakeholders, and the necessity to respond effectively and in a timely fashion to emerging issues.
5. Professional advocacy skills: core to public health nutrition practice, utilising effective communication to maximise opportunities to advance strategic policy or programme agendas.
6. Developing professional and organisational support: enables the public health nutrition practitioner to maintain their professional expertise and the public health nutrition agenda to become core to the business of the organisation. This will provide ongoing support for public health nutrition related activities, enabling public health nutrition practitioners to focus on achieving public health nutrition outcomes.

Leadership

Improving nutrition in populations requires that key public health nutrition issues are on the public policy agenda, to enable leverage of funding and support for programmes. This will occur through leadership within the profession and champions for public health nutrition. Without such leadership, other groups with vested interests or market forces will determine directions for nutrition.

Public health nutrition issues are affected by many factors, social, cultural, economic and political, as well as biological and physical. This has two main implications for public health nutrition practitioners. First, they require a unique knowledge set – knowledge of food systems, food security, food and health practices and health systems (Beaudry & Delisle 2005), together with basic nutritional sciences and public health practice. Second, the work by Kingdon (1995) on influencing the policy agenda identifies that they need to be able to not only understand this broad range of issues, but also to identify key influences and leverage points for taking action, be able to identify favourable opportunities for action, and have targeted strategies to recommend for implementation. These are the traits of leadership, or in Kingdon's terms, policy entrepreneurs. In relation to public health nutrition, such leadership may be demonstrated by sole practitioners in regional public health units or individual public health nutritionists working within teams championing specific public health nutrition issues within more complex organisations such as State departments of health. More recently Yngve (2006) has stated that public health nutrition leadership characteristics are related to personal and professional experiences giving rise to a state of mind. They are not a set of principles to be followed.

Personal leadership attributes

Different types of leadership are possible, depending on the personal traits of individuals and the environment within which leadership is required (Xirasagar et al. 2006). Transformational leadership is the ability to be directive and solve problems. Transactional leadership is the ability to motivate others and embrace change. Fertman (2003) also has identified the following attributes of leadership: practitioners who strive for excellence, are responsive and flexible, have the confidence to challenge established ideas or ways of practice, and can communicate a shared vision for improving nutritional status. Different styles of leadership can be directed to achieving changes in the behaviour of others (for example, team building or motivation), or it can be directed to leadership of a policy agenda (such as ensuring public health nutrition is integrated within organisational goals or government policy). Thus, leadership requires people skills and policymaking skills.

Leadership that utilises people skills can foster a culture of innovation and increased productivity (Cleary et al. 2005). It focuses on maximising staff productivity through the development of well-functioning teams and a shared vision of strategies and outcomes. A positive outcome from leadership would be the ability to create a consensus (Yngve 2006). There are many studies that seek to define the personal traits of leadership. Personal attributes of leaders considered important have been identified by research on nurse executives by Carroll (2005) as:

- personal integrity, including high ethical standards trustworthiness and creditability
- strategic vision/action orientation, including the ability to set goals and change practice
- developing partnerships/communication skills, while being able to delegate
- management and technical competencies
- developing a collaborative team and enabling others to act
- people skills that encourage and inspire others
- personal survival skills – being politically sensitivity, having self-direction and self-reliance.

There are many personal benefits for taking on a leadership role. Cleary and colleagues (2005) report on five benefits, including gaining more satisfaction at work, pursuing areas of personal interest, seeing your work come to fruition, overseeing the development of colleagues, and having a sense of contributing to the workplace and ultimately the public health nutrition profession.

Leadership requires the development and consolidation of skills and knowledge. In the area of policymaking, the range of skills required includes analytical thinking, priority-setting and negotiation, building partnerships via networks and coalitions, effective oral and written communications, and skills in advocacy for public health nutrition. Also crucial for public health nutritionists is training or education in the process of policymaking. Public health nutritionists need to be informed about political interests, approaches to policy development and potential points of influence, and to understand different ways to work together to bring about changes. Other ways to develop professional leadership skills are included in Table 15.1.

There is little written about leadership in public health nutrition. Hughes (2003) reports on advanced level Australian practitioners' views on their own competency development. The sample interviewed was selected due to identified leadership in senior positions. Hughes identified that leadership skills were developed through exposure to mentors, on-the-job experiences, postgraduate training in public health, and committee work.

While little has been reported on leadership in public health nutrition, it has been identified that greater and more rapid progress can be achieved in public health when leadership and vision are provided at a national level to complement local initiatives in skilling up existing practitioners (Brocklehurst et al. 2005).

Table 15.1 Ways to develop professional leadership skills

Individual level	Organisational level
• Identify a key public health nutrition issue of concern to you, research the latest information about it and effective approaches to dealing with it, and then use all opportunities to talk about it with others.	• Identify two or three nutrition issues of relevance to the organisation's mission, and regularly talk with your manager/ chief executive officer about what the organisation can do about them.
• Join a committee that is involved in policymaking, and provide nutrition expertise to the processes. Examples include your children's school canteen committee, a committee of your professional association that is involved in responding to policy papers, or a local government's community consultative committee.	• Take on leadership roles within the organisation – this can be leader of a particular project, chairing a committee, or even a fund-raising activity. Whatever the role, it helps to develop your profile within the organisation.
• Negotiate with your local newspaper to provide regular short news articles on current nutrition issues.	• If you manage a small (or large) team, identify a series of nutrition issues that individual staff members can champion within the organisation.
• Identify a recognised leader and ask him/her to mentor you.	• Foster links with the local media, to provide access to reliable information or comment by contacting you or your unit.
• Make a time to meet with your local elected (and opposition) members to talk about nutrition issues in the local community.	• Meet with key organisational and community leaders to discuss nutrition issues and how it affects them.
• Facilitate a series of professional or community seminars addressing local nutrition issues and presented by energetic and entertaining speakers.	• Foster activities that encourage other units or external organisations to participate in public health nutrition events.

Organisational level

Leadership skills needed at the organisational level are strategic planning and operational management.

Healthcare systems are in constant organisational change, and studies have identified different factors that affect the outcome of such changes (Riley 2003). Organisational leadership can be demonstrated through the championing of public health nutrition issues, effective timing of initiatives, and minimising the impact on individual enthusiasm and performance.

Champions are a key influence on the affect of organisational change processes. They are usually internal to the organisation and act to advocate and support an issue. Champions for public health nutrition can be developed by ensuring open communication; establishing transparent, accessible systems; and supporting internal advocates.

The timing of ideas for change is important, as a good idea might be rejected one year, only to become the right idea the next. To be effective in advancing public health nutrition goals, programming requires attention to the long-term visions of what the environment could be, while also satisfying the immediate needs of management within the organisation and/or needs of the community.

Organisational change has been found to have an effect at the individual level through demoralising staff, resulting in health professionals and their teams losing their perspective (McMaster 1999). One way identified as addressing this risk is for organisational leaders to celebrate small successes during the change process (Kerfoot 1997). Building on these findings, public health nutritionists and their teams can maintain/restore their enthusiasm and direction through rewarding small and large contributions as part of positive organisational change. There is a need to be proactive: to predict or adapt to radical change rather than trying to play catch-up or being reactive to organisation change. Managing teams and people, team-building and development, conflict resolution and mentoring are critical strategies.

Working in partnerships

Working in partnerships with others can be formal or informal, advocacy or technically based, long or short term, focused on outcomes or on achieving an intermediate goal, such as building capacity within a community. The concept of partnerships is one that has taken on many forms in the literature. The primary focus is to work with others to influence policymakers and public health nutrition outcomes. This recognises there are many factors that can influence nutrition in sectors other than health. The development of intersectorial partnerships is an important way to progress public health nutrition by developing public opinion and relationships with peers (Lansing & Kolasa 1996). Partnerships may also be formed within public health nutrition networks, enabling public health nutrition practitioners to exchange information, work together, share resources and solve public health nutrition problems. Today's public health nutrition challenges required networking and collaboration on a broad scale (Yngve 2006). Margetts (2006) urges public health nutritionists to build stronger partnerships between all sectors with a stake in public health nutrition.

Successful partnership principles

Public health practitioners either work with others at an individual level, or develop organisationally based relationships. Acting as an individual, the practitioner takes on the role of a champion or advocate, working with individuals or organisations having similar goals or the potential to influence public health nutrition outcomes (Riley 2003). Organisationally based partnerships are more challenging, as they require not only the organisational commitment to an issue but also the internal capacity and structures to enable it to happen. For example, even though health departments and departments of primary industry both have a commitment to outcomes related to healthy food, it is a very challenging task to identify where their core activities may overlap or support each other (Tillotson 2003). The public health nutritionist can have a key role in engineering the organisational processes and policies that support such collaboration. It takes a long time to develop the necessary shift in procedures and activities to enable mutually supportive activities to occur (McDonald 2005). However, once achieved, an organisational partnership is more sustainable, whereas partnerships based on the actions of individuals may well dissipate when the individual moves on to other responsibilities.

Conceptually there are many aspects to partnerships. Lansing and Kolasa (1996) describe various aspects of productive partnerships. The basis for successful partnerships is the need for shared goals and mutual benefit. Strategic plans will help provide a framework for decisions about which partnerships to develop in order to achieve goals.

Partnerships in public health nutrition have been successfully developed using a research-based partnership framework that recognises every member of the partnership is knowledgeable and therefore significant (Gillespie et al. 2003). Explaining the success of public health nutrition partnerships requires a paradigm shift in what many might see as the key principles. This shift is described in Table 15.2.

Table 15.2 Paradigm Shifts in Partnership Principles

Typical Assumptions of Partnerships	Reality of Successful Partnerships
• The missions and motives of partner organisations must be closely aligned to justify collaboration.	• Partners can have mutual goals even if their missions and motives are different.
• Partner suitability is judged by personal opinions, perceived public opinion, or by non-profit/for-profit status.	• Partners are selected on the basis of objective criteria related to the fit of the partnership's goals with those of the organisation.
• Relationships are established to further goals of one partner.	• Relationships are based on mutually beneficial goals.
• One partner works for the other.	• Partners work with one another.
• Money is the only valued resource.	• Valued resources include technical expertise, influence, credibility, marketing kills, new insights, communication channels, etc.
• Power in the relationship is tied to who contributes money.	• Power is balanced among all partners, each of whom contributes valued resources.
• Non-profit partners bear all the risk in relationships with for-profit organisations.	• Risks may be different, but all partners assume some risk to their organisations.
• For-profit partners cannot be trusted because of their for-profit orientation; motives of public or voluntary sector partners are not suspect because they are non-profit.	• Partnerships depend on mutual trust based on relationship experience irrespective of partner's for-profit/non-profit status.
• One partner pre-empts the other, constraining communication and compromising independence in decisions and actions.	• Partners foster understanding of and respect for each other's views; growing trust encourages rather than constrains straightforward communication and independent thinking and action.
• One partner dictates processes and controls outcomes.	• Partners share responsibility for process and share control over outcomes: control issues are clearly stated and agreed to by the partners upfront as a condition of the partnership.

Source: Adapted from Probert 1997

Types of partnerships

Greater impact can be achieved through the development of a range of partnerships. Public health nutritionists should strive to build a range of working relationships, with a diversity in membership to ensure the greatest outcomes for nutrition. Developing partnerships will mean that outcomes are most likely to be more successful, particularly the private/public partnerships (Donato 2006). Partnerships can further be broken down into different types with separate names, and with specific purposes. The type of partnership you develop will depend on the outcomes required.

Probert (1997) represents the types of partnerships in the following figure, with partnership being the umbrella term. These partnership types are:

- Networks: A loose-knit group of individuals/organisations connected via communication links. Example: Special Interest Groups in professional organisations (see Case study 15.1).
- Alliance: A union of interests that have similar character, structure or outlook. Example: A community-based alliance around a specific public health nutrition issue (see Case study 15.2).
- Consortium: A group with similar interests who are prepared to work together for common outcomes/advantage. Example: Several organisations

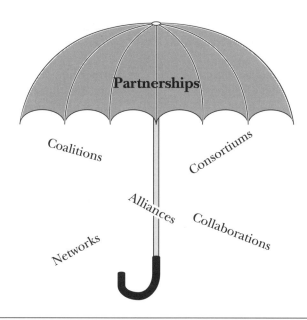

Figure 15.1 Types of partnerships that can be considered for public health nutrition

---

CASE STUDY 15.1

FOOD AND NUTRITION SPECIAL INTEREST GROUP OF THE
PUBLIC HEALTH ASSOCIATION OF AUSTRALIA

The objectives of the Food and Nutrition Special Interest Group are to:
- provide a focal point for discussion of and action on public health food and nutrition issues
- provide a formal vehicle for networking, advocacy and collaboration in public health nutrition
- promote development of a framework for education and professional development of public health workers interested in public health nutrition
- ensure that public health nutrition is represented in the affairs of the Public Health Association of Australia Inc.

Source: <www.phaa.net.au>

---

may develop and implement a community-based programme (see Case study 15.3).
- Collaboration: A joint effort that represents the most intense way of working together while still maintaining the separate identity of participants. Example: The Parents Jury (see Case study 15.4).
- Coalition: A temporary alliance of parties for some specific purpose. This may be to solve or monitor a problem or special event that an individual organisation with limited resources may not be able to undertake. Coalitions have become the most popular partnership for improving health and nutrition (Zakocs & Edwards 2006). They can be very focused, and people/organisations can commit for limited periods of time. Coalitions are successful at influencing the policy agenda and an example would be the Food Policy Coalition in Penrith, New South Wales (see Case study 15.5).

Developing Partnerships

There is certainly an art to developing partnerships, but more importantly the development of effective partnerships that will progress public health nutrition goals further than working alone. Probert (1997) has identified several elements essential to the success of partnerships:

- staff and organisational support
- a focal point of coordination

CASE STUDY 15.2

WORLD ALLIANCE FOR BREASTFEEDING ACTION

The World Alliance for Breastfeeding Action (WABA) was formed on 14 February 1991. The WABA is a global network of organisations and individuals who believe breastfeeding is the right of all children and mothers, and who dedicate themselves to protect, promote and support this right. The WABA acts on the Innocenti Declaration, and works in liaison with UNICEF. The WABA is like an umbrella that encompasses all working at the international, regional, national, and community level to protect, promote and support breastfeeding. Everyone who is committed to a breastfeeding culture can be part of WABA: non-governmental organisations, community activists, healthcare workers, professional associations, university teaching staff, researchers, health officials and others. The goals of WABA are:

- re-establish and maintain a global breastfeeding culture
- eliminate all obstacles to breastfeeding
- promote more regional and national level cooperation
- advocate for breastfeeding in development, women and environmental programmes.

The roles that WABA plays are:

- information sharing and networking
- to strengthen and coordinate existing activities to create more momentum
- to build bridges among all breastfeeding advocates: grass roots groups and individuals, UN agencies, governments and international non-government organisations
- stimulate and support new and collaborative efforts.

- specific system of communication, such as email, teleconferences, face-to-face meetings, regular minutes of meetings
- actively involved community leaders
- strong relationships between private and public sector groups
- communication networks within the community
- constituency for public health nutrition that can advocate for resources and for attention of politicians and/or funders.

Skills needed by public health nutritionists to build effective partnerships include:

CASE STUDY 15.3

FOOD FAIRNESS ILLAWARRA AND THE WARRAWONG COMMUNITY KITCHEN

A food security forum in October 2005 brought to attention the fact that many services and groups were seeing people experience hunger in the Illawarra community. A consortium was established between individual community members, Wollongong Wesley Mission, South East Sydney Illawarra Area Health Service, Wollongong City Council, Healthy Cities Illawarra, Warrawong Community Kitchen, and University of Wollongong. Food Fairness Illawarra has been active in a number of activities, supporting its members to work toward food fairness. Achievements include:

- applying and receiving Healthy Local Government Grant funding to coordinate a food access project, which will build the alliance infrastructure as well as coordinate food access research and programs
- developing promotional material in regards to food safety
- mapping data on food providers, outlets, distributors, alongside housing and transport information to show the need of fairer food access in Wollongong
- linking with other Food Security programs in New South Wales and Australia.

Source: Food Fairness Illawarra <http://www.healthycitiesill.org.au/foodfairness.htm>

- identifying individuals/organisations that deal with the issues and the specific roles they undertake
- bringing people together to discuss an issue and identify their purpose and define problems
- relationship building, where everyone has equal opportunity to give their perspectives, which are listened to by the rest of group. This may take several meetings and different strategies to achieve. Skills to negotiate and use group process techniques, for example, facilitation, brainstorming and nominal group processes and consensus-building
- negotiating a consensus about purpose and/or problem, requiring agreements, memoranda of understanding (MOUs) and contracts
- facilitating each member of group to identify to their contribution to the purpose and/or problem. A 'RACK' analysis could be helpful, assessing the Resources, Access, Constraints and Knowledge of each individual or organisation (Landers 2006).

The success of partnerships will also contribute to the overall professional development of the public health nutritionist by accomplishing more than acting

CASE STUDY 15.4

THE PARENTS JURY

The Parents Jury is a web-based network of parents who wish to improve the food and physical activity environments for children in Australia. As explained in chapter 9, the Parents Jury originally developed in the United Kingdom (see <http://www.foodcomm. org.uk/parents_jury.htm>). The Parents Jury now has been established in Australia (see <http//www.parentsjury.org.au>).

The Parents Jury provides a forum for parents to voice their views on children's food and physical activity issues, and to collectively advocate for the improvement of children's food and physical activity environments (for example, reduced marketing targeted at young children, more healthy choices for school canteens, and making neighbourhoods safer and more child-friendly).

The Parents Jury enables parents to nominate and vote for the biannual Parents Jury Awards for people or organisations that affect, positively or negatively, the availability and promotion of healthy food and physical activity choices for children.

The Parents Jury in Australia is a collaboration of Diabetes Australia–Victoria, The Cancer Council Australia and Australasian Society for the Study of Obesity, which together have a major interest in improving children's nutrition and levels of physical activity, and reducing overweight and obesity in Australia.

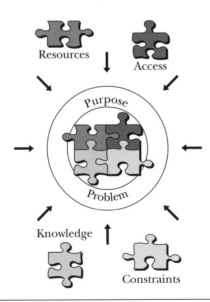

Figure 15.2 Elements of a RACK analysis
Source: Landers 2006

CASE STUDY 15.5

PENRITH FOOD POLICY COALITION

The Penrith Food Project was a ten-year evolution of a local intersectoral project aimed at improving components of a community's food system as an approach to improving nutrition. The project demonstrates aspects of innovation in collaborating for health promotion. Key initiators of the project were a university public health department, a community health service and a local government authority. Players brought into the process included the agricultural sector and food retailers. An intersectoral project working party was established with the city council, which led to the establishment of food policy committee. This committee planned and oversaw the project implementation. In establishing the committee, seniority of members was considered important for community credibility as well as implementation of policies and plans. Located in the local government, the committee operated on a constitution that outlined the requirements for accountability, annual general meetings and decision-making processes. Monthly business meetings were a mix of information, sharing, planning and decision-making. The project's success in achieving policy and system level changes was due to a specific focus on organisational development and capacity building many key partners and the use of formative evaluation methods to improve the collaborative nature of the partnership.

alone and being a collection of ideas and resources. Partnerships work to create healthy environments, as illustrated in Case study 15.6.

However, after the initiation of a partnership such as a coalition, sustaining, re-energising or merging and collapsing coalitions become complex tasks that require leadership skills. Strong leadership is a key factor identified in a recent review of coalition effectiveness (Zakocs & Edwards 2006). Also important for success identified in their review were formal governance procedures, specified roles and agreed timeframes, active participation by members, diverse membership and group cohesion.

It is worthwhile taking time to consider and develop effective partnerships for programme delivery in public health nutrition. Sharing common goals provides the opportunity to capitalise on the benefits of identifying skills and contributions required for the effort and combining resources. Effective partnerships will contribute to the overall productivity of the public health nutritionist and integrate nutrition into broader health objectives or other organisations.

CASE STUDY 15.6

THE EAT WELL SA PROJECT

The term 'capacity building' is used in the health-promotion literature to mean invest-ing in communities, organisations and structures to enhance access to knowledge, skills and resources needed to conduct effective health programmes. The Eat Well (South Australia) project aimed to increase consumption of healthy food by children, young people and their families (Smith et al. 2004). The project evaluation demonstrated that awareness about healthy eating among stakeholders across a range of sectors, coalitions and partnerships to promote healthy eating and sustainable programs had been devel-oped. The project achievements were analysed further using a capacity building framework. This analysis showed that partnership development was a key strategy for success, leading to increased problem-solving capacity among key stakeholders and workers from education, childcare, health, transport and food industry sectors. It was also a strategy that required concerted effort and review. New and ongoing programmes were initiated and institutionalised within other sectors, notably the child-care, vocational education and transport sectors. A model for planning and evaluating nutrition health promotion work is described.

Source: <http://chdf.org.au/eatwellsa/index.html>

Professional ethics and conduct of interest

Professional ethics and conduct are particularly pertinent to public health nutri-tion, as there are many situations where conflicts of interest (perceived or otherwise) can function to undermine the achievement of public health nutri-tion outcomes. In addition, as public health nutritionists often work in professionally sole situations, diligence must be given to maintain a current and comprehensive public health nutrition knowledge and skill base, to ensure that professional advice is soundly based.

Public health as a discipline works to address the social determinants of disease. The concept of social determinants of health implies the need for social justice or a commitment to fairness and/or equity in the delivery of public health nutrition practice (see chapter 7). Ethics for public health nutrition practice are similar to other professions, such as dieticians (American Dietetic Association 1999). Public health nutrition practice, including the delivery of services and other specific actions, needs to be conducted with honesty, integrity and fairness. In addition, public health nutritionists must accept the responsibility and accountability for their actions.

The following is a list of key ethical considerations for a public health nutritionist.

- Respect the rights of individuals in the community. Respect diverse values, beliefs and cultures; seek input from members by providing communities with information they can make decisions on; do not discriminate against particular subgroups; and provide for equitable distribution of resources. Act in a timely manner, protecting the confidentially of information that may bring harm to an individual or community, and engage in collaborations or partnerships that build trust. Respect others and their points of view even when they are opposed to your own. Do not take conflicts personally. Learn from your opposition's opinion, as you may be able to strengthen your own position. It is necessary to learn to accept viable solutions even when they are less than ideal.
- Take responsibility for your own competence and be accountable for continually building skills and knowledge to improve practice and provide high-quality services. Provide objective evaluations of the performance of others and make an effort to avoid bias in any kind of professional evaluation. A practitioner's scope of practice will depend on an individual's education and training and the competencies that have been developed. The type of service delivery undertaken will depend on these skills and the resources available.
- Be alert to situations that might cause a conflict of interest within and across organisations.

Public health nutritionists focus on improving the food and nutrition system. There are partnerships between those stakeholders in the food and nutrition system that could lead to conflict of interests. Nestle (2001) describes the potential for conflicts of interest when corporations such as the food processing industry establish financial relationship with practitioners, academics or researchers. It may be difficult therefore to accept food industry support of projects even if both parties maintain that the relationship does not comprise the view of nutrition issues or the common goal of improving the health of populations. Many peer-reviewed journals require authors to declare any potential conflicts of interest, and these can provide a starting point for public health nutritionists to consider any potential conflict of interest (see Box 15.1).

Implied endorsements are a potential risk of partnerships (Lansing & Kolasa 1996). This is particularly the case when the partnerships are between the food

---

Box 15.1

QUESTIONS POSED TO AUTHORS IN PEER-REVIEWED JOURNALS

Have you accepted the following from an organisation that may gain or lose financially from your work:

- received reimbursement for attending a symposium/conference
- fee for speaking
- funds for research
- fees for consulting?

Have you been employed or held shares in an organisation that may gain or lose financially from your work?

Have you had any other competing interests like:

- relative with a link to a person or organisation whose interests may be affected by your work
- membership of a political party or special interest group whose interests may be affected by your work
- deep personal or religious convictions that may affect your views?

---

industry and a nutrition organisation (see case studies 15.7 and 15.8). Good planning, effective communication and skilful negotiation of messages minimises the possibility of implied endorsements. It is also essential to specify use of name or logos, or to use a disclaimer statement whenever collaborations with others occur.

Public health nutrition practice involves the collection and collation of data to design nutrition programmes (see Case study 15.9). There are international and national rules on how data collection or research should be conducted. It may be necessary to consult a human research ethics committee of a health department, hospital or university, which would follow rules guiding research from organisations like the National Health and Medical Research Council in Australia.

The public health nutritionist needs to follow ethical principles in practice that require honesty, integrity and fairness (Moran 2006). The public health nutritionist need to provide sufficient information to individuals, groups or partnerships to enable people to make informed decisions and to treat any information collected confidentially.

CASE STUDY 15.7

LESSONS TO BE LEARNED: WORKING WITH PRIVATE
PARTNER ORGANISATIONS

The National Heart Foundation (NHF) (Queensland Division) entered into a partnership with a large catering company with the aim of providing a healthier food service for its clients. The clients of the catering company had asked for the provision of healthy food options and the NHF was seen as a credible organisation to assist in achieving this aim. The partnership existed from April 1997 to August 1999, when both parties agreed to withdraw from the project. One of the critical factors contributing to the final outcome was the non-systematic approach to the partnership itself. The authors describe how many of the issues experience could have been prevented with clear partnership planning, an evaluation process of policy, development of mutual purpose, and agreed decision-making and project management strategies.

Source: Ashton & Hehir 2002

Personal communication skills

Effective communication by the public health nutritionist is the ability to draw on a range of communication styles and behaviours to transmit a message so that it is received in a manner consistent with the original intent. This will apply both at the individual level and also within an organisation.

Public health nutrition practice requires multidisciplinary work and strong advocacy skills. Strong communication competence for public health nutrition requires recognition of the role of the public health nutritionist within a team (specialist contributions) and identification of individual abilities and limitations (personal contributions). The team may have as its primary goal a public health nutrition outcome, in which case the contributions of the public health nutritionist is central, and he/she should be taking a leading role, or public health nutrition may be a secondary outcome, in which case the public health nutritionist can make strategic contributions regarding issues that are considered important to public health nutrition goals. Two examples illustrate this:

1. Meals-on-Wheels: A committee that focuses on the delivery of nutritional meals via home-delivery services for the aged or infirm should have a core concern about nutrition and the factors that may affect the nutritional status of the recipients, such as length of time of delivery of meals, types and

---

CASE STUDY 15.8

HEALTH WORKING WITH INDUSTRY

In 1990, the Department of Health (DOH) in Western Australia initiated a five-year multilevel, state-wide, social marketing campaign to increase adult awareness of the need to eat more fruit and vegetables. Fruit and vegetable growers, marketing, processing and retailing groups were solicited as campaign partners. The strengths of this partnership were the need and opportunity for the DOH and industry to work together to promote the increased consumption of fruit and vegetables. DOH had the commitment, expertise and resources to plan, implement and evaluate many aspects of the campaign. The industry had established channels of communication within the fruit and vegetable supply chain from agricultural advisers to consumers. The initial expectations of the DOH to generate significant industry resource input into a generic campaign was modified by grower needs to promote their own specific product, and retailer expectations of product promotions resourced and organised by suppliers. Partnership weaknesses arose when action taken by enthusiastic individuals without formal commitment by their sponsoring organisations. Difficulties arose in sustaining organisational relationships and action when staff changes occurred. Establishment of a broader-based campaign advisory group with formal representation from key industry and health organisations may have helped to sustain consultation, relationships and action. This case study highlights the potential, but also the weaknesses that must be overcome for effective intersectorial action between industry and health.

Source: Miller & Pollard 2005

---

quality of foods provided, and temperature of foods. The public health nutritionist should take a leadership role on such a committee.

2. Preventing overweight in primary school-age children: A committee may be focused on preventing overweight with primary school children. Nutrition is important, but so too are physical activity and the social and emotional development of children. Clearly, the public health nutritionist has an essential contribution, but others also have important roles, and it may be more appropriate for the public health nutrition not to take a leadership role, but be an effective team member.

Partnership communication skills

The following partnership communication skills are essential to furthering the public health nutrition agenda. Within teams, minutes of meetings which reflect discussions, proposed actions and outcomes to be achieved are kept. Taking the minutes may appear tedious, but it is an effect mechanism for influencing how the issue or problem is being portrayed. Talking with team or committee members outside of official meeting times allows common understandings of issues to be developed, and more time to negotiate ways of dealing with challenging situations. If official communication is to occur around important items, ensure that people agree to specific wording at the time — set a few people the task of writing the letter or petition during the meeting time, so it is ready to sign or be agreed while all people are still present. Get input from others and recognise inherent resistance to change. A public health nutritionist may plant an idea and eventually let others take the credit.

Personal communication skills are often a reflection of your own individual learning style; however, there are a few tips to ensuring that you make maximum use of a team or committee situation. It is important to be clear about your requirements and be honest about your ability to meet requirements. Offering a lot but delivering little only leads to others ignoring your potential contributions. Consider the public health nutrition expertise you have to offer, the resources available, and whether you have any potential conflicts of interest, or just potential conflicts with other tasks. Listen carefully to what others are saying, and be empathetic to their situation. Focus on the task, not the people, and try to offer suggestions that identify a way forward, rather than merely reflect what has already been discussed. Study the resistance and learn to overcome and be persistent. In your communications, be positive and continue to demonstrate ways to improve or build on the task.

Emotional intelligence skills

Researchers in public health have looked into the social sciences and business fields in an effort to improve health professionals' communication skills. The construct called emotional intelligence (EI) has been identified as a desirable competency in a number of fields that require effective communication skills and leadership (Buchler et al. 2006). The EI is sometimes referred to as a gut instinct or an innate sense about what others are feeling, but it is generally recognised that there is more to it than that. It was first introduced to the scientific literature by Mayer and Salovey (1990).

EI is defined as the ability to understand feelings within oneself and in others, using these feelings in guiding thought and action. It relies on the four cognitive abilities of identifying, using, understanding and managing emotions.

The descriptions of EI have been further described as:

- the ability to motivate oneself
- persist in the face of frustration – resilience
- regulate one's moods, emotions and behaviours
- allows one to empathise with others
- gives people the ability to maintain an above-average level of leadership and social skills.

More recent research in this area has focused on the capacity of emotional intelligence to enhance leadership skills (Wieand 2002) and to predict transformational leadership amongst individuals (Barbuto & Burbach 2006).

The EI can be useful to a public health nutrition practitioner at several levels. On a very basic level, EI has been linked to people's capacities to obtain good nutrition – so the concept can be integrated into nutrition education approaches (Webb 2001). On a professional level, it can contribute to increased motivation and an ability to focus on a goal rather than demanding instant gratification. A person with a high EI is also capable of understanding the feelings of others, and is better at handling relationships of every kind. Relationships like the partnerships already described are particularly important in public health nutrition practice. Practitioners with high EI will strengthen internal and external networks, and some healthcare organisations also promote teams with complementary emotional intelligence attributes (Freshman & Rubino 2004).

On the level of public health nutrition practice, emotional intelligence requires practitioners to work in a range of different contexts. In a multicultural society, communication with culturally and linguistically diverse groups is very important. Developing high EI helps to develop a high degree of cultural sensitivity or cultural intelligence, and will effectively bridge potential differences in communication. It will enable the public health nutrition practitioner to acquire knowledge and respond quickly and productively to a new situation, especially in the face of knock-backs or slow progress towards goals.

High EI can be developed, but it takes training. A number of strategies have been used to develop EI, particularly as it relates to leadership. Journaling or reflective practice are processes that develop self-awareness. This self-awareness is the first step in becoming emotionally intelligent. Answering 'yes' to any of the questions in the checklist below will give you some indication as to whether you have some of the characteristics of EI:

Emotional intelligence checklist

- Are you able to read others individual feelings and behaviours?

- Are you able to look beyond the behaviour to recognise hidden motivations or agendas?
- Are you able to receive criticism from others without taking it personally?
- Are you able to give criticism without making it personal?
- Do you behave and speak appropriately?
- Are you able to stay on tasks?
- Are you able to separate the cause of the emotion (another person) from the emotion?
- Do you later reflect on the situation that led to the emotion?
- Are you able to grow and learn from the experience?

No one person can do all the self-regulation aspects at one time. Self-talk shapes feelings and actions, and teaches practitioners to reframe negative self-talk into a constructive format. Development of an awareness of others, and also the development of empathy through actively listening to others, will foster empathy (Reeves 2005; Consortium for Research on EI in Organisations n.d.).

It is important for public health nutritionist to develop skills in EI because the behaviours associated with EI further public health nutritions' goals to improve health outcomes.

Mass media skills

How the media frames an issue will often determine public opinion. It is important for public health nutritionists and related organisations to build credibility, educate the public on nutrition and discuss current issues. The media itself is a frequently quoted source of food and nutrition information (Keenan et al. 2002). There is a need to think about the role of media in supporting consumers' understanding of nutrition issues via accurate reporting and the concept of using the media to promote events in public health nutrition. The amount of misinformation or conflicting information in newspapers, television and on radio provides a compelling reason for public health nutritionists to develop effective skills in using the mass media (Miller et al. 2006). Public health nutritionists can work proactively with the media to identify groups with extremist ideas.

Undertaking media training enhances working effectively with the media. Some professional organisations offer this, and it is worth taking up if the opportunity arises. Before accepting invitations or using the mass media for promotion, it is worth thinking about the general public's best interest: who do you represent — yourself or the organisation or the profession, and whether you are the best spokesperson. There have been enough experiences with the mass media to develop a range of tips for working effectively with the mass media. The skills you need as a public health nutritionist may depend on whether you are using newspapers (most common), or radio through to television and the skills include:

- get to know who are the main contacts at your local newspaper, radio and television stations — some of these contacts may have more interest in health and nutrition than others and this will increase your chance of getting your story or article in the media
- select points will make your story or article newsworthy — consider if the information is new and significant and relevant to the readers or listeners
- think about the human interest in the story or article, how is it relevant to ordinary lives
- prepare what you want to say — use the concept of 'sound bites', short, clear, precise statements based on the topic (McCaffree 2006; Hahn-Nowlin 1994) — in radio or television, you may only have five to ten seconds to make your point, so it may help to write out one to three points beforehand and have these in front of you when speaking to journalists
- if you are interviewed plan your 'spontaneity', rehearse your responses — practice makes perfect
- don't get sidetracked from your main points when being interviewed, and always work your answer back to your original point
- defuse loaded questions: answer calmly and politely.

Working with the mass media may involve being reactive to stories. Write letters to the editor of newspapers in relation to published articles that are inaccurate and biased. Public health nutritionists need to express concern when mis-information is reported, and be able to direct the media to reputable sources of nutrition information and to provide constructive criticism. The key to this type of writing is to write as actively or persuasively as possible and include important facts.

From an organisational perspective, a policy on communications will involve an outline for publicity. Many organisations have an active media policy that uses the media to support the goals and objectives of the policy. Public health nutritionists may work for organisations that have a communications or public relations department who would direct all media content. In the case of organisations who don't have this type of arrangement, it would be important for a public health nutritionist to discuss what is acceptable to managers.

Organisations may use the media routinely to publicise events. This may involve using the media to promote a nutrition story or getting the media to attend events. The basic tool used to achieve this is to issue a press release. This is basically a statement outlining what is happening, who you want to attend, and quotes from professionals or important people that can be used in media stories. This press release is emailed or faxed to editors of all media. The press release is often included in a 'media kit'. There are a range of other additions to the press release that will be worth considering to get maximum exposure for your message or event. The common inclusions in a media kit are:

- press release
- invitation to attend events
- background information on organisation
- biographies of important people with quotes on the topic or event
- photos that can be used in media stories
- links to important websites that support your cause
- fact sheets or journal articles
- name and address of personnel to call for more information.

Writing skills

The importance of good writing skills should not be underestimated, nor taken for granted. Professional writing can include a range from briefing papers, position statements, ministerials (responses to letters sent to ministers for health), research reports (see Box 15.2), grant applications, newspaper articles and much more. Each purpose requires a different type of writing style.

- Writing for advocacy must contain your position upfront, and have active facts and solutions. Using common language and short sentences, and sticking to one or two main points are the key.
- Writing to secure funding for programs is important when limited funds in public health can mean that obtaining external funding increases a programme's sustainability. Being able to write a successful grant proposal as a mechanism to increase revenue also increases stability and capacity of a nutrition section, and reflects positive initiative. It is time-consuming and requires some support from the agency. Potential funding sources include the government, foundations, corporations or chargers for services rendered. Some funding bodies will run seminars on their funding rounds, and discuss key issues to consider when applying. Sometimes it is useful to read prior successful funding applications or to secure the services of a writer who has a strong track record in the relevant field.
- Writing grant proposals requires time, patience and skills that come with experience. Starting with small grants for demonstration projects is a useful

---

Box 15.2

READER-FRIENDLY WRITING

The Canadian Health Services Research Foundation has simple rules for writing research reports to ensure they have an impact and are easy to read and understand called 1:3:25:

- 1 page: of main messages (the significance of the findings—the lessons learnt)
- 3 pages: executive summary of the main findings
- 25 pages: presenting the detail of the findings, using language that someone not familiar with the field would understand.

Source: <www.chsrf.ca/knowledge_transfer/pdf/cn-1325_e.pdf>

---

first step. These outcomes can then be used for expanded funding. Ask for feedback on unsuccessful grants.

- Report writing is another key communication skill that should not be under-estimated. A clear, concise report that catches a decision-maker's attention is far more likely to receive positive attention than one poorly written, not to the point or including unnecessary detail.
- Programme reports describe the success of various activities in achieving their goals, and they provide continued feedback and assist with development of new priorities. Too often, project reports are not written or they are not circulated widely. Use a number of avenues to ensure wide circulation of a programme's results, including the report itself, conference presentations, internal newsletters, briefing for the manager or minister concerned, and also internal staff workshops or seminars.
- Consumer materials for nutrition education are a key use of writing skills for public health nutritionists. It is worthwhile establishing your expertise when writing for the general public. The main point when writing for the public is to think about using commonsense language and avoiding jargon. The general age range to write for is from eleven years of age (year 6 at school) to not more than thirteen years (year 8) (Paul & Redman 1997b).

The Australian Bureau of Statistics (ABS) assessed the literacy skills of adults in 1996 and the results show that most adults have average (35 per cent) or poor

literacy skills (47 per cent) (ABS 1996). Literacy skill was defined as the information processing skills necessary to use printed materials found at work, home
and in the community. The implication for public health nutrition practice is
that the majority of target groups will require education materials that are
simply written and presented.

There are over 60 characteristics of printed materials that have been linked
with their effectiveness (Paul & Redman 1997a). These include content characteristics such as the use of short words, short sentences and design
characteristics such as the use of headings, choice of fonts and colours. One way
the content characteristics can be assessed objectively is to measure the readability of the material. Generally patient health education materials are higher
in readability than the reading levels of the consumer groups they target (Paul
& Redman, 1997b). A lower level of readability can be achieved by dropping
technical language, abbreviations and simplifying words such as using 'eat more
food' instead of 'overconsumption'.

Writing for consumers needs to use positive language, active rather than
passive voice, needs to take abstract nutrition concepts and turn them into
concrete examples. Use stories, examples, metaphors or analogies (Leff 2004).

Public health nutrition practice involves working with a range of different
individuals and communities in diverse settings. This practice requires a broad
range of personal communication skills. The information presented here should
be considered a starting point from which to develop skills. Personal improvement will come through trying out the ideas, doing further reading and
researching and finding out what works best for you and your practice area.

Professional advocacy skills

Advocacy is concerned with working as proactively as possible. Good advocacy
requires having a set of principles and values, and knowing your priorities.
Advocacy requires the public health nutritionists to work consistently and
continuously to get nutrition issues on higher agendas (Patrick 2005). It may
work to change the policies, positions and programmes of any type of organisation or to draw a community's attention to an important issue and direct
decision-makers towards a solution (WHO 2005). There are natural advantages
to advocacy in the nutrition area, as everyone eats and eating affects health.
Public health nutritionists have the moral high ground in advocacy.

Advocacy can work to change a decision-maker's perception or understanding of a problem or issue, influence choices that will be considered in

formulating decisions, and change decision-making behaviour. Advocacy may be needed because there are unequal power relations and the usual communication channels have been ineffective. The best opportunity is when a problem or issue is being identified, or at least trying to influence the issue before a decision is made. A last resort in advocacy for nutrition would be attempting to reverse a decision that has already been made.

Types of advocacy

There are a range of levels to advocate on public health nutrition issues, depending on your personal levels of confidence and on employment limitations:

- low profile: negotiation, meeting ministers/civil servants, sharing information, providing briefings
- medium profile: continued negotiation, public briefings, 'feeding' opposition, representations, politician communication, and alliances with other groups, letters and articles to newspapers, media releases
- high profile: public criticism, PR and ad campaigns, release of information, letter writing, demonstrations and rallies.

Developing effective advocacy

Advocacy involves lobbying. Lobbying is seen by many as the process or use of activities for advocacy. Public health advocacy can be the strategic use of news media to advance a public policy initiative, often in the face of opposition (Chapman 2004). Chapman poses a series of questions for advocates that have been developed from tobacco advocacy:

1. What are your public health objectives with this issue?
2. Can a 'win–win' outcome be first engineered with decision-makers?
3. Who do the key decision-makers answer to, and how can these people be influenced?
4. What are the relative strengths and weaknesses of your and your opposition's position?
5. What are your media advocacy objectives?
6. How will you frame what is at issue here?
7. What symbols or word pictures can be brought into this frame?
8. What sound bites can be used to convey 6 and 7?
9. Can the issue be personalised?
10. How can large numbers of people be quickly organised to express their concern?

Public health nutrition can lead from advocacy experience in other areas such as tobacco (Yach et al. 2005) and physical activity (Shilton 2006). Nutrition needs to develop an effective model of advocacy involving all interested organisations. There is a perceived lack of advocacy for nutrition often due to a lack of leadership.

The WHO (2005) have identified a ten-step process for nutrition advocacy for countries in the western Pacific region, where malnutrition is a priority. These ten steps were developed from points around targeted actions, focused communication and systematic planning for advocacy:

Step 1:   identify the issue
Step 2:   collect relevant data — develop your evidence base
Step 3:   define your advocacy goal and objectives
Step 4:   consider all the stakeholders and their agendas, consider potential partners
Step 5:   identify the target audience
Step 6:   develop your message
Step 7:   build support from partnerships
Step 8:   prepare for resistance
Step 9:   create an action plan or strategy
Step 10:   monitor and evaluate the progress.

Advocacy for nutrition should be viewed as a dynamic process that can be approached in different ways (see Case study 15.9, for instance), such as developing coalitions or networks, and educating organisations, as well as influencing decision-makers like politicians via a campaign. The action plan or strategy may target and use media, community mobilisation, professional mobilisation, advocacy from within the public health nutritionist's own organisation, and political advocacy, such as in Case study 15.10.

Cannon (2006) urges public health nutritionists to get out of their comfort zones and work with citizen-based action groups for nutrition advocacy. Cannon cites examples of advocacy in breastfeeding and salt for health in the United Kingdom as having the basis of their success in working with what he calls 'civil society' organisations.

Public health nutritionists need to seriously consider new approaches, new strategies and new partnerships to combat issues like obesity. Long-term effectiveness will depend on practitioners who employ strong advocacy skills in their day to day practice.

CASE STUDY 15.9

THE FRUIT AND VEGETABLE CABINET PROJECT

It is common practice in many Aboriginal community stores to see fruit and vegetables in the bottom of soft drink fridges or cool rooms. Fruit and vegetables stored in these locations are not easily accessible or visible to the consumer and the quality of the produce is severely compromised due to inadequate or inappropriate storage facilities. Funding was secured from the Lotteries Commission for three fruit and vegetable chilled display units for use in community stores. The cabinets cost $6000 each to purchase. The Lotteries Commission granted $10 000 for the purchase, location and installation of each unit and for the collating of sales data to assess the impact of the sales of vegetables and fruit. The Office of Aboriginal Economic Development in Western Australia initiated a study to analyse the effect on the sale of foods in collaboration with the Gascoyne and Kimberley Public Health Units. There is potential for a large health benefit from improved infrastructure in community stores with funding provided from a non-traditional health organisation.

Source: adapted from Department of Health, Western Australia, 2003

Developing professional and organisational support

Developing professional and organisational support enables the public health nutrition practitioner to maintain their professional expertise, and for the public health nutrition agenda to become core to the business of the organisation. This will provide ongoing support for public health nutrition-related activities, enabling public health nutrition practitioners to focus on achieving public health nutrition outcomes. Public health nutritionists have the responsibility to make a commitment to lifelong learning to continually advance the field of public health and to remain current with ongoing advances in the field, an attribute highly valued by employers (Hughes 2004b).

Continuing professional development (CPD) is one way to contribute to competency development in public health nutrition. Traditionally, the competency development of advanced level public health nutritionists in many countries has been due to the intrinsic motivations of practitioners rather than any planned CPD push. It is the responsibility of the workplace to undertake a review or audit of practitioners and to provide regular supervision linked with performance appraisal. CPD needs to be planned, and a mix of informal and formal CPD is available. The growth of electronic resources and information technology enable practitioners to participate on a regular basis.

CASE STUDY 15.10

AUSTRALIAN SCHOOL CANTEENS

The quality of the food and drink sold to children via school canteens in Australia has been a controversial issue for many years. The obesity debate has focused the contribution of school canteens to the obesogenic environment (Bell & Swinburn 2005). There are increasing advocacy attempts to influence the nutrition content of the food and drink sold to children. There are calls for governments to develop accreditation and training schemes for those who work in canteens (and for mandatory nutrition criteria to be in place). The New South Wales Healthy School Canteen Strategy was a major result of the NSW Government Childhood Obesity Summit in 2002. It is now mandatory for state schools to provide food and beverage choices consistent with the dietary guidelines. NSW Health is also supporting the NSW Canteen Association so that it is able to support schools to operate economically viable, nutrition-oriented school canteens. Advocacy for this initiative came from parents, canteen managers, some food companies and, increasingly, local health and education services. In Western Australia, the Minister for Education convened an expert review panel in 2006 to investigate the potential for mandatory nutrition criteria in government schools. Zimmet and James (2006) call for regulatory measures that include strict food and physical activity requirement for schools. Continued and expanded advocacy efforts will result in changes in the school nutrition environment.

Informal continuing professional development

There are many informal or workplace-related CPD opportunities. Workplaces need to support and encourage practitioners who may cite time and financial constraints as barriers to CPD. Passive dissemination of information is generally ineffective in changing workplace practice. There are several informal or workplace-related CPD activities that can be considered:

- Reflective practice, building emotional intelligence to enhance performance: This involves a process of doing, learning and critically reflecting. From this process we can improve our practice by putting time aside for reflection or to keep a diary or journal. Further discussion with colleagues or professional reading will add to the process of improving practice.
- Workshops: Discussion groups with colleagues or other professionals can be used to facilitate change in practice.
- Local Nutritionist networks: Most professional organisations or states have informal networks of those interested in public health nutrition. These

networks may meet on a regular basis to share solutions to public health nutrition problems or to describe innovative programme development. Many of these networks maintain an email link and group meetings which enable informal CPD.

- Mentoring schemes: Mentoring is a process where a less skilled and experienced person is linked with a more skilled person from whom they are willing to obtain advice (APHNAC 2005). Mentoring can be informal based on individual rapport or as a structured and formalised mentoring scheme.
- A professional association: These will provide activities for CPD, newsletters, professional journals, conferences, special interest groups and networks, including listserve networks. Special interest groups in these associations will enable practitioners to contribute to teleconferences, email discussion, participation in development of position statements or policies, contribute to advocacy – that is, input to letters or press releases from organisations on topical issues.
- Short courses: In recognition of time poverty of professionals, many academic instituitions may offer short courses (several days) that enable a public health nutritionist to up-skill. In some circumstances it may also be possible to convert the short course into part of a higher degree qualification by completing assignments (see Case study 15.11).
- Journals (peer reviewed): Professional memberships will often include the association's related journal, but many journals have alerting services that enable you to receive the table of contents by email and allow you to then seek out an article of interest.

Formal continuing professional development

CPD can take the form of a more formal approach, such as completing a higher degree – coursework degree or higher degree by research. Most postgraduate degrees involve opportunities for flexible learning that enable the public health nutritionist to continue working and either study after hours or by distance from the university (see Case study 15.12). There are also many opportunities to integrate further study into existing work responsibilities; for example, a research project required for a higher degree can be based around an existing project at work or be an extension of an idea or project that will contribute to work output. Traditionally the most internationally recognised degree in the public health field is a Master of Public Health, which is designed to assist practitioners from a range of backgrounds to meet the challenges of complex health issues faced by populations. In recognition of the need for advanced and specialised competencies in public health nutrition, degrees such as a Master of Public Health

CASE STUDY 15.11

OBESITY PREVENTION SHORT COURSE—DEAKIN UNIVERSITY

The Obesity Prevention Short Course has been developed by Deakin University to provide health service managers and practitioners working in the fields of nutrition and physical activity a fundamental understanding of the obesity epidemic and the determinants of obesity, as well as approaches for addressing the obesity epidemic.

The course is marketed through electronic networks to health service managers and practitioners employed in the areas of health promotion, community health, public health, nutrition, physical activity and local government. It is presented as an intensive mode three-day programme made up of lectures, activities and a workshop. The course is divided into three modules, each building on the knowledge and skills gained in previous modules. A comprehensive workbook provided to each participant contains information on the facilitators, a timetable for the three days, the three modules containing a copy of the presenters' slides and space to make notes, as well as some journal articles and reference materials. The final day allows participants to workshop their new skills to develop an action plan for obesity prevention in their area of work. The participants' action plans are collated and distributed to each participant.

Source: <http://www.deakin.edu.au/hbs/who-obesity/short-course/course-index.php>

Nutrition are offered by some universities and are rapidly growing in popularity. A higher degree can add to your credibility and employability.

Research opportunities should be considered as adding to professional knowledge on the effectiveness of public health nutrition interventions, as well as part of the public health nutritionist's ongoing work. Data collected at the local level may be transferable to a larger population group. Research evidence can drive policy and, in turn, policy directs future strategies. It is important that a public health nutritionist has basic research skills and access to other research professionals for advice. Public health nutritionists have the responsibility for dissemination of lessons learned from practice. The lessons learned from building partnerships, programme planning and evaluation should be shared with all who have a vested interest in public health nutrition, and help kick-start future research.

There is much talk about how evidence-based research applies to public health nutrition, but learning from others' experiences will help future programmes. Conference presentations, viewpoint articles or research papers submitted for publication to peer-reviewed journals are the formal avenues for reaching a larger audience with information about your work. Most professional

---

CASE STUDY 15.12

AUSTRALIAN PUBLIC HEALTH NUTRITION
ACADEMIC COLLABORATION

The Australian Public Health Nutrition Academic Collaboration (APHNAC) is a national initiative that aims to strengthen capacity to educate and train Australia's public health workforce. APHNAC is a collaboration linking together academic units offering postgraduate, post-entry level public health nutrition topics available by distance education.

Most of the university members of APHNAC are members of the Australian Network of Academic Public Health Institutions, which receive funding from the Australian Government Public Health Education and Research Program (PHERP) to teach public health degrees. APHNAC was funded by PHERP to develop advanced level units or topics.

The project has primarily focused on developing a set of advanced level, peer reviewed university units or topics in public health nutrition. These are available as electives in post-entry level degrees and are offered by flexible delivery. Students who enrol may, depending on the rules and with the permission of the degree coordinator at their home university, cross-enrol in public health nutrition topics. Individual topics can also be accessed for continuing professional development by those with an appropriate background.

Source: APHNAC <www.aphnac.com>

---

organisations will run workshops on how to publish a paper or how to put together a conference abstract, oral and/or poster presentation. Take advantage of experience of those who present at these types of events to increase your skills in publication. Watch out for dates for conference abstract submissions, as this is usually many months before the conference. Seek feedback from experienced conference presenters on your abstracts and presentations.

The development of public health nutrition requires greater interaction between research and practice. Continued identification of effective personal and organisational practice skills will considerably enhance the training of public health nutritionists and the delivery of public health nutrition programmes.

Conclusion

This chapter has reviewed the personal and organisational supports that are critical to public health nutritionists in their current professional practice. Effective professional practice includes the use of these supports alongside knowledge of public health nutrition. Individual practitioners should challenge themselves to expand on their skills in all the areas covered in this chapter.

References

American Dietetic Association 1999, 'Code of ethics for the professional of dietetics' in *Journal of American Dietetic Association*, vol. 99, no. 1, pp. 109–13.

Ashton, B. and Hehir, A. 2002, 'Working with private partner organisations to address public health nutrition issues: A case study' in *Nutrition & Diet*, vol. 59, no. 1, pp. 43–47.

Australian Bureau of Statistics (ABS) 1996, *Aspects of Literacy: Assessed skill levels Australia*, catalogue no. 4228.0.

Australian Public Health Nutrition Academic Collaboration (APHNAC) 2005, *A Mentoring Framework for Public Health Nutrition Workforce Development*, cited at <www.aphnac.com>.

Barbuto, J. and Burbach, M. 2006, 'The emotional intelligence of transformational leaders: A field study of elected leaders' in *Journal of Social Psychology*, vol. 146, no. 1, pp. 51–64

Beaudry, M. and Delisle, H. 2005, 'Public('s) nutrition' in *Public Health Nutrition*, vol. 8, no. 6a, pp. 743–48.

Bell, A.C. and Swinburn, B.A. 2005, 'School canteens: Using ripples to create a wave of healthy eating' in *Medical Journal of Australia*, vol. 183, pp. 5–6.

Brocklehurst, N.J., Hook, G., Bond, M. and Goodwin, S. 2005, 'Developing the public health practitioner workforce in England: Lessons from theory and practice' in *Public Health*, vol. 119, pp. 995–1002.

Buchler, P., Martin, D., Knaebel, H.P, and Buchler, M.W. 2006, 'Leadership characteristics and business management in modern academic surgery' in *Langenbecks Archives of Surgery*, vol. 391, pp. 149–56.

Cannon, G. 2006, 'Dear friends and collegues, let's get real' (Letter to the Editor) in *Public Health Nutrition*, vol. 9, no. 4, p. 531.

Carroll, T.L. 2005, 'Leadership skills and attributes of women and nurse executives: Challenges for the 21st Century' in *Nursing Administration Quarterly*, vol. 29, no. 2, pp. 146–153.

Chapman, S. 2004, 'Advocacy for public health: A primer', *Journal of Epidemiology of Community Health*, vol. 58, pp. 361–65.

Cleary, M., Freeman, A. and Sharrock, L. 2005, 'The development, implementation, and evaluation of a clinical leadership program for mental health nurses' in *Issues in Mental Health Nursing*, vol. 26, pp. 827–42.

Consortium for Research on Emotional Intelligence in Organisations (no date), Emotional competence training program—American Express, cited at <http://www.eiconsortium.org/model_programs/emotional_competence_ training.pdf> on 19 September 2006.

Department of Health (WA) 2003, 'Food for health in Australia', Department of Health, Western Australia, pp. 70–71.

Donato, K.A. 2006, 'National health education programs to promote healthy eating and physical activity in *Nutrition Reviews*, vol. 64, no. 2, pp. S65–70.

Fertman, C.I. 2003, 'Health educators are leaders: Meeting the leadership challenge' in *Health Promotion Practice*, vol. 4, no. 3, pp. 336–9.

Freshman, B. and Rubino, L. 2004, 'Emotional intelligence skills for maintaining social networks in healthcare organizations' in *Hospital Topics*, vol. 82, no. 3, pp. 2–9.

Gillespie, A.H., Gantner, L.A., Craig, S., Dischner, K. and Lansing, D. 2003, 'Productive partnerships for food: Principles and strategies' in *Journal of Extension*, vol. 41, no. 2, cited at <http://www.joe.org/joe/2003april/a8.shtml> on 19 September 2006.

Hahn-Nowlin, B. 1994, 'Keep it short and simple' in *Journal of American Dietetic Association*, vol. 94, no. 9, pp. 971–73

Hawe, P. and Stickney, E.K. 1997, 'Developing the effectiveness of an intersectoral food policy coalition through formative evaluation' in *Health Education Research*, vol. 12, no. 12, pp. 213–25.

Hughes, R. 2003, 'Competency development in Australia: Reflections of advanced level practitioners' in *Nutrition & Dietetic*, vol. 60, no. 3, pp. 205–11.

— 2004a, 'Employers expectations of credentials and competencies of the community and public health nutrition workforce in Australia' in *Nutrition & Diet*, vol. 61, pp. 105–11.

— 2004b, 'Competencies for effective public health nutrition practice: A developing consensus' in *Public Health Nutrition*, vol. 7, no. 5, pp. 683–91.

Johnson, D.B., Eaton, D.L., Wahl, P.W. and Gleason, C. 2001, 'Public health nutrition practice in the United States' in *Journal of American Dietetic Association*, vol. 101, no. 5, pp. 529–34.

Keenan, D.P., AbuSabha, R., and Robinson, N.G. 2002 'Consumer's understanding of the Dietary Guidelines for Americans: Insights into the future' in *Health Education Behavior*, vol. 29, no. 1, pp. 124–35.

Kerfoot, K. 1997, 'The people side of transformations' in *Pediatric Nursing*, vol. 23, no. 6, pp. 643–4.

Kingdon, J.W. 1995, *Agendas, Alternatives, and Public Policies* (2nd edition), HarperCollins College Publishers, New York.

Landers, P. 2006, 'Networking for nutrition' in Edlestein, S. (ed.) 2006, *Nutrition in Public Health: A handbook for developing programs and services*, Jones and Barlett Publishers, Sudbury, MA.

Lansing, D. and Kolasa, K.M. 1996, 'Applying a new model, principles and processes in nutrition intervention partnerships' in *Journal of American Dietetic Association*, vol. 96, no. 8, pp. 806–09.

Leff, D. 2004, 'How to write for the public' in *Journal of American Dietetic Association*, vol. 104, no. 5, pp. 730–32.

Margetts, B. 2006, 'Leadership and responsibility in public health nutrition: Time to get serious' in *Public Health Nutrition*, vol. 9, no. 5, pp. 533–39.

Mayer, J.D. and Salovey, P. 1990, 'Emotional Intelligence' in *Journal of Imagination, Cognition and Personality*, vol. 9, no. 3, pp. 185–211.

McCaffree, J. 2006, 'Promote yourself and your profession with sound bites' in *Journal of American Dietetic Association*, vol. 106, no. 5, pp. 661–62.

McDonald, R. 2005, 'Shifting the balance of power? Culture change and identity in an English health-care setting' in *Journal of Health Organization and Management*, vol. 19, no. 3, pp. 189–203.

McMaster, R. 1999, 'Institutional change in UK health and local authorities' in *International Journal of Social Economics*, vol. 26, no. 12, p. 1441.

Miller, D.G., Cohen, N.L., Fulgonim, V.L., Heymsfield, S.B. and Wellman, N.S. 2006, 'From nutrition scientist to nutrition communicator: Why you should take the leap' in *American Journal of Clinical Nutrition*, vol. 83, pp. 1272–75.

Miller, M. and Pollard, C. 2005, 'Health working with industry to promote fruit and vegetables: A case study of the Western Australian fruit and vegetable campaign with reflection on the effectiveness of inter-sectorial action' in *Australian and New Zealand Journal of Public Health*, vol. 29, pp. 176–82.

Moran, M.B. 2006, 'Ethical issues in research with human subjects' in *Journal of American Dietetic Association*, vol. 106, no. 6, pp. 1346047.

Nestle, M. 2001, 'Food company sponsorship of nutrition research and professional activities: A conflict of interest' in *Public Health Nutrition*, vol. 4, no. 5, pp. 1015–22.

Patrick, M.S. 2005, 'Knowing when to hold and when to fold in advocacy' in *Journal of American Dietetic Association*, vol. 105, no. 11, pp. 1714–15.

Paul, C. and Redman, S. 1997a, 'The development of a checklist of content and design characteristics in printed health education materials' in *Health Promotion Journal of Australia*, vol. 7, pp. 153–59.

—— 1997b, 'A review of the effectiveness of print material in changing health-related knowledge, attitudes and behaviour' in *Health Promotion Journal of Australia*, vol. 7, pp. 91–99.

Probert, K.L. (ed) 1997, 'Moving to the future: Developing community-based nutrition services' in *Training Manual & Curriculum*, Association of State & Territorial Public Health Nutrition Directors, cited at <http://www.vahealth.org/ wic/course.htm>, p. 7.

Reeves, A. 2005, 'Emotional Intelligence: Recognising and regulating emotions' in *American Association of Occupational Health Nurses Journal*, vol. 53, no. 4, pp. 172–76.

Riley, B. 2003, 'Dissemination of heart health promotion in the Ontario Public Health System: 1989–1999', *Health Education Research*, vol. 18, no. 1, pp. 15–31.

Shilton, T. 2006, 'Advocacy for physical activity: From evidence to influence' in *Journal of the International Union for Health Promotion and Education*, in press.

Smith, A., Coveney, J., Carter, P., Jolley, G. and Laris, P. 2004, 'The Eat Well SA project: An evaluation-based case study in building capacity for promoting healthy eating' in *Health Promotion International*, vol. 19, no. 3, pp. 327–34.

Tillotson, J.E. 2003, 'Pandemic obesity: Is it time for change in economic and development policies affecting the food industry?' in *Nutrition Today*, vol. 38, no. 6, pp. 242–45.

Webb, J. 2001, 'Emotional rescue' in *Better Nutrition*, vol. 63, no. 2, p. H6.

Webb, K., Hawe, P. and Noort, M. 2001, 'Collaborative intersectoral approaches to nutrition in a community on the urban fringe' in *Health Education & Behaviour*, vol. 28, no. 3, pp. 306–19

Wieand, P. 2002, 'Drucker's challenge: Communication and the emotional glass ceiling' in *Ivey Business Journal*, May/June 2002, pp. 32–37.

World Health Organization (WHO) 2005, 'Asia-Pacific Workshop on Raising the Profile of Nutrition: Meeting report', *WHO Western-Pacific Region, Report Series* RS/2005/GE17.

Xirasagar, S., Samuels, M.E. and Curtin, T.F. 2006, 'Management training of leadership executives, their leadership style and care management performance: An empirical study', *American Journal of Managed Care*, vol. 12, no. 2, pp. 101–08.

Yach, D., McKee, M., Lopez, A.D. and Novotny, T. 2005, 'Improving diet and physical activity: 12 lessons from controlling tobacco smoking' in *British Medical Journal*, vol. 330, pp. 898–900.

Yngve, A. 2006, 'Challenges for public health nutrition are immense: To be a good public health nutrition leader requires networks and collaboration' in *Public Health Nutrition*, vol. 9, no. 5, pp. 535–37.

Zakocs, R.C. and Edwards, E.M. 2006, 'What explains community coalition effectiveness? A review of the literature' in *American Journal of Preventive Medicine*, vol. 30, no. 4, pp. 351–61.

Zimmet, P. and James, W.P.T. 2006, 'The unstoppable Australian obesity and diabetes juggernaut: What should politicians do?' in *Medical Journal of Australia*, vol. 184, pp. 187–88.

16

Project management

MARTIN CARAHER
GILL COWBURN
JOHN COVENEY

Many public health nutrition books deal with project management from the perspective of evaluation and research, and thus ignore the important aspects of how to actually set up and run a programme. This chapter adopts the view that good programme planning and management is the key to good evaluation and research.

A template for programme planning and management is set out, including indicators of barriers and opportunities to implementation. This covers the range of public health nutrition activities, as illustrated in Figure 16.1, representing a public health continuum. The different responsibilities a practitioner may have in relation to programme planning and management, such as setting up, running, implementing and evaluating all aspects of the programme, are also discussed.

This chapter provides a step-by-step guide to planning, implementing and evaluating food-based programme/projects, whether large or small. The chapter presents the activities in chronological stages, but in the real world the stages interrelate, and will happen concurrently. In essence, this chapter will help address the following overarching questions that provide a framework for public health nutrition action:

- What is the public health nutrition intervention trying to achieve?
- How is it going to do this?
- How will success be judged or gauged?

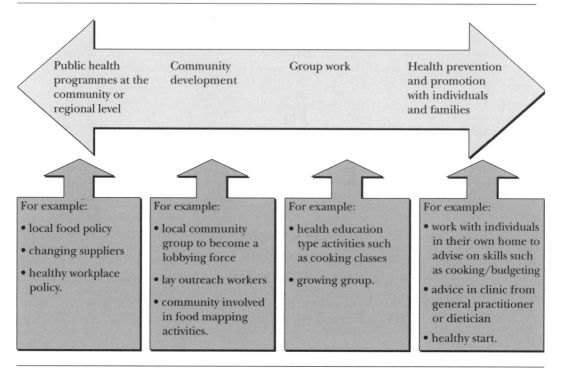

Figure 16.1 A public health continuum model as applied to food

The first part of the chapter focuses on thinking through the planning and implementation steps. This provides answers to the first two of these questions. In the remaining part of the chapter, the focus is on evaluation that will help to assess the success of plans and programmes.

Background

Much that has been written on public health nutrition jumps to discussing evaluation and outcomes (see, for example, Margetts 2004). There are, of course, some good reasons for this. For example, it is important to know if something has worked or not, to assess value for money, and also to add new evidence. But there is value in first examining the development of ideas for public health nutrition, the planning of public health nutrition programmes, and the management of interventions, as well as focusing on evaluation. Only by taking a broad view of these activities, and by ensuring that quality is built into them from the start, can there be confidence in the development of an integrated approach.

The term 'public health nutrition' is used to describe those activities — projects, programmes and interventions — that are designed to improve the nutritional health of populations, communities and groups. The focus can be national, regional or local, and Figure 16.1 provides an overview of the scope of public health nutrition activities, ranging from individual patient/clinical interventions to population interventions. Such activities do not exist in isolation, but are part of a larger-scale plan whose activities contribute to an overall purpose.

Where to start — What is the problem?

Almost all public health nutrition projects or programmes start with a problem. It may be one that a group or a community recognise and want to address, or it may be a problem that has been identified from other sources, for example surveys, epidemiological data, research or evaluations from earlier work. Regardless of how it has arisen, any problem will benefit from a problem analysis, or a series of questions to assist in defining the dimensions and basis of the problem. The following questions can form the basis for the start of public health nutrition programme or project:

- What is the problem that the programme/project seeks to address?
- Why and for whom is it a problem? Different data sources may shed light on different aspects of the problem.
- What might be the causes of the problem?
- What are the various aspects of the problem (such as the region, the local area, the local policies, etc.)?
- Does the problem appear to be solvable (given the available resources)?
- Has anyone else done similar work?
- Would a food/nutrition-based intervention help?
- Should complementary, non food-based interventions (such as income support) be considered?

This first phase involves elucidation and clarification of the problem, which will help make clear the rationale behind the proposed action, so it is worth spending some time addressing the issues in the bullet points above, including talking to other people. It also helps to define the context in which the intervention will be working. This will be useful in later stages of programme/project development and implementation. There is a need to be clear about this first phase before moving on to devise the intervention strategy that should meet and fit with the definition of the problem. This is important because problems are often perceived or experienced in different ways by different groups. Once the problem has been defined, the next step is to see if anybody else has done similar work.

What evidence is already out there?

'Evidence-based practice' is a term that has arisen from a drive across sectors to ensure that public money is not spent wastefully or haphazardly. This concept has been discussed in chapters 1, 2 and 14 of this book. Put simply, it means current practice is based on past practice that has been observed and known to have worked (Booth 1997). 'Evidence' in this context can take many forms, including both quantitative data (such as statistical data, which tells us how many) and qualitative data (such as interviews that tell us the why and what) (Punch 1998; Valente 2002). This means that it is likely that some of the public health nutrition initiative can be premised on existing practice rather than having to start from scratch. For many programmes or projects, the discovery of an existing evidence base has three possible implications:

- provide sufficient data/information on which to base the initiative
- guide the new initiative into new or unexplored areas
- shift the focus from a full evaluation of the proposed project to monitoring against criteria established from other studies.

The existing literature, drawn from the fields of general health promotion, public health and public health nutrition, cannot yet tell us conclusively that nutrition prevention action works (see Box 16.1 for some examples). There are many reasons for the lack of evidence about what works, including the poor design of and assumptions behind many nutrition programmes or projects (International Union for Health Promotion and Education 2000; Oliver & Peersman 2001; Summerbell et al. 2005).

In collecting the information, it is a good idea to keep a record of the sources, type of study, findings and their relevance to the project and the quality of the evidence. Table 16.1 sets out a series of criteria against which to judge a study. These can be made more detailed and/or more specific according to the needs of the proposed intervention. A systematic review of the area is generally taken to be the gold standard, but still needs interpretation and application to the work context and setting. Many reviews are based on the principle of evidence-based clinical practice, and as such have what is called 'high internal validity' (what they measure and find is accurate for the setting under study), but often poor application to the real world (poor external validity).

Box 16.1

EXAMPLE OF LESSONS FROM EXISTING PRACTICE

Example 1 public health nutrition targeted at lower socioeconomic groups

In summarising twenty years of evidence, the International Union for Health Promotion and Education reports that lower socioeconomic groups get cheap energy from foods such as meat products, full-cream milk, fats, sugars, preserves, potatoes, and cereals. There is, however, little intake of vegetables, fruit, and wholewheat bread. They conclude that dietary interventions should be aimed in the first place at increasing the knowledge of the short-term and long-term effects of a healthy diet and acquiring the skills for changing them. Second, but equally important, interventions should include improved accessibility to healthy foods, and should incorporate involvement of the social environment. Differences in behaviour are often generated by elements of the social position itself (such as housing and working conditions) or by characteristics that are closely related to this social position. It can be seen from this that any initiative targeted at lower socioeconomic groups should aim at increasing vegetable and fruit intake, and address issues of access and affordability alongside knowledge and attitude.

Source: International Union for Health Promotion and Education 2000

Example 2 Review of interventions for preventing obesity in children

Conclusions from the review included:
- the current evidence suggests that many diet and exercise interventions to prevent obesity in children are not effective in preventing weight gain, but can be effective in promoting a healthy diet and increased physical activity levels
- the programmes in this review used different strategies to prevent obesity, so direct comparisons were difficult. Also, the duration of the studies ranged from twelve weeks to three years, but most lasted less than a year.

Source: Summerbell et al. 2005

More extensive ways of doing this exist, and these can be found on the following websites:

- EPPI centre <http://eppi.ioe.ac.uk/CMS> has details of evidence-based work on social interventions (see Oliver & Peersman 2001)
- ScHARR <http://www.shef.ac.uk/scharr/ir/netting/> has details on searching, appraising and implementing evidence as well as databases (Booth 1997).

Table 16.1 Checklist for documenting existing evidence

Name of study/ authors/date	Where published/ how discovered	Type of study	Lessons for my work	Strengths/ weaknesses
'A survey of food projects in the English NHS regions', Caraher and Cowburn, 2004	*Health Education Journal*, found on electronic search	Evaluative study of support for local food projects looking back on what had happened	Way in which study was conducted	English-based; some questionnaires in appendix could be of use
'Taxing food: Implications for public health nutrition', Caraher and Cowburn, 2005	Learned of from colleague then requested journal article	Review of the literature on food taxes and policy	Hints for what I can do in a school setting in introducing food taxes and subsidies	Policy research based on others' work; no clear guidelines what to do in a school setting, just broad principles
'Differences in lay knowledge of food and health', Coveney, 2005	Recommended by colleague	Qualitive study with parents	Reminder of need to tailor information for different social groups	Qualitive research so not necessarily generalisable

Both these sites contain evidence of effectiveness, mainly from a clinical or interventionist perspective, so-called evidence-based practice. This takes evidence from (research) studies and applies them to practice. This is not the same as practice-based evidence, which is concerned with evidence that has been built up in practice, and comes largely from evaluative studies.

What if there is a gap in the evidence?
Many nutrition prevention projects face the problem of a lack of existing evidence of effectiveness. In this case, there are two options: do nothing or intervene. Taking the findings from the systematic review by Summerbell and colleagues (2005) in Box 16.1, it appears that little can be done to prevent childhood obesity. In common with other areas of prevention work, public health

nutrition work suffers from a lack of evidence-based, well-designed intervention projects (Oakley 1998, 2000; Peersman et al. 1999). One way of addressing this is by adopting what Robinson and Sirard (2005) call a 'solution-orientated' approach. This means that past orientation or lack of evidence of cause can be overruled in favour of future orientation. They give the example of soft or carbonated drinks, and say that:

> *What is the justification for skipping over the requirement to prove soft drinks cause obesity and jump directly to an experiment testing elimination of soft drink sales? In the case of childhood obesity, it is universally accepted (and has been for at least eight centuries) that energy imbalance results in changes in weight. Therefore, without knowing the true underlying cause(s) of any individual's or any population's obesity or risks for obesity, any intervention that produces a deficit in energy balance, by increasing energy expenditure and/or decreasing energy consumption, will lead to prevention or reduction in weight gain. As described, there is face validity to the hypothesis that eliminating soft drink sales in schools will result in a negative energy balance (future orientation) regardless of whether soft drink consumption was the cause of obesity (past orientation).*

In essence, this moves the focus of future work away from developing more descriptions of the problem to working on solutions, and hence the importance of a strong evaluation strand. As mentioned earlier, as well as evidence-based practice, there is also a need to be mindful of generating practice-based evidence. This is evidence that arises from actually trying to solve a problem from first principles, as in the example above (we are grateful to Professor Boyd Swinburn for this distinction).

Involving stakeholders

The importance of assessing the needs of the different groups who will be affected by the public health nutrition action has already been noted. Identifying all the different groups of people (or stakeholders) who have a view about the problem that it is hoped to address is a vital step because, to be successful, public health nutrition programmes/projects need community involvement or investment.

Just because food and nutrition professionals see a problem does not mean that groups or communities do. Indeed, quite a lot of work in public health nutrition involves creating awareness of a problem. The analysis of the problem should also involve the analysis of needs, or a needs assessment. A needs assessment (which can be incorporated as a part of formative evaluation, dealt with in more detail later) is a set of activities undertaken before or at the start of an intervention to shed light on what the problem is and how it is experienced, interpreted or manifested by different groups. This helps inform programme development. For example, there may be good quality existing data on the poor availability of fruit and vegetables in a community, gathered through survey research. But this might not tell us what people's views or perceptions are of the problem – what they know about and think about it or where it sits in their priorities. So this type of evidence is needed, and the methods used to collect it should be rigorous and systematised in order for the data to be credible.

Take public health nutrition action in a school setting as an example. Schools are communities: they comprise students, teachers, parents, funders, regulators, volunteers, and other groups. Any work with schools would need to include some or even all of these groups. It is now well known that working with communities has a number of important characteristics that can facilitate or mitigate against success. Some of these are included in Table 16.2. In order to maximise success there is a need to ensure an increase in those factors known to facilitate involvement and reduce those known to be barriers.

Funding priorities sometimes provide a dilemma for food and nutrition community-based activities; for example, national or regional funding is sometimes made available to target specific problems. It may be to reduce overweight and obesity, or increase consumption of certain food groups. However, the communities who are believed to benefit from them do not always share these concerns, starting points, beliefs or goals. This leads to the question of how to maximise community involvement in initiatives that were conceived elsewhere. Clearly, part of the early activity would be to enlist the community's involvement and create ways of working to sustain this participation (see Table 16.2). The process of planning a public health nutrition initiative and the need to discuss it with a wide range of people in the early stages is as important as using existing evidence to help direct the activities.

What is the baseline?

Finding a 'baseline' at the outset of a project provides a picture so that, throughout a project's life, and at its end, measurement can indicate how far from the original situation there has been movement (if at all). It may be that existing research findings relevant to the project have already been collected by someone locally or even nationally, and may form the basis for action as well as doubling as baseline data. For example, findings that 30 per cent of the population in an area consume 2.6 portions of fruit and vegetables per day or that three out of five children consume no green vegetables at lunchtime, can

Table 16.2 Summary of key issues that help and hinder food-based community initiatives

Characteristics that facilitate community projects	Possible organisational constraints and barriers
• area- or community-based focus • given sufficient time to develop, establish and consolidate the project (two years) • based on community participation and needs assessment, and is credible to staff, funders and local community • needs assessment and ongoing evaluation are used to fine-tune and change programme delivery • contributes to enhancing community capacity • reconciling different agendas • funding that spans set-up and establishment periods • has community support and involvement • the focus extends beyond single issues and addresses wider issues of the food supply chain • professional support • shared ownership and involves local residents, workers and professionals • dynamic worker • ability to respond to changing agendas • properly conducted evaluations can prove the worth and thus influence future funding of projects or programmes • the process includes understanding the systems in one's community, and gaining a sense of being able to manoeuvre within them, and is not solely on counselling and educating about consumer choices • investing and supporting local food systems in community and public spaces — schools, community facilities, social housing complexes, health centres.	• opposing agendas • funding inadequate or uncertain • meeting limited needs • lack of support • changing agendas • exclusive ownership • lack of time to set up and develop • evaluation (especially that which is overly-complex) can be a hindrance to project delivery • changes in policy dictate changes in public health nutrition prevention initiatives midstream. The focus is exclusively on skills, with no accounting for the reasons for deskilling • overemphasis on self-help.

Source: Adapted from McGlone et al. 1996; Dobson et al. 2000; Caraher & Reynolds 2005; McGlone et al. 2005

act as the starting point for action and a baseline for a project designed to increase fruit and vegetable consumption in a community.

Sometimes needs assessments can provide baseline information and can help refine the problem; other times this information has to be sought elsewhere. More often than not, it is a series of different activities that build together to contribute to the baseline picture. It is necessary to be as sure as possible that the work is based on sound data and that the baseline data is chosen carefully. The nature of the baseline must be linked to the problem the intervention is seeking to change; it must also be amenable to measurement at different stages to ensure compatibility. In other words, the baseline information must be related to the project's aims. If the existing evidence is based on research studies that have no direct lessons for the setting of the programme, then there is a need to translate the implications into practice-based evidence. The checklist in Box 16.2 is designed to help in the process of programme planning.

Box 16.2

CHECKLIST . . . ARE YOU READY TO PLAN?

- Has the problem been analysed?
- Have the needs of the audience been assessed?
- Is a food-based project approach the best way of meeting the audience's needs?
- If the issue is lack of material resources to buy food or lack of access to shops, then a programme based on knowledge transfer (for example, one that provides information about which foods to include in a healthy diet) is not likely to be effective.
- Has there been clear identification of what has already been done in this area?
- Do you know what the baseline data is/or should consist of?

Bringing about change

It is obvious but worth remembering that public health nutrition projects and programmes are generally designed to bring about change, either increases in some behaviours and decreases in others. There may be a need to see differences in the populations and groups with whom the intervention is working. Here are some areas in which change is usually sought (the seven 'As'):

- awareness — for example, the importance of eating more fruit and vegetables
- acceptability — for example, eating green vegetables or eating fruit in place of a sweet snack
- appropriateness — the foods on offer to the individual, household or groups in the evaluation
- affordability — food to people on low incomes
- availability — food to people through a breakfast club, local food co-op or shops
- accessibility — to healthy food choices in shops that are convenient and affordable
- advocacy — community groups through better lobbying and policy development.

Each of these is amenable to change, and public health nutrition projects or programmes often aim to change either one of these or several in combination. However, as already said, some idea of what exists already is necessary in order to assess the impact of the intervention and/or contribution to change.

The extent of change a public health nutrition intervention is aiming for is important to consider. Depending on where measures are pitched, there is a danger that wider influences may mask the impact of the public health nutrition intervention. For example, in running a school programme to increase fruit intake and measuring overall fruit intake, the effects of the programme may be hidden within wider environmental influences. If there is a decrease between the intervention and the end, then this may be due to external influences. On the other hand, if there are increases, how can these be related to the specific intervention? Small campaigns run on the back of and in conjunction with national ones run this danger. How can the effect be attributed to the programme intervention and not background noise? The general advice is to stick to effects that the programme can have a direct influence on; for example, the amount of fruit eaten/sold in the school setting or increase in knowledge or attitudes due to the intervention.

How to work with a clear purpose: Setting aims and objectives

Once the problem has been defined, the next step to consider is the best way to address it. This leads to the development of aims and objectives. Project aims and objectives provide a planning framework onto which the project's phases can be hung. More importantly, a good set of aims and objectives will not only help to guide and govern the project, but also to measure an intervention's or a project's overall success.

A programme of work should have a purpose, normally arrived at by directly addressing the problem faced. This is often called an 'aim' (sometimes also referred to as a 'goal'). The plan of action designed to achieve the overall aim is contained in the objectives. These specify action time and activities, whereas the aim can be defined as a broad pious hope (Baker & Caraher 1999). All this may seem obvious — there is a certain familiarity with the term 'aims and objectives' — so it is surprising to note that many public health nutrition prevention programmes do not start with a clearly defined purpose. The absence of clear and concise aims and objectives is a feature of the findings of many systematic reviews of prevention activities (Oakley 1998; Caraher & Cowburn 2004).

Formative evaluation

Formative evaluation is a way of ascertaining needs and developing an understanding of what people want and feel. Needs assessment has already been discussed, and this can sometimes double up as formative assessment, although the two are not always the same. Formative evaluation can contribute to outcome evaluation (which will be discussed later) because it can help to establish and clarify prevention aims and objectives, and establish knowledge or attitude baselines for the target population (see Box 16.3). Formative evalua-

---

Box 16.3

Formative evaluation can

- contribute to clarifying and refining programme aims and objectives
- discover how the target audiences view the problem and suggest solutions
- indicate whether the intended approach is appropriate to the audience
- verify the intervention has identified the most appropriate audience and have targeted the most appropriate subdivisions
- identify the best ways of accessing the target audience, whether face-to-face or through existing programmes or through local media
- identify stakeholders and gatekeepers and how to get them involved
- ascertain whether there are other audiences (intermediaries) who would be better placed to deliver the programme.

---

tion sometimes identifies barriers to the implementation of a project. Well-designed formative evaluation can identify issues such as the project direction, and be useful in providing insights into ways forward based on the perceptions and demands of the groups involved, and can be useful to test out hunches and find out the needs of a proposed client group, or to indicate possible effects of different interventions. Determining audience needs, wants and perceptions is one of the key principles of good quality health-promotion work in helping create supportive environments for health and strengthening community action for health (WHO 1986). Formative evaluation can also be used to help establish knowledge levels or other baselines for the target population by which post-intervention outcomes can be measured. The formative evaluation can and should inform and contribute to the refinement of the public health nutrition aims and objectives, but is not itself a substitute for arriving at these.

A project or programme, however big or small, will benefit from formative evaluation. Sometimes a research or evaluation study is found that has been conducted with the same, or similar audience, which may provide baselines suitable for use in the intervention. In these circumstances, it is still advisable that such data be verified on a small scale. Formative evaluation can be carried out by straw-polling a small number of the audience the public health nutrition intervention is trying to reach. For example, this may involve telephone interviews using a pre-set questionnaire or setting up a series of focus groups. Qualitative reporting methods are better suited for small-scale initiatives like these because such small numbers will not have (nor are intended to have) any reliable statistical significance.

What are public health nutrition prevention aims and objectives?

As noted, the aims and objectives devised at the outset of a project are called 'prevention aims and objectives'. These are distinct from evaluation aims and objectives (which will be discussed later). In general, prevention aims and objectives describe the desired effect in terms of improving nutrition or food consumption through the seven As set out earlier. Prevention aims are not generally well stated or defined; for example, it is easy to confuse a prevention aim with a process aim. The aim 'to produce a leaflet' is not a prevention aim in itself: it does not give any information that can help measure the leaflet's effect. Producing a leaflet to impart information on healthy eating could be a (process) objective that derives from an overall aim, and is informed by a theoretical model of operation that contributes to the attainment of the aim. Writing good aims and objectives is a skill in itself, and it is worth spending time on getting them right at the outset.

How to set public health nutrition prevention aims
Put simply, the prevention aim can be established by asking a series of questions:

- What is the problem?
- What needs to change?
- By how much?
- Who or what do we want to change?
- When do we want to change it?

Here are some examples of prevention aims.

- To reduce the demand for carbonated drinks among young people aged forteen to eighteen in School Area X over the six months of the project.
- To reduce fat consumption in the school population by 25 per cent by the year 2007.
- To increase the availability of fresh fruit and vegetables by 10 per cent in Community Y within twelve months.

These aims may seem ambitious, but they provide a vital base on which any project or programme of work can be developed. They provide a sense of direction and a time scale. A project's aim needs to be related to the chosen prevention theory or model. Remember, at the outset there is a need to ensure everyone involved in a project agrees with the project's aim and approach. Indeed, the process of setting prevention aims can be one way of increasing involvement and commitment to the project by ensuring everyone is in agreement with the overarching strategy and philosophy.

As aims are formulated, bear in mind that baseline data needs to be related to the purpose of the project so that evaluation can measure whether or not there has been any difference at the project's end. In other words, don't set an aim that cannot possibly be measured. It's no good having an aim 'to reduce the demand for chocolate in workplace vending machines' if there is no indicator of what the present demand for chocolate is. If the aim is to increase knowledge, then there should be some information that establishes what people already know (baseline) against which to compare any increase in knowledge over the period of the intervention. If the aim is to change attitudes, then there is a need to have a baseline that reflects current attitudes and a way of measuring them. If the aim is to improve access to healthier foods, then it is necessary to have an understanding of what current levels of access are.

How to set public health nutrition prevention objectives
Each aim will usually have a number of objectives attached to them. Objectives are the steps by which the aims or the purpose will be achieved. These can be set by asking, 'How is the aim to be achieved?' Here are examples of some objectives that have been developed from an aim:

Aim: To reduce the demand for carbonated drinks among young people aged fourteen to eighteen olds in school X over a school year.

Objective 1: To develop a multi-component food prevention programme aimed at young people aged fourteen to eighteen by month three.
Objective 2: To deliver the programme developed in objective 1 to all fourteen to eighteen year olds between month three and month six of the intervention period.
Objective 3: To establish and run ten training sessions for teachers and cookery workers involved in delivering the programme in the first six months.
Objective 4: To reformulate school policies concerning products sold in school canteen.

Here too there is a need to be mindful of the importance of being able to measure or assess the extent to which an objective has been met. Set SMARTER objectives for the project. SMARTER stands for:

- **S**pecific rather than vague – be concise and don't leave the objective open to interpretation
- **M**easurable – frame the objective so that it can be measured
- **A**ccepted (by programme team and the community) and **A**chievable as worthwhile, realistic and attainable within the timeframe
- **R**ecorded and **R**eliable – that is, written down as the basis of a contract with yourself and durable so that with repeated use it will produce similar results
- **T**ime-constrained – with specific time limits
- **E**valuated – with progress monitored regularly
- **R**evisible – in the sense that goals should be able to be revised in the event of setbacks (like injury) or failure to achieve a goal that was over-ambitious to begin with.

Table 16.3 may help to work out aims and objectives. The process has been started in the table so you can continue to fill it in or use it as a template for a specific public health nutrition project or programme.

Table 16.3 Prevention aims and objectives

Project title:	Fruit intake among year 6 students in school X
Project workers:	Angela Davies
Dates:	
Start	Oct 2007
Finish	March 2008
Prevention aim (broad, overriding purpose):	To increase fruit intake among year 6 students during the school day
Does it specify:	
What?	Fruit
By how much?	Three portions per week in the intervention period
Who?	Year 6 students 11- to 12-year-olds
When?	Over six months
Where?	In the school setting
Prevention objectives (plan of action to achieve aim):	
Objective 1	
Objective 2	*(Continue to work through the example)*
Objective 3	

How could the aims and objectives be
    measured or judged against a baseline?
Are there some you can routinely collect?
Are there some that require special systems of
    data collection?
Which objectives are a priority?
Can you identify which ones you might need to
    know more about?
What methods could you use?
Can you identify which ones you already know
    a little/lot about? (What in the existing
    literature is well documented or what local
    knowledge is there?)

Once the public health nutrition prevention aims and objectives have been set, then it is possible to sort out the aims of project evaluation, but before that the theoretical basis of the intervention should be clarified.

Working with a model in mind

A model, theory or underlying principle is an essential part of planning, developing and evaluating any intervention, and a key to its success. It provides a rationale for activities and sets out how in public health nutrition prevention terms the intervention is expected to change or influence the impact or outcomes. Underpinning objectives with a model allows work towards a set of consistent activities.

Using a model or theory can also help contribute to what is called theory-based evaluation – that is, evaluation with an underlying basis for action. Many public health nutrition projects fail to have a clearly identified model or theory underpinning the intervention. The theory used to underpin programme activities is useful in helping structure the planning framework, and is essential for evaluation purposes. A small-scale project might simply set out to influence awareness without any commitment to changing attitudes or behaviour. This means that the evaluation methods should focus on changes in awareness, not behaviour (Valente 2002). A more ambitious project might set out to influence long-term behaviour based on changes in awareness and attitude, and thus measure all three aspects.

For some commentators, models come after the setting of aims and objectives; others claim that a model helps inform aims and objectives. The former argument is based on the premise that the model chosen should help deliver the aims and objectives, and the purpose is to match appropriate methods with the achievement of aims and objectives. The latter line of reasoning is based on a principle of 'horses for courses' and that what the intervention aims to achieve has to be tailored to the resources, which include skills as well as time and finance.

There are numerous models in the health promotion literature that can aid the development process. The choice of which one to use is a matter of 'fit for purpose'. A simple model that helps guide the process where little resources are available is adequate for most purposes. Table 16.4 presents a range of models that may help guide in this respect, but be aware that these are just examples from the plethora available.

Margetts (2004) sets out Beattie's framework of health promotion as a model (Beattie 1994, 1995) suitable for public health nutrition programmes. A more comprehensive approach and methods are set out in Egger and colleagues (1999). The choice of a model not only influences the programme planning in terms of what activities will be carried out, but can also have a direct bearing on the evaluation measures or indicators. For example, an approach based on

Table 16.4 Some examples of health promotion models

Area of change	Theories or models that underpin change
Changing health behaviour by focusing on the individual	• health belief model • theory of reasoned action • transtheoretical model • social learning theory

Changing health behaviour in communities and community action for health	• community mobilisation including
	  – social planning
	  – social action
	  – community development
	• diffusion of innovation theory

Communication strategies to changes to promote health	• communication for behaviour change • social marketing
Models applied to organisations and the creation of healthy settings	• theories of organisational change • models of intersectoral action • whole-systems approaches
Healthy policy models	• ecological; frameworks • tackling inequality • determinants of public health nutrition policy

Source: Adapted from Nutbeam & Harris 2001

one of the individual behaviour models means that the data collected will focus on awareness, attitudes and behaviour. If using a whole-systems or (healthy) settings approach, the focus could be more on process and outcomes, and be less concerned with changes in individual awareness and attitudes.

Another way of approaching the issues is to have a set of principles that underpin the actions. One such set can be found in the Ottawa Charter (WHO 1986), which identifies three basic strategies for health promotion:

1. advocacy for health to create the essential conditions for health
2. enabling all people to achieve their full health potential
3. mediating between the different interests in society in the pursuit of health.

From these come five priorities:

1. building healthy public policy
2. creating supportive environments for health
3. strengthening community action for health
4. developing personal skills
5. reorienting health services (WHO 1986).

Public health nutrition programmes can use some or all of these five priorities, but structural policy and advocacy areas are often missing from the equation (Caraher & Reynolds 2005).

Whether the decision is taken to base the actions on a model or principles, it all leads to helping decide the evaluation methods and priorities.

Why bother evaluating?

A simple answer to this question is, because this is a requirement of most interventions. But there are several purposes for evaluation. Everyone involved in the project needs to know whether the project has succeeded in doing what it set out to do. Project workers will need to know that what they're doing has worked; the community involved need to know that action has been taken to achieve a change they wanted; funders will need to know their money has been put to good use, and policymakers will need to know government targets have been met. Evaluation provides knowledge about what works and what does not, and helps fine-tune public health nutrition implementation. Also, if the project makes a positive contribution to the existing evidence base, and others would like to replicate it, there is a need to build in some degree of evaluation. Even if the project is to be a one-off that cannot be replicated, it is still important to build in some degree of evaluation or monitoring, if only to account for the expenditure of public money.

Whatever the scale of the intervention, programme evaluation should try to find out what has been achieved. There is a relationship between evaluation and project implementation, as can be seen in figures 16.2 and 16.3 show the relationship between formative evaluation, process evaluation, and impact and outcome evaluation.

Evaluation should not be seen as an activity separate from programme delivery; it is not about standing back and watching if things change or are not going in the direction sought. Evaluation and programme or project planning are cyclical processes that feed into one another. Those running projects who

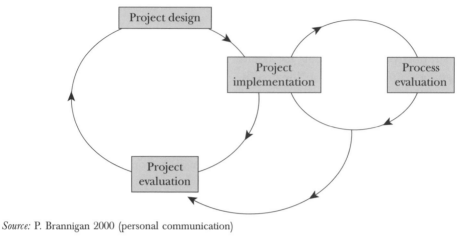

Source: P. Brannigan 2000 (personal communication)

Figure 16.2 Relationship of evaluation and programme implementation

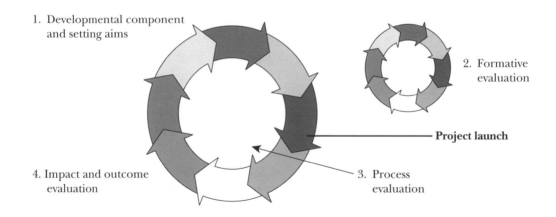

Source: P. Brannigan 2000 (personal communication)

Figure 16.3 Formative, process, impact and outcome evaluation

understand evaluation are in a position of power and have the opportunity to negotiate the utility of the evaluation and shape it to meet their own needs and requirements.

The purpose of the evaluation may be defined by what the implementing organisation or the funders value about the public health nutrition initiative. Relying on instinct that something has worked (or not, as the case may be) is not enough — others, such as funders, may be less convinced. Every project, on whatever scale, will benefit from evaluation and dissemination of evaluation findings to help convince policymakers and funders that the investment has been well spent, and also to inform the work of others.

The question of evaluation and its relationship to and distinction from research are all-important points. Evaluation differs from research in a number of important respects: it is generally short term and tied into specific programmes or projects. The following working definitions distinguish between the two:

- evaluation — a formal and systematic activity where assessment is linked to original intentions and is fed back into the planning process
- research — a formal and systematic activity where the intervention, method and context of activity are constructed by researchers.

Evaluation is primarily about addressing the utility of intervention programmes or projects. It is not a lesser activity than research, just different. Good evaluations, like good research, should be systematic, rigorous and applied to the conceptualisation, design and implementation of programmes. Research can often set out what the problem is and provide details of how a problem was tackled, but often does not address issues of utility or repeatability or replication of the intervention. Evaluation is located in the real world, and Pawson and Tilley (1998) call for realistic research designs in evaluation.

Box 16.4 shows the characteristics of a good evaluation plan. Many of these are also aspects of a good programme or project plan (Egger et al. 1999; Valente 2002).

Evaluation is not an add-on . . .

As has already been noted, evaluation is often something that happens at the end of a project. Just as an evaluation chapter has not been tagged on at the end of this book, it is not advisable to view evaluation as the last step in the project process. It is easy to see evaluation as a cumbersome extra — an onerous task that must be tackled once the excitement of project activity is over. All too often the momentum of a project fizzles out before a proper evaluation is set in place. Interestingly, most projects allocate a budget to cover costs like travelling expenses, but too few allocate specific resources for evaluation as it is often considered to be an expensive extra. As most in the field are working on limited budgets, it is easy to see why it is often not prioritised.

Box 16.4

The characteristics of a good evaluation plan

The project evaluation and the methods used should:
- be built in at the start of the project
- be based on clear evaluation aims and objectives that should clearly come from the nutrition prevention aims and objectives
- involve the community or target of the intervention
- be informed by a needs assessment/formative evaluation
- allow enough time if changes in impact, behaviour and attitudes are to be established (sometimes referred to as 'evaluability assessment').

Source: Hawe et al. 2000

Another reason evaluation is seen as an add-on is that projects may not be perceived as large enough to measure significant health behaviour change. In the commercial world results are based on sales and it is easy to claim success if sales are boosted or income increased. But social interventions like those in the area of public health nutrition almost never have the benefit of a sales sheet by which to measure their efficacy. It is often claimed that behaviour change is impossible or too costly to detect. Of course, it is important to be realistic about what the project can achieve, but this does not mean that evaluation or monitoring is pointless.

Evaluation planned at the outset of the project – and as an integral part of the project – can help tackle some of these negative perceptions. As a general principle, you need to set aside ten per cent of the resources for evaluation. One way of subsuming evaluation into a project, both in terms of cost and effort, is to gather data as the project progresses and make this aspect of evaluation an intrinsic part of the project. In this way, evaluation can be viewed as an indispensable part of the whole rather than an extra job that requires extra time, effort and resources all at the end. Using the ten per cent rule-of-thumb means that, in project plans, staff time should be allocated to monitoring/evaluation activities such as data gathering, data entry and analysis. This is also a useful way to indicate to funders who and by whom evaluation activities are to be carried out. In bigger projects (those over US$100K) ten per cent of the budget can be set aside, for example, for commissioning an outside evaluation team.

Components of public health nutrition evaluation

A public health nutrition prevention intervention may undergo one, a combination of, or all of the following types of evaluation:

- process evaluation
- impact evaluation
- outcome evaluation (see figures 16.2 and 16.3).

Each stage of evaluation has a separate purpose and therefore has separate aims and objectives, although these relate closely to the overall programme/project aims and objectives. Each of these evaluation types are described in turn below.

Process evaluation

Process evaluation examines the processes adopted to implement and disseminate a project or programme. It judges the planning, implementation and appropriateness of a project in relation to its outcomes, and is an important part of any intervention. Review guidelines produced by the EPI-Centre (1997) define process evaluation as one which 'examines the acceptability and feasibility of an intervention, studies the ways in which the intervention is delivered, assesses the quality of the procedures performed by the programme staff, etc.' It is designed to describe what goes on, and may suggest ways in which the programme design and implementation could be improved.

Collecting information about the reach of the programme activities (for example, are the right groups getting involved?), acceptability of programme material (such as, do pamphlets contain relevant information in the right format?) and satisfaction with programme intentions (as in, are partner groups satisfied with the way in which the project is being rolled out?) are common elements in process evaluation. Process evaluation can use both quantitative and qualitative methods. Getting first-hand knowledge of what people think and experience in the project is important for process evaluation, especially in terms of improving and refining the processes used to implement the project. The knowledge gained is invaluable because it allows others to replicate the project (or aspects of it) and to learn from the mistakes. It also allows plans to be adapted for subsequent rounds of a project. Figure 16.3 shows the role of formative evaluation and its relationship to the other stages. The article by Kafatos and colleagues (2004) on interventions in Cretan primary schools shows how process measures such as observations and ongoing interviews can contribute to the overall evaluation, including adding value to impact and outcome measures. Similarly, Kreisel's (2004) evaluation of a computer-based nutrition tool used qualitative and observational processes in gauging process and impact.

Impact evaluation

Impact evaluation assesses the immediate effect of an intervention, and can use a combination of both quantitative and qualitative measures. It may involve measuring a reaction to an intervention and the intervention's 'acceptability', at post-intervention stage. It can also include proxy indicators that may imply behaviour change; for example, did anyone say they had learned something after they were exposed to the intervention that may make them behave differently, or that they were persuaded by the message and expressed an intent to change their behaviour? A good example of proxy indicator is consumption of fruit and vegetables, where changes in the consumption of fruit and vegetables are proxy indicators of healthy or unhealthy eating.

Of course, none of this guarantees that an intervention has any long-term effect or that it actually changed behaviour, or that individuals or groups maintained any change, but it does reflect the impact upon those who have been exposed to the intervention. Knowing how many people recall seeing the poster on key messages about a five-a-day fruit and vegetable intervention, for example, may well be an important part of the evaluation, but it is probably not all that is needed to assess whether the intervention has achieved its aims and objectives. Knowing how many people enjoyed looking at a leaflet or appreciated its colour scheme won't establish whether the leaflet succeeded in its prevention aims. It is unlikely that the project aim is simply to produce materials that are seen by X per cent of the population. It may be important to measure the message assimilation and whether it has resulted in increased knowledge and behaviour change among those who have seen the poster or leaflet. Make sure measurements are related to what it has been set out to achieve.

One mistake often made in evaluation is to use inappropriate methods to measure impact. At the pre-testing stage or during formative evaluation, interviews are best done individually or by using group techniques (such as focus groups) for the initial formation of plans, resources or training. Using such methods to gauge the impact or effectiveness of the intervention may not be appropriate. If you want a leaflet to be understood and to communicate a message, and the objective is that exposure to the leaflet results in an increase in answers about five-a-day to six out of a possible ten (from an initial base of three correct responses), then this is what is measured. If post-exposure 60 per cent of the audience can now answer five questions correctly (from a base of three) and the cost of the leaflet is $1, then this means that for every $100 spent, $60 is effectively used or targeted in meeting the objective. If, however, only 30 per cent understand or correctly identify five answers, then $70 out of every $100 spent is not being used wisely. All this of course depends on the target audience; street homeless people are a hard-to-reach group with varying needs, and for this group the decision may be that 30 per cent is in fact a reasonable uptake of the message for this audience compared to other options available. Although a crude measure, this example moves from purely subjective measures such as colour preferences and likes to making transparent the decision-making process. The study by Eriksen and colleagues (2003) shows the value of impact evaluation in gauging the success of a school fruit and vegetable subscription scheme.

Outcome evaluation

Outcome evaluation (in the United States, this is sometimes referred to as summative evaluation: Valente 2002) assesses the effectiveness and efficiency of an intervention. It establishes the extent to which an intervention's aims and objectives have been met. If the original aim was to change behaviour, then it should assess whether the audience's behaviour has been changed, and can assess, in the longer term, whether the audience's change of behaviour has been maintained. It can use a combination of quantitative and qualitative measures. The EPI-Centre (1997) defines outcome evaluation as being: '. . . designed to establish whether an intervention works or not, whether or not the intervention changes the outcomes (for example, knowledge, attitudes, intentions, behaviour, service use) specified in the aims of the study.' A study may include process, impact and outcome evaluation, but analysis shows that there is a tendency in health promotion-type initiatives to rely on process and to a lesser extent on impact evaluation, often without reference to outcome evaluation (Caraher & Cowburn 2004; McGlone et al. 2005). This is often due to the short-term nature of interventions and the lack of resources to follow up the sustainability of outcomes. As Valente (2002) points out about health promotion programmes, many 'are created to generate specific outcomes or effects in a relatively well-defined group, within a relatively short period of time'. Experiences in evaluation suggest this is true of many public health nutrition programmes.

Outcome evaluation is generally of a long-term nature, costly and requires specific skills. As a general rule of thumb, outcomes from an intervention are judged to be stable six months post-intervention, so by this stage the number of those who will have relapsed and those who have maintained the behaviour are established. Very often programmes that measure short-term effectiveness do not measure long-term sustainability. The six-month post-intervention measure is often outside their time reference, funding, and staffing. So do those in the target group who increase their fruit and vegetable consumption after exposure to a programme still maintain this increase six months later? This is a question often left unanswered in evaluation programmes. The study from Crete on nutrition education and the Mediterranean diet combines all the elements of a good evaluation, ranging through process and impact to an outcome measure eleven months after the intervention had ended (Kafatos et al. 2004). Box 16.5 shows some important elements of a sound evaluation.

One important question to ask at this stage is whether findings were as a direct result of the programme. Those involved in intervention may also be all subject to a wide range of different messages about food, from various social contexts, from mass media and the use of food imagery in advertising campaigns, and it is difficult to separate out the specific impacts of an intervention from everything else. Experimental research (one type of which is known as a randomised controlled trial, or RCT) is an approach to evaluation that attempts to maximise certainty and minimise guesswork. The simplest example of experimental evaluation is one in which the target population is randomly allocated to two groups, one of which is exposed to or involved in activities, and one that is not (this latter group is called the 'control'). The difference between the two groups is then measured. In the real world of public health nutrition prevention, such an evaluation approach is not often an option for a variety of reasons, including feasibility and cost, and may be questionable from an ethical perspective.

Box 16.5

Important elements of a sound evaluation (gold standard)

A sound evaluation:
- reports pre-intervention and post-intervention data for individuals/groups
- has some means of comparing and contrasting before and after data
- reports on outcome measures as described in the aims of the study
- has a clear underlying model, theory or rationale for action
- has clearly defined prevention aims and objectives
- describes the intervention and the evaluation design well enough for both to be replicated
- process and impact evaluation indicators are robust and contribute to internal validity
- reports numbers involved with some description of who might have been missed or who dropped out.

Source: Adapted from Valente 2002; McGlone et al. 2005

Using the right tools for the job

Evaluation methods are generally divided into two kinds: qualitative and quantitative approaches; although there is clearly an overlap between the two. There are many textbooks on methods, and it is not intended to go into detail here on the various methods and approaches. Qualitative methods include techniques such as focus group interviews and one-to-one interviews. They are well suited for investigating in-depth issues such as attitudes, perceptions, beliefs of a target audience and, in evaluation terms, for providing a commentary on why something has, or has not, worked. Quantitative methods include techniques such as questionnaires and surveys, and, as the term implies, are better suited to providing information about quantity. For example, quantitative methodologies (on their own) may be insufficient for developing an understanding of complex local needs and workings of a local community. Quantitative and qualitative data both offer useful and differing perspectives on research and evaluation (Oakley 1998) — it is not a case of one being better than the other. As noted above in Box 16.5, consideration should be given to the means of comparing and contrasting before and after data, so that it is can demonstrate change and compares like with like, as well as using data from process and impact findings to show public health nutrition development over the period of intervention. There are also existing validated resources developed by others that can be used (see McGlone et al. 2005; Nelson 1998). More creative ways to collect the information can be used, especially if the evaluation is part of the work with young people — techniques such as group brainstorms, storytelling, video, quizzes, photos, collages, or creative writing and drawing (see Caraher et al. 2004).

There is value in using multiple methods and approaches to evaluation to provide a complete picture. This is called triangulation and involves looking at the problem from different perspectives. So using interviews with students, empirical observation of food choice in a school canteen, and questionnaires to gauge changes in knowledge/awareness is an example of triangulation (of methods) to report on the changes to influence healthy food choice. A common pitfall is to use qualitative research to establish what are clearly quantitative baselines. For example, one of the prevention objectives may be to increase knowledge, but the formative work employs qualitative methods to elicit perceptions and needs of the target audience. These findings may well be useful in refining the programme and developing an information campaign to suit the audience, but it may do little to establish baselines of existing knowledge, attitudes or skills, which will be needed to evaluate whether the objective to increase knowledge has been achieved.

What is important is that the evaluation methodology chosen should be informed by what is expected from the project, and emerge from the evaluation aims and objectives. It is common to find a mismatch between aims and objectives and the evaluation methodology of a project.

Who do you collect information from?

It is often not feasible to collect information from everyone. In this case, common evaluation practice is to define a sample group. This group could be chosen to be representative (that is a group of people selected from a definitive population, for example a school or general practitioner client list), purposive (a group of people chosen for a particular reason, for example because they are all male, or all live in a particular street) or opportunistic (a group of people chosen because they just happen to be around at the time, for example, on a busy high street or attending a club). What is vital is that, if an unrepresentative selection has been used, then it is not possible to claim to have discovered indisputable facts that can be applied to other groups or populations.

One of the issues with evaluation is the setting of priorities and deciding what is most useful to know. While it may be possible to evaluate everything, it is rarely feasible. So from the existing knowledge and formative evaluation, what are emerging as priorities? There are two ways of collecting data. One takes a broad and shallow approach, which means that a variety of data at many stages in the project/programme is collected. The second a deep and narrow approach, exploring fewer issues in more depth (see Figure 16.4). Another way of conceptualising the collection of data can be seen in Figure 16.5, where the emphasis is on depth, but in project 1 an in-depth approach is taken at one point in time, whereas in project 2 numerous samples or measures are undertaken, perhaps at different times with the same group or with different groups. The point is to decide which approach best addresses the evaluation aims and objectives and can be managed within the resources available. The reality is that the approach taken is often dictated by the limitations of resources.

Think of the utility of the evaluation. As a general principle, if it is not possible to identify how the answers will be used, then it may be better not to ask the questions.

The second-biggest weakness of evaluation projects after poor design is attempting too much. Those responsible for evaluation need to give themselves permission not to do everything and to focus on the interests of quality and rigour. Think of the questions and utility of the evaluation. There is not a need to — and more than likely, no requirement to — have to evaluate every aspect of the public health nutrition project or programme.

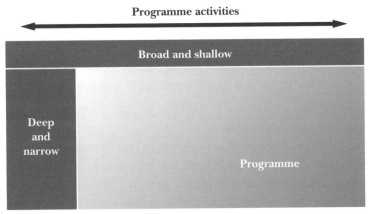

Source: Foster et al. 2000

Figure 16.4 Relationship of evaluation focus and depth of focus

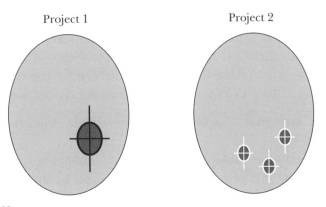

Source: Foster et al. 2000

Figure 16.5 Comparative evaluation focus

Who can do the evaluation?

Evaluation can be conducted internally (that is, by those doing the project work) or it can be commissioned from outside specialists. The advantages of inside evaluation is that people are familiar with the project and sensitive to the needs of project partners, stakeholders and users, and findings from process and impact evaluation can be fed back into the work quickly. On the other hand, the potential disadvantages of evaluating internally are that those doing the work may not be able to take an objective standpoint on work with which they have been personally involved. Outside evaluators may offer improved objectivity, but may also bring their own biases and perceptions of how the project should have been run. They also come at a cost, and commissioning outside researchers may not work within the timescale. This is especially so with small projects that have to be run quickly and have a short life-span.

Write-up and dissemination

Once the project is finished, it is really important to make time to disseminate the findings so that others may learn from the experience. For example, a feedback or celebration event for local community groups involved in the project might be held, the full written report presented to funders and/or at conferences, and the results written up for formal publication.

Ethics and evaluation

It is important to consider the ethical implications of any evaluation activities. Ethics are not about right and wrong but about ensuring that public health nutrition evaluation is focused on improving wellbeing of a group or community. This means there is a need to consider the responsibility in protecting the interests of those partaking in the evaluation. On what grounds and basis are they agreeing to be part of the process? Consider the following:

- Issues of anonymity – will groups, area or individuals be identified in any write-up?
- How will data be collected–face-to-face, questionnaire, etc.?
- Are the proposed evaluation methods intrusive in any way?
- Have the implications of data protection acts, copyright and libel laws, which may affect the conduct of any evaluation, been considered?
- Are physical safety measures in place for evaluators?
- Are resources adequate for the planned evaluation?
- Will evaluation data be stored in a secure way?

This list is not exhaustive, and it is recommended that this be supplemented by seeking advice on local situations and circumstances.

Conclusion

Project management is a process that offers a number of advantages to any programme and those implementing it. In particular:

- it can be fun — this is often forgotten in the mayhem of day-to-day activities
- it can be creative
- it can help improve the quality of the programme for all concerned — funders, workers and clients
- it can be dynamic and feed directly and within project time back into project delivery
- for those engaged in the delivery of programmes, it can facilitate a process of standing back from day-to-day activities and seeing solutions where none were previously seen to exist — in this sense, it can be reflexive
- well-designed and managed projects can also contribute to securing future funding.

REFERENCES

Baker, H. and Caraher, M. 1999, *Do It Yourself: The process of developing a drugs information resource for children*, Home Office, Central Drug Prevention Unit, London.

Beattie, A. 1994, 'Healthy alliances or dangerous liaisons? The challenge of working together in health promotion' in Leathard, A. (ed.) 1994, *Going Inter-Professional: Working together for health and welfare*, Routledge, London, pp. 109–22.

—— 1995, 'Evaluation in community development for health: An opportunity for dialogue' in *Health Education Journal*, vol. 54, pp. 465–72.

Booth, A. 1997, *The ScHAAR Guide to Evidence-Based Practice: Occasional paper no. 97/2*, School of Health and Related Research, University of Sheffield, Sheffield.

Caraher, M. and Cowburn, G. 2004, 'A survey of food projects in the English NHS regions' in *Health Education Journal*, vol. 63, no. 3, pp. 197–219.

—— 2005, 'Taxing food: Implications for public health nutrition' in *Public Health Nutrition*, vol. 8, no. 8, pp. 1242–49.

Caraher, M. and Reynolds, J. 2005, 'Lessons for home economics pedagogy and practice', *Journal of the Home Economics Institute of Australia*, vol. 12, no. 2, pp. 2–15.

Caraher, M., Baker, H. and Burns, M. 2004, 'Children's views of cooking and food preparation' in *British Food Journal*, vol. 106, no. 4, pp. 255–73.

Coveney, J. 2005, 'A qualitative study exploring socio-economic differences in parental lay knowledge of food and health: implications for public health nutrition', *Public Health Nutrition*, vol. 8, no. 3, pp. 290–97.

Dobson, B., Kellard, K. and Talbot, D. 2000, *A Recipe for Success? An Evaluation of a Community Food Project*, Centre for Research in Social Policy, Loughborough University.

Egger, G., Spark, R., Lawson, J. and Donovan, R. 1999, *Health promotion strategies and methods*, McGraw-Hill, Sydney.

Eriksen, K., Haraldsdottir, J., Pederson, R. and Flyger, H.V. 2003, 'Effect of a fruit and vegetable subscription in Danish schools' in *Public Health Nutrition*, vol. 6, no. 1, pp. 57–63.

Foster, C., Kaduskar, S. and Cowburn, G. 2000, 'Evaluation Training Programme', cited at <http://www.dphpc.ox.ac.uk/bhfhprg> on 1 December.

Hawe, P., Degeling, D., Hall, J. 2000, *Evaluating Health Promotion: A health workers guide*, McLennan Petty, Sydney.

International Union for Health Promotion and Education 2000, *The Evidence of Health Promotion Effectiveness: Shaping public health in a new Europe; Part Two Evidence Book: Assessing 20 years evidence of the health social economic and political impacts of health promotion*, International Union for Health Promotion and Education, Paris.

Kafatos, I., Peponaras, A., Linardakis, M. and Kafatos, A. 2004, 'Nutrition education and Mediterranean diet: Exploring the teaching process of a school-based nutrition and media education project in Cretan primary schools' in *Public Health Nutrition*, vol. 7, no. 7, pp. 969–75.

Kreisel, K. 2004, 'Evaluation of a computer-based nutrition education tool' in *Public Health Nutrition*, vol. 7, no. 2, pp. 271–77.

Margetts, B. 2004, 'An Overview of Public Health Nutrition' in Gibney, M., Margetts, B., Kearney, J.M. and Arab, L. (eds) 2004, *Public Health Nutrition: The Nutrition Society textbook series*, Blackwell Publishing, London, pp. 1–25.

McGlone, P., Dallison, J. and Caraher, M. 2005, *Evaluation Resources for Community Food Projects*, Health Development Agency, London.

McGlone, P., Dobson, B., Dowler, E. and Nelson, M. 1996, *Food Projects and How They Work*, York Publishing Services Ltd for the Joseph Rowntree Foundation, York.

Nelson, M. 1998, 'The validation of dietary assessment' in Margetts, B.M. and Nelson, M. (eds) 1998, *Design Concepts in Nutritional Epidemiology* (2nd edition), Oxford University Press, Oxford, pp. 241–72.

Nutbeam, D. and Harris, E. 2001, *Theory in a Nutshell: A practitioners guide to commonly used theories and models in health promotion*, University of Sydney, Sydney.

Oakley, A. 1998, 'Experimentation in social science: The case of health promotion' in *Social Sciences in Health*, vol. 4, no. 2, pp. 73–89.

—— 2000, *Experiments in Knowing: Gender and method in the social sciences*, Polity Press, Cambridge.

Oliver, S. and Peersman, G. 2001, *Using Research for Effective Health Promotion*, Open University Press, Buckingham.

Pawson, T. and Tilley, N. 1998, *Realistic Evaluation*, Sage, London.

Peersman, G.V., Oakley, A.R. and Oliver, S. 1999, 'Evidence based health promotion? Some methodological challenges' in *Journal of the Insitute of Health Education Promotion and Education*, vol. 37, no. 2, pp. 59–64.

Punch, K. 1998, *Introduction to Social Research: Quantitative and qualitative approaches*, Sage, London.

Robinson, T.N. and Sirard, J.R. 2005, 'Preventing childhood obesity: A solution-oriented research paradigm' in *American Journal of Preventive Medicine*, vol. 28, no. 2S2, pp. 194–201.

Summerbell, C.D., Waters, E., Edmunds, L.D., Kelly, S., Brown, T. and Campbell, K.J. 2005, 'Interventions for preventing obesity in children' in *Cochrane Database, Systems Review*, July, issue 3, Review Manager 4.2.3.

Valente, T.W. 2002, *Evaluating Health Promotion Programs*, Oxford University Press, New York, pp. 3, 34.

World Health Organization (WHO) 1986, *Ottawa Charter for Health Promotion*, First International Conference on Health Promotion, Ottawa, 21 November, WHO, Geneva.

17

Promotion and communication

TONY WORSLEY

Public health nutrition promotion and communication are widespread activities around the world that have been in existence since nutritional deficiencies were first observed in North America and Western Europe at the end of the nineteenth century. Then, the problems faced were of deficiencies of energy, protein and micronutrients; today, micronutrient deficiencies and overconsumption of energy are principal problems that vary from region to region and locality to locality.

Much of the emphasis in the past hundred years has been on the nutrition education of mothers and children. In the past twenty years, however, this has broadened to include nutrition promotion, as it has become clear that knowledge and individual action, while important, are not the only ways to raise the nutrition status of populations. Nutrition promotion, then, can be broadly defined as any set of coordinated actions designed to make a population's food consumption and nutritional status healthier. The population concerned may be small, such as the members of a local rural community, or large, for example, a nation state. It is useful to consider nutrition promotion as including supply and demand side approaches. We can educate and motivate consumers to demand different foods, and we can influence food suppliers – farmers, distributors, manufacturers to provide healthier foods through a variety of methods, ranging from education of the workforce, through marketing of healthier foods, to government regulation of sales and marketing.

How does nutrition promotion relate to health promotion?

Originally these two subsets of public health were initiated by different groups of people. The former were usually nutrition scientists who applied their science to a variety of problems produced by industrial capitalism, such as starvation arising from low wages, compulsory mass education that exposed the effects of nutrition deficiencies in primary schools, and the militarism associated with the two world wars, which again exposed nutrient deficiencies in recruits. The home economics movement of late ninteenth- and early twentieth-century North America, associated with what became known as the 'Cult of True Womanhood' (in New Zealand) and emphasising the supposed primary domestic responsibilities of women, also promoted healthy eating and nutritional principles.

Health promotion, on the other hand, has mixed roots in school health education (often of a nonphysiological sort), the nineteenth century public health movement and community development movements. Today, nutrition promotion might be regarded as a subset of health promotion. However, unlike health promotion, which is firmly based in the health system, its main context is the food system and, to a lesser extent, the health and education systems. Knowledge of human physiology, nutrition and the structure and working of the food system are central to nutrition promotion. At one extreme, this is often seen as a strong focus on individuals' health and, at another, on issues of ecological and economic sustainability. The latter focus is important for the maintenance of the long-term nutritional status of the population; food supplies must be sustained for future as well as present generations.

What is a healthy diet? The behavioural basis of eating and drinking

Public health nutrition differs from nutrition science in that it recognises the importance of individuals' food behaviours such as shopping, preparation and consumption as the basis of population nutrition status. If people eat lots of high-energy foods, for example, then their nutrition status is likely to be compromised. So in nutrition promotion a lot of attention is given to influencing the population's food behaviours through persuasion, communication and education, regulatory and food policy measures, or through some combination of these approaches.

This raises the question of what exactly is a healthy diet? What sorts of foods and beverages are compatible with optimal health? These are behavioural questions because they are recommendations about the foods people ought to select in order to be healthy. These questions are discussed in chapter 3 in relation to nutrient reference values, dietary guidelines and food group taxonomies. For now, it is important to note that a healthy diet depends on the culture a person belongs to, with its normative expectations of what the average person should be capable of doing (for example, a capability for manual labour is regarded as essential in agricultural societies − if you cannot do it, then you may be judged as being 'unhealthy'). Life stage is the other key moderator of food consumption patterns − babies and children undergo growth and so require foods that foster growth; at the other end of the age spectrum, older people require nutrient-dense foods along with regular resistance, flexibility and endurance exercise to prevent frailty and its associated conditions.

Why nutrition promotion?

It is often claimed, with some justification, that in hunter–gatherer societies people discovered which foods were health promoting and which were danger-ous, and how they could process dangerous foods into safe foods (Fischler 1980; Tansey & Worsley 1995). This knowledge was passed from generation to generation, mainly through family transmission (that is, mother to daughter, father to son). Jarrod Diamond describes the extensive botanic knowledge of the average tribal person in Papua New Guinea in his book *Guns, Germs and Steel* (1998). With the rise of agriculture, the lines for the supply of food became longer − people didn't always know who produced their food, and with industrialisation these lines became even longer, with scores of people from all around the world having some part on the production of the foods we eat (Tansey & Worsley 1995). So we have to trust manufacturers and food retailers regarding the safety of our foods, and we need food and nutrition education in order to understand how this complex system works so we can maintain our health and safety. This is essentially the argument for nutrition education.

The argument for nutrition promotion includes this view, but it is broader since it is centred on population health. So the reasons for having a lively set of nutrition promotion professionals in today's society include the promotion of several societal 'goods', including:

- the prevention and amelioration of diseases such as heart disease, cancers and type 2 diabetes, among many others (including the prevention of obesity and other risk factors) − this is associated with the prevention of over-nutrition and excess energy intake (which lead to non communicable disease) in the general population and in sub-populations such as children, older people and those with disabilities (as outlined in chapters 1, 2, 5, 6 and 9)

- the prevention and treatment of undernutrition, frank malnutrition and starvation, especially among women and children — increasingly, older people may be at risk of undernutrition (referred to in chapters 4, 6, 7, 8 and 10)
- the promotion of access to safe, healthy food at a reasonable price is a major aim, even in affluent countries — put another way, this is the prevention of food insecurity, often occurring in marginalised communities (chapters 7 and 8)
- the promotion of food safety through the safe preparation and distribution of foods. While this usually refers to microbiological safety, it can also refer to the promotion of the chemical safety of foods, such as the detection and prosecution of the adulteration of foods and beverages — an emerging challenge in many countries is the prevention of life-threatening allergic reactions such as peanut allergy, which, though low in prevalence, have severe consequences for an unfortunate minority
- the promotion of social health and positive social interactions, which has been an age-old benefit of food consumption — people coming together to enjoy food — and it remains the same today, though the rise of the individual high-energy snack that can be swallowed in seconds (to save time — for what?) is a threat to social cohesion
- the prevention of environmental degradation associated with food production and distribution. The negative effects of a fossil-fuel, water-guzzling society are becoming clear through global warming and desertification of land — it is no longer possible to tolerate production methods that lead to land degradation or distribution methods that waste fossil fuel through unnecessary transport of foods (unnecessary 'food miles'). Public health nutritionists have to safeguard future food supplies for later generations as well as the nutritional status of the present inhabitants of earth (see chapter 11).

These issues can be found in all countries, though they differ in their impact for societies at different stages of the nutrition transition (chapter 10). Within countries they affect people from special population groups differently and with more or less importance; for example, babies, infants, children and adolescents have need for food that enables them to grow, and they experience lifelong problems if they are denied to them (described in chapters 4 and 5). Older persons, disabled people and hospital patients have special requirements relating to possible undernutrition; and members of minority, indigenous and socially disadvantaged groups are likely to have problems of access to healthy food and perhaps combinations of over- and undernutrition (see chapters 6, 7 and 8).

Nutrition education or nutrition promotion?

These two terms are not the antithesis of each other; nutrition education is just one approach used in nutrition promotion. The area started out as the education of mothers and children in the late nineteenth century in the new science of nutrition. This has now extended to other groups such as preschool children attending long daycare centres. The aims of nutrition education, outlined by Gussow and Contento (1984) and Johnson and Johnson (1985), are similar to those of general education – that is, to provide learners with sufficient knowledge and skills so that they can make healthy food choices or decisions that benefit rather than harm them. In order to do this, learners assimilate some basic cognitive frameworks or principles ('schema' in psychological jargon) so that they can understand and make sense of the food world. An example of a central nutrition schema is the concept of 'energy balance', which enables us to understand quite different phenomena such as children's growth and body-weight maintenance. Other important nutritional schema include:

- chemical energy (thus energy balance)
- antioxidants and free radicals
- vitamins and minerals as essential 'enzymatic' factors, for example, the role folate plays in the inflammatory process, the role of calcium in bone growth
- proteins, and growth and repair concepts
- concepts of nutrient sufficiency and excess
- saturated fats, serum cholesterol and heart disease.

Nutritionists take these basic schema very seriously. However, food consumers have to use additional food schema in their daily lives (which nutritionists do not) – and nutrition promoters need to be aware of these consumer issues, for example:

- What sort of variety of foods should they eat?
- How often should they consume foods from particular food groups, for instance, 'Do I need to eat fruit every day or every week, or even less often?'
- Are some foods better choices than others? And if so, what are they?
- How are energy intakes and energy outputs kept in balance?

Stakeholders

The decision over what should be taught to school children or other targets of nutrition education, as well as the decisions about the design and implementation of any nutrition promotion programme, does not emerge out of thin air. It is taken by interested stakeholders — people with a vested interest in the outcomes of the programme (Wass 1994). Take school children's nutrition education as an example. There could be many stakeholders, including the children themselves, who hold views about what they should learn about food. The children's parents have views of what their children should learn; the teachers have views about the capability of children; as does the school principal, who may have a limited budget and face pressure from politicians about the state of numeracy and literacy education: the nutrition scientists want to ensure that their discipline is taught 'correctly' (that is, in the ways they like — often with a strong emphasis on quantification); local food companies want the children and their families to bring their custom to them (Tesco in the United Kingdom has provided nutrition education programmes for children); members of ethnic communities may want their food traditions to be taught at school; branches of national health promotion foundations (such as the Cancer Council, National Heart Foundation, drug awareness groups) and many more groups and individuals, all have a stake in school education. Sound nutrition promotion ensures that all the stakeholders are consulted, and, if appropriate, enlisted before any programme is undertaken. Failure to do so may see the programme derailed by protests from powerful stakeholders soon after the programme begins.

Demand or supply side?

While nutrition education is concerned mainly with the demand side in its emphasis on the education of consumers, other nutrition promotion approaches include:

- mass and tailored communication often aimed at motivating people rather than just informing them
- micro-environmental approaches, such as the development of food policies in kindergartens about the types of foods that may be served to children
- government policy approaches that regulate the supply and marketing of foods; for example, in Japan large supermarkets are discouraged since the government wishes to foster small retail businesses; in the European Union and the United States, some farmers (such as dairy farmers) are paid subsidies

to produce products that are relatively low-priced. Often government supply-side policies are not enforced for nutritional reasons, rather they are implemented to shore up political support among sections of the community; nevertheless, they do affect the supply of food, and thus the nutritional status of the population

- middle-level supply side approaches include worksite programmes, for example, some American companies provide inexpensive healthy food in worksite cafeterias (Biener et al. 1999), often as part of a broader employee health programme.

In summary, nutrition promotion uses the same variety of approaches used by other health promoters enshrined in the WHO's Ottawa Charter (1986), a worldwide source of guidance through the five essential strategies to:

1. build healthy public policy
2. create supportive environments
3. strengthen community action
4. develop personal skills
5. reorient health services.

Paradigms and Theories

Paradigms

Our views of society (and nutrition promotion) are examples of worldviews or paradigms. This term was popularised by Thomas Kuhn in his book *The Structure of Scientific Revolutions* (1962) in his attempt to understand the nature of science. He defines a paradigm in terms of the basic axioms or assumptions that scientists (and all humans) use to explain the world about them. Euclid, for example, assumed that there are points, lines and angles — he didn't prove that they exist, but he showed that they are useful concepts for understanding geometric phenomena.

Theories

These are generalisations about the main processes that are believed to cause phenomena which are the subject of study. Nutrition promotion uses a number of diverse theories to try to understand how to influence human food production and consumption. Most are taken from the social and behavioural sciences (often without much consideration of the special nature of food behaviours). In this chapter it is only possible to refer briefly to theories that are in common use. We can broadly divide them into theories based on individual-level social psychological processes, and those that emphasise the primacy of environmental influences. Most of the theories used by health and nutrition promoters were not designed to explain change processes; instead many of them were invented to explain human behaviours. These two goals are not the same.

Individual-level models

These tend to have a narrow focus on specific food choice behaviours. One of the few that have been designed specifically for understanding food choice behaviours is the Food Related Lifestyle model (Grunert et al. 1997) depicted in Figure 17.1. This is very much concerned with individuals' food-purchasing behaviours, though not exclusively so. Its main advantages are that it is fairly simple, having seven components, and it incorporates aspects of several other models, especially attitude-behaviour models.

The main components of the Food Related Lifestyle Model incorporate:

- the food's concrete characteristics, such as its appearance, shape, mouth feel, aroma, taste, and price. All these features have to be 'right' — what the consumer expects — if the consumer is to accept the food.
- the positive consequences of buying (and consuming) the foods or drinks have to outweigh any negative consequences. Indeed, certain possible negative consequences like the possibility of becoming ill, will completely abort the buying process. Typical desired benefits include saving money, better health, relatives liking the purchase, friends being impressed when it is served, etc. Nutrition promoters can highlight likely positive consequences, not only the health consequences.
- quality expectations ('higher order attributes') is shoppers' expectations of food quality and these vary. For example, some consumers may look for foods that are healthy while others want foods that are slimming, or natural or organic or luxurious. Most consumers want convenient foods or foods that are good value for money. Health benefits may not rank among the shopper's priorities.
- shopping and cooking scripts and skills are the procedural knowledge (the 'how-to' knowledge) that enables people to buy and make enjoyable foods. Scripts (learned procedures) that incorporate healthy eating principles are likely to enable children (and adults) to eat more healthily.
- usage situations are the settings in which foods are bought or consumed. Usage situations have social, temporal, and physical aspects. Consumers act

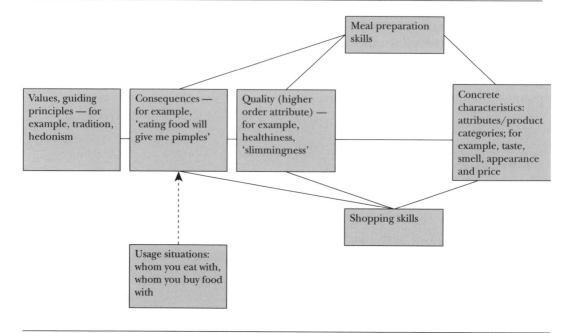

Figure 17.1 The Food Related Lifestyle Model

according to demands of the usage situation, for example, teenagers may avoid drinking with straws because their friends (present in the usage situation) would disapprove (it's too 'childlike'). Like marketers, nutrition promoters need to understand the social situations in which foods are purchased and consumed.

- values, motivations and goals. Many food behaviours are performed to attain implicit or explicit goals that are congruent with a person's values (guiding principles). Often, these behaviours are quite unconscious and habitual, for instance, buying breakfast cereals, packaged bread, milk, etc. Most consumers do not consciously seek health as a goal (unlike nutrition promoters), though many do. Nutrition promoters have to consider the likely range of goals that are likely to be pursued in typical usage situations, and then examine the extent to which these goals are consistent with nutrition promotion's goal of facilitating healthy food choices. Foley and Pollard designed the FoodCents programme in this way (Foley and Pollard 1998).

Other individual models include:

- learning theories, which employ concepts such as 'exposure' (to new foods, for example), 'modelling' of behaviours (for example, parents regularly eating fruit and vegetables – happily – in front of their children), and 'reinforcement' (that is, rewarding examples of healthy eating with hugs, smiles and other non-food rewards). Birch (1999) has shown the power of learning theories in shaping children's diets, her work often used in kindergarten healthy eating programs. The UK Food Dudes programme is a good example of the application of learning principles in children's nutrition promotion (Tapper et al. 2003).

- cybernetic and self-monitoring approaches are derived from learning theories. Simple self-monitoring approaches were used more than twenty years ago in the South Australian Body Owner's programme (Worsley et al. 1987). The assumption is that the learner has power to influence their behaviours by setting goals and assessing the degree to which they meet them and then taking remedial action.

- Attitude–Behaviour models such as Social Cognitive theory (Bandura 1986), the Health Belief Model (Janz & Becker 1984) and the Theory of Planned Behaviour (Ajzen 1991) have been very widely used, especially in intervention projects (below). Their basic assumption is that people have expectations of the consequences of their behaviours (expectancies); for example, that chocolate eating will lead to pimples, and that these perceived consequences are evaluated by them with varying degrees of goodness or badness ('value', hence the term 'expectancy-value' theories). The sum of these expectancy-values forms an attitude toward the behaviour that is moderated by intention, by the opinions of other people close to the person, and by the person's perceived self-efficacy (the confidence that they can do the behaviour). These models work best for one-off utilitarian behaviours like buying a vacuum cleaner, but not for habitual behaviours (such as eating fruit) or behaviours that involve personal values (like eating meat, Allen et al. 2000).

- the Transtheoretical Theory or Stages of Change Model (Prochaska & DiClemente 1984) was designed to understand behavioural change (unlike attitude–behaviour models). It was derived from studies of drug- and tobacco-addicted patients, not studies of food use. It suggests that when people change their behaviours, they go through a series of stages or steps at each of which the person has to alter the 'decisional balance'. Counsellors try to encourage them to ensure that their perceptions of the advantages of changing their behaviours outweigh the disadvantages of change. It can be a useful model, which has led to tailored interventions (Horwath 1999), but there are varying accounts of how many stages apply to food behaviour change.

[431]

There are several other important individualist and social models, such as decision-making, education and adult learning, social diffusion, organisational and social marketing models, for which there is not space here. Many of them, including those alluded to above, have been well reviewed for health promoters by Nutbeam & Harris (2003).

Environmental models

Environmental theories are many and varied. Furst and colleagues have provided an excellent broad model of the main environmental influences on food consumption that should be considered by all nutrition promoters (1996). These range from the climate and soil conditions through to economic and social policy influences. However, we can go a little further by dividing environmental influences into internal and external (to the person) influences, as suggested by Swinburn and colleagues (1999).

Among the internal or physiological influences are satiety and sensory processes. It is a rule of thumb among food marketers that if a food doesn't taste or look good, people won't eat it. The processes underlying this generalisation are complex and largely outside human consciousness. For example, taste preferences are partly genetically endowed and partly learned, but most people are usually unaware of the sensory learning that they undergo until they suddenly find that they don't like a food. Satiety or feelings of satisfaction during and after eating or drinking is moderated by complex physiological processes; for example, foods rich in protein or dietary fibre tend to switch off eating for several hours after a meal, while those rich in simple sugars or fats often encourage prolonged eating. These internal environments are highly relevant to nutrition promotion (as distinct from health promotion, in which non-conscious processes may have little importance apart from drug addiction). There is evidence to suggest that men who have large breakfasts containing large amounts of dietary fibre and meat (such as muesli, bacon and eggs) tend to be slimmer than other men (Kent & Worsley 2005), perhaps because starting the day with a large meal prevents nibbling on high-energy snacks between meals. So the promotion and presentation of high-satiety meals may help prevent obesity without people being particularly aware or having to make agonised decisions about what to eat.

Examples of environmental influences that impinge on the individual include the effects of family socialisation (for instance, the opinions and example of parents and siblings, or classmates at school), the proximity of food sources (such as soft drinking vending machines placed in schools so that children buy them rather than drink water); the convenient placement of fast food outlets in low socioeconomic areas, and the pricing and marketing of foods.

Table 17.1 Microenvironmental and macroenvironmental settings that might be targeted in the prevention of obesity

Microenvironmental settings	Macroenvironmental sectors
• homes	• technology/design (e.g. labor-saving devices, architecture)
• workplaces	• media (e.g. women's magazines)
• schools	• food production/importing
• universities/tertiary institutions	• food manufacturing
• community groups (e.g. clubs, churches)	• food marketing (e.g. fast food advertising)
• community place (e.g. parks, shopping malls)	• food distribution (e.g. wholesalers)
• institutions (e.g. hospitals, boarding schools)	• food catering services
• food retailers (e.g. supermarkets)	• sports/leisure industry (e.g. instructor training programs)
• food service outlets (e.g. lunch bars, restaurants)	• urban/rural development (e.g. town planning, local councils)
• recreation facilities (e.g. pools, gyms)	• transport system (e.g. public transportation systems)
• neighbourhoods (e.g. cycle paths, street safety)	• health system (e.g. Ministry of Health, medical schools, professional associations)
• transport service centres (e.g. airports, bus stations)	
• local health care (e.g. GP, hospital)	

Source: Swinburn et al. 1999

Merging individual and environmental approaches — the PRECEDE-PROCEED model and the social–behavioural–biological model

This model was derived from the Health Belief Model (HBM), an individual expectancy-value model (Green & Kreuter 1991). Although the HBM worked well within defined clinical situations, it did not account for the environmental influences on change. The PRECEDE-PROCEED model includes a combination of individual factors such as beliefs and attitudes, perceived barriers and triggers combined with environmental factors (see Figure 17.2). It is a useful health promotion planning tool as it requires the health promoter to consider up to six environmental diagnoses that help identify the problems faced by a group of people or community. For example, the epidemiological diagnosis concerns the population's health and disease status, the behavioural diagnosis examines behaviours that may contribute to the disease risk (such as cigarette smoking or overconsumption of fast foods), the social diagnosis looks at the

[433]

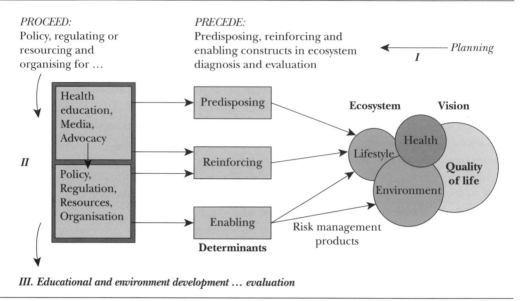

PROCEED:
Policy, regulating or resourcing and organising for …

PRECEDE:
Predisposing, reinforcing and enabling constructs in ecosystem diagnosis and evaluation

III. Educational and environment development … evaluation

Figure 17.2 A schematic of the PROCEED/PRECEDE model

Source: Green & Kreuter 1991 (see <http://lgreen.net/precede.htm>)

social conditions fostering the behaviours, and so on. A recent development of the environment–behavioural nexus is the social–behavioural–biological model put forward by Glass and McAtee (2006). In particular, its specification of 'risk regulators' that may moderate populations' likelihood of exposure to noxious environmental exposures and health risk behaviours provide useful conceptual tools for health promoters (see Figure 17.3).

Change methods: Designs and Evaluation

Contrary to many learned people's opinion, there is much scope and opportunity for nutrition promotion, so long as appropriate methodologies are employed. Useful questions to keep in mind are:

- Who or what do we want to influence?
- What do *they* want to do?
- What do *we* want them to do?

The aims of any programme must be consistent with the culture of the various settings in which the promotion takes place. The levels of social organisation and the settings in which food activities occur place practical limitations on

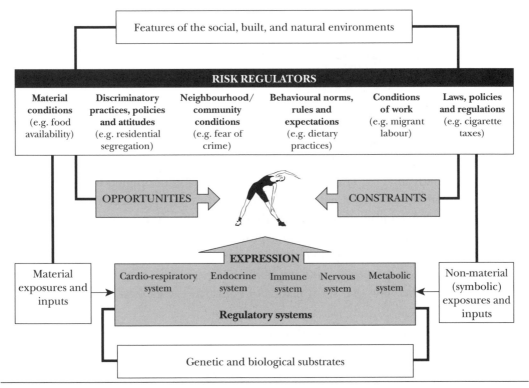

Figure 17.3 The social–behavioural–biological model

Source: Glass & McAtee 2006

nutrition promotion aims and the methods that can be employed to achieve them. However, a wide range of nutrition promotion and communication activities can be conducted across several levels of society using diverse methodologies at the level of:

* individuals and the small groups to which they belong
* organisation or system, such as a company or an educational or hospital system
* locality or region
* nation and international community.

The various theories can be applied to match the levels of social organisation. For example, at the level of the individual, personal and group counselling (and related approaches such as health coaching) can be used along with learning models and decision-making models. At the level of the organisation, similar models can be used, but in addition so can environmental and policy models

[435]

since the organisation has the power to use them. Finally, at national and international levels, economic policy and mass communication approaches can be combined with community development models.

Three methodological paradigms

There are considerable tensions and disagreement about the best approaches or methods to use. Each of the paradigms described below has its advantages and disadvantages. Traditionally, the main division of opinion has been the split between those who use top-down approaches in the belief that their expert knowledge combined with clear theoretical direction is likely to yield fairly precise results versus those who aspire to bottom-up approaches, who are suspicious of overarching theory and wish to involve the targets of nutrition promotion in its design and implementation as fully as possible. (They often aspire to the view that short chains of command work best.)

Paradigm 1: The intervention project

The intervention project is a very common form of nutrition promotion. Thousands of nutrition interventions have been conducted around the world in the past century, but very few of them have been reported, and fewer still have been well designed (Worsley & Crawford 2005). Typically, a group of people, such as pregnant women or school children, are exposed to a series of messages that may encourage them to change their behaviours by researchers ('content experts'). In well-designed projects, some form of comparison group(s) is included in the design, and a set of outcome variables (for example, indices of healthy eating) is measured before and after the trial, and sometimes they are measured during the trial too. Most studies have been of very short duration, rarely more than three months, and follow-ups longer than a few weeks, if any, are very rare (Ciliska et al. 2000).

The interesting thing is that many of these interventions do work — in the sense that short-term changes in the targeted behaviours occur, as in the number of serves of fruit consumed per week may increase in the treatment group (Johnson & Johnson 1985; Ciliska et al. 2000). The key question, however, is: How long do their effects persist after the intervention ceases? The evidence suggests that it is not for long. Continued effort and resources are usually required to maintain long-lasting change, and the typical intervention project is externally funded for a short period. Several quasi-experimental designs have been created over the past half century to take advantage of natural experiments (such as comparing schools' nutrition promotion programmes with those that do not have them). Various threats to validity are likely to confound the interpretation of such uncontrolled studies, but clever designs may be capable of accounting or minimising these artefacts (Shaddish et al. 2002).

The intervention project has a number of uses, advantages and disadvantages. It is useful for the examination of factors that are likely to bring about changes in outcome variables. This is usually the reason for university and government researchers designing the project, typically to test hypotheses about ways to change behaviours. The main advantage of intervention designs is that they can tell us precisely which are important factors for change and which are not – so they test and extend behavioural theories. When well designed, they can act as excellent demonstrations of what might be achieved by health and education workers like teachers, nurses and community personnel (given sufficient funding). They can act as centres of innovation, enabling health promoters to learn new ideas and techniques; for example, the SHAPE daily physical education project in South Australia in the late 1970s, though far too intensive for use in schools, clearly showed that children's cardiovascular health could be substantially improved by non-specialist primary teachers. As such, it was used as a model for the introduction of daily physical education programmes throughout South Australia and beyond (Worsley et al. 1987).

Unfortunately, the intervention project has some disadvantages. These are largely due to its top-down nature – experts find funding and persuade members of a community or organisation to take part. These experts often have narrow aims that may or may not coincide with the needs and wants of the local community, for instance, they may want to lower children's serum cholesterol concentrations, whereas the community might want better transport services. Pursuit of such expert goals may cause resentment and serious disruption to the normal workings of an organisation. For example, if due care is not taken, daily physical education and nutrition programmes may displace other activities in a school (such as, there may be no time for lessons about philosophy or arts). The result may be that the subjects of an intervention may be very relieved when it is over!

Perhaps the main drawback relates to lack of long-term commitment – often no provision is made for the community to continue to bring about the desired project aims when it has ceased – people may have changed their diets during a programme, but that really doesn't help them if they are not enabled to do it in the long term. A further disadvantage is that expert goals are often influenced by scientific fads and fashions; for example, many nutrition promotion interventions in the 1980s were focused on lowering cholesterol levels and reducing total fat intakes. We now know that the latter is inappropriate — not all fats are bad. These criticisms do not negate all intervention projects, but they do highlight the need to offset their disadvantages through greater commitment to community concerns. Institutionalisation of intervention projects so that they become a permanent normal aspect of particular settings is a key goal.

Paradigm 2: Action research or community participatory research

Action Research is a bottom-up approach that takes the view that problems are to be identified and fixed by members of the local community or organisation, according to their wishes. Usually, it does not employ strong experimental or quasi-experimental designs, but instead it relies on needs assessment processes to identify common problems and consensual goal-setting. A good example is the establishment of food and nutrition policies in kindergartens, which vary according to the problems perceived by the kindergarten community. Once goals have been agreed, action researchers then aim to achieve them using a variety of methods such as advocacy, communication and community building. They tend to use methods that will achieve their goals, and they may change both goals and methods as circumstances change (unlike the rigid protocol-driven approach of the intervention project). The aim is to fix the problem, though if initial goals prove to be unworkable they may be modified or abandoned.

The main advantage of the action research project is that it focuses on problems that are relevant to people who are most affected by them. It often brings a sense of ownership and community cohesion. However, it may encounter difficulties associated with lack of resources and the use of volunteers. For instance, community management groups may have diverse memberships and can encounter problems in group dynamics, often because authority structures are weak. The original goals may become blurred or may shift radically away from the original goals. For example, goals to increase fruit and vegetable use may become engulfed by more urgent food safety and food-handling goals. A further disadvantage is that even if a local programme is successful, it may be difficult to replicate elsewhere (because solutions to problems often depend on highly specific local circumstances). The North Karelia Project was a hybrid of the intervention project (it was heavily influenced by Stanford University staff) and by the community participatory approach since it was initiated and funded by locals living in North Karelia (Puska et al. 1983).

Paradigm 3: Total quality management — systemic change in organisations

This is a relatively recent paradigm, which focuses on the sustainability of change. It is concerned with systemic change within settings and organisations. It assumes that social systems ought to be engineered to produce health (and nutrition) outcomes as part of their normal functioning. For example, schools should supply appropriate amounts of healthy food to their children, and the quantity and quality of these foods can be monitored regularly, and action be taken if certain quality and quantitative criteria are not met. This is very similar to hazard analysis critical control points (HACCP) systems used in industry. This approach involves the redesign of organisational and job specifications. For example, schools and teachers are expected to foster the health of their children, as well as educate them. While this has always been the case, the difference is that health goals are operationalised and measured. Changing organisations' and professions' normal functions involves goal-setting, monitoring of performance, and continuous nutrition promotion activities.

There is considerable tension between health promoters who advocate top-down and bottom-up approaches. Fortunately, in recent years, there has been some rapprochement between the two positions, greater emphasis being placed on formative and process evaluation and the use of a wider range of theories to guide interventions (Sorenson et al. 1998, Thompson et al. 2003, Dooris 2005). Indeed, recent developments emphasise the importance of achieving sufficient dosages of interventions through the use of multiple methods, multiple components at multiple societal levels (individuals, small social groups, settings and systems like regions and states) to reach as wide a section of population as possible in order to change the prevalence of disease and health indices Thompson et al. (1993). The outlook in community health (and nutrition) promotion has become more optimistic with the realisation that small changes in social health norms have cumulative effects over decades (Sorenson et al. 1998) and seemingly small changes in individuals' behaviours and health are, as Rose (Rose 1985) noted long ago associated with major changes in population health.

Criteria for change

Whichever paradigm is employed (or a mix of all three), there are several criteria that can be used to judge the adequacy of any nutrition promotion programme. The various paradigms differ in the ways they meet these criteria. Glasgow and colleagues (1999), have described some of these criteria which are outlined in Box 17.1.

Box 17.1

The RE-AIM Framework

There are five dimensions in this framework that should be present in a public health or health promotion programme:

1. *Reach:* The proportion of individuals in a population that are involved in the programme as well as their degree of disease risk. Ideally, everyone in the population at risk should be reached, but especially those at high or moderate risk.

2. *Efficacy:* The degree to which the intervention brings about effects. There can be negative as well as positive outcomes. The side effects of drugs for example are well known, but even the labelling of someone as 'at high risk of heart disease', say, can have negative social or psychological consequences. Promoters have to be certain that the harm caused by a programme does not outweigh its benefits, or that the harm caused is not too large.

3. *Adoption:* The proportion of individuals and settings (like worksites) that adopt a programme. Barriers to adoption need to be examined when non-participating settings or individuals are assessed.

4. *Implementation:* The extent to which a programme is delivered as intended. It is distinguished from effectiveness, which is how well the programme is conducted by individuals who are not specialised research staff in real-life settings. Effectiveness can be defined as implementation × efficacy. At the individual level, this is called 'adherence' to programme regimens. At the setting level, it is the extent to which staff members deliver the programme as intended by the designers.

5. *Maintenance:* The length of time that the changes brought about by the programme last. At the individual level, this is indicated by relapse rates. At the setting level, it is the extent of institutionalisation, which Glasgow and colleagues define as 'the extent to which a health promotion practice or policy becomes routine and part of everyday culture and norms of an organisation'.

The product of these five dimensions is the public health impact score.

Source: Glasgow et al. 1999

Settings for nutrition promotion

Nutrition promotion, like other forms of health promotion, generally takes place in social and physical settings. Like the swings and roundabouts in a fairground, it is likely that sooner or later most people will enter the influence of several settings. Therefore, it is important to make as many relevant settings as possible that are supportive of healthy food choices. Ideally, actions taken in different settings should be congruent with each other (Dooris 2005), for example, food polices adopted by preschools should be reinforced and supported by those adopted in schools, retail outlets, the mass media and health services, among others. This rarely happens — it requires some degree of government leadership and statewide policymaking. Most health promotion, then, occurs only within specific settings, not between them.

By far the most studied settings include places where pregnant women, lactating mothers and children receive health or education services, such as antenatal clinicians, hospital outpatients, childcare centres, preschools and schools. However, nutrition promotion also takes place in a huge variety of additional settings, such as worksites, local government centres, retail shops and food service outlets, transport hubs and community centres of various types (as in scout halls, refuges, churches, libraries, etc.). Finally, the mass media and the internet reach people in their own homes, and can have a strong influence that may interact with that of other settings.

Antenatal clinics, maternity hospitals and birthing centres, and the care of pregnant and lactating women

The nutritional quality of the maternal can have life-long effects on the child's health (Moore & Davies 2001). Pregnancy is a life stage when many women try to improve the nutritional quality of their diets. Therefore, this is a useful stage of life full of teachable moments. There is strong evidence that education programmes conducted during this period bring about changes in attitude and in lactation practices (Worsley & Crawford 2005). This stage of life and its associated professional settings have much potential for nutrition promotion. This should elicit the support of fathers and other adult family members, as well as changes in the external transport and food services environments (McIntyre et al. 1999). The Australian government, for example, provides kits for businesses to help them provide wholesome places for mothers to breastfeed their babies. The kits provide signs to identify business such as restaurants and transport hubs as baby friendly (that is, they allow breastfeeding).

Maternal and child health centres, and professional and industry nutrition information services

Many parents, especially new parents of young infants, ask for advice from these agencies to help them deal with problems such as food refusal and fussy eating. The communication of basic behavioural and nutritional principles can do much to help parents establish healthy eating habits in their children. The

British Food Dudes programme (Lowe et al. 2001) is a good example of such communication. Commercial nutrition information services operated by food companies have come under a cloud recently because of their possible conflict of interest (such as the promotion of the companies' products). However, many people access their helplines, and many provide sound information. A good example of a non-profit internet site is <www.healthyeatingclub.com>.

Long daycare centres, preschool centres and kindergartens

Staff in these centres know the concerns of parents and, unlike many other prac-titioners, they usually feed the children. The Western Australian Department of Health's carer training and accreditation programme enables carers to provide parents with practical behavioural and nutritional advice about feeding children (Pollard et al. 2001). This has been taken up in Victoria through the Start Right, Eat Right programme. There is a great need in these settings for strong nutrition promotion among staff and parents.

Primary and secondary schools

Interventions that directly involve parents or which change the food school supply are probably more effective than those, which are based solely on class-room activities. However, even short-term interventions can alter children's food choices (Worsley & Crawford 2005). In most countries, national nutrition educa-tion curricula are implemented in many primary schools, but usually their long-term effects have not been evaluated. The amount of effort spent on nutri-tion education, food preparation and tasting experience varies widely.

School settings are ripe for the implementation of total quality management (TQM) techniques. The development of the Health Promoting School (Nutbeam & St Ledger 1997) and of school food and canteen policies related to the WHO FRESH programme (Focusing Resources on Effective School Health <http://www.freshschools.org/>) are perhaps the beginning of this approach. The school support network developed by the New South Wales School Canteen Association is a useful model <http://www.schoolcanteens.org.au/>. The rising numbers of out-of-school-hours' care programmes are excellent vehicles for nutrition and physical activity promotion (van Herwerden et al. 2006). Recent changes in the United Kingdom, mandating healthy eating skills education for schoolchildren and healthy eating programmes and resources for school canteen managers may signal major changes in the settings.

American research suggests that there are major opportunities to promote healthy eating in secondary schools, particularly through adolescent-directed programmes. French's study of the content and prices of vending machine foods in Minnesota schools illustrates the importance of school food services (French et al. 2001).

Community settings — sports and leisure clubs

There are major opportunities for community network building between food producers, food markets, retailers, schools and consumer and ecology groups. Nutrition promoters can rapidly build effective partnerships within local communities for a variety of purposes. Local councils can foster food markets, community gardens, and local horticultural production. A good example is the South Australian Eat Well network.

Workplace settings

Many employees who consume foods and beverages during working hours wish to eat healthier meals. Excellent worksite programmes have been developed in the United States, partly because of favourable company tax regimes (Sorenson et al. 1999). Worksites present major opportunities for effective nutrition promotion.

Retail outlets such as supermarkets and fruit and vegetable markets

The nutritional quality of populations' diets reflect the food products stocked in local supermarkets (Cheadle et al. 1995). Prominent examples of retail nutrition promotion programmes include Tesco in the United Kingdom and Giant Foods in the United States. Supermarket tours, signage, cooking demonstrations and product formulation are some of the ways in which retailers can guide shoppers to healthier purchases.

The mass media

The media are pervasive and persuasive. There are major issues over the regulation of children's food advertising and marketing in many countries (Story & French 2004). A recent study suggests that most Australian consumers would prefer reductions in confectionery and fast-food advertising, and increases in the advertising of healthier foods (like fruit and vegetables), perhaps via government subsidies (Worsley 2006).

Communication and the food consumer

There are many influences on food consumers' daily behaviours that are integral to nutrition promotion. In this overview, it is only possible to indicate them and to suggest further reading. Key issues to understand are as follows.

[443]

Consumers' knowledge and beliefs about food and health
An example of this would be parents of young children are highly concerned about the effects of possible pesticide contamination on their children's health. Table 17.2 shows lay people's typical food and health concerns in South Australia in 1991 and 1999.

Consumers' sources of information about nutrition and their trust in these sources
Table 17.3 shows that they trust orthodox sources a lot (though not completely), and also that they use many sources. Nutrition promoters have opportunities to influence these opinion leaders.

Table 17.2 Consumers' rankings of the importance of food and health concerns in 1999 and 1991, South Australia

Food concerns	1999 importance ranking	1991 importance ranking
Clean handling of food in shops	1	3
The honesty of food labels	2	4
Harmful bacteria in food	3	2
The microbiological safety of imported foods	4	12
The safety of drinking water	5	10
Enforcement of food regulations	6	6
The safety of takeaway foods	7	18
Animal cruelty in food production	8	19
Chemical additives in foods	9	1
TV advertising of junk food to children	10	16
Eating too many fatty foods	11	9
Genetic modification of foods	12	—
Uncertainty about what is in foods	13	15
The cost of basic foods	14	5
Poverty in Australia	15	11
The links between food and cancer	16	8
The irradiation of foods	17	14
The links between food and heart disease	18	13
Importing of foreign food products	19	17
Driftnet fishing	20	7

Source: Worsley, unpublished data

Table 17.3 Consumers' trust in sources of nutrition information

	% Trust women	% Trust men	p
Mass media sources			
Advertising (TV, radio, magazine ads, etc.)	22	15	0.047
Television programmes	36	31	ns
Radio programmes	26	29	ns
Articles in women's magazines	33	18	0.0001
Newspaper articles	33	27	0.039
Articles in cooking magazines	54	49	ns
Food labels	46	37	0.008
Social sources			
Friends	43	36	ns
Family	55	57	ns
Workmates	23	14	0.0001
Teachers/school/higher education	29	21	0.052
Alternative sources			
Health food shops/staff	39	26	0.0001
Alternative health practitioners	39	34	ns
Articles in vegetarian magazines	29	29	ns
Articles in health magazines	54	49	ns
Slimming clubs	17	10	ns
Articles in cooking magazines	54	49	ns
Articles in women's magazines	33	18	0.0001
Specialist sources			
Articles in science magazines	37	39	ns
Articles in sports magazines	18	20	ns
Books	49	42	ns
Articles in health magazines	54	ns	ns
Radio programmes	26	29	ns
Newspaper articles	33	27	0.039
Orthodox health sources			
Dietitians/nutritionists	74	69	ns
National Heart Foundation/Anti-Cancer Foundation	85	80	ns
Doctors (medical)	83	81	ns
Food labels and other sources			
Food labels	46	37	0.008
Internet	4	5	0.04
Slimming clubs	17	10	0.0001
Teachers/school/higher education	29	21	0.052

Source: Worsley & Lea 2003

The primary influence of social ideologies

Food consumers are engaged in social discourses that encompass values, beliefs, and social practices. These social ideologies are likely to influence consumer's use of foods (and thus their responses to nutrition communications). Common examples include equity and gender egalitarianism; nature and the environment; the cult of appearance and the tyranny of slenderness; purity and cleanliness; and materialism. Each of these social ideologies appears to be associated with different dietary patterns, for example people who strongly believe in gender equity tend to adopt diets containing little meat, those who subscribe to the tyranny of slenderness may be more likely to adopt slimming diets (Worsley & Skrzypiec 1997). Nutrition promoters need to take these worldviews into account in design of communications.

The status and role of food and nutrition knowledge

In dietary change this requires careful consideration; greater emphasis on the communication of procedural knowledge (how-to information) appears to be indicated rather than accurate declarative knowledge that may not be relevant to consumers' daily needs (Worsley 2002a; Worsley 2002b).

Conclusion

Promotion and communication is an integral and rapidly developing component of public health nutrition. It is changing as the evidence base for nutrition science develops in a number of directions. The advent of functional foods and eco-nutrition present two divergent directions challenging nutrition promotion. As one theme in the broader health promotion and public health disciplines, nutrition promotion and communication is becoming increasingly methodologically sophisticated and effective. The challenge it faces is to provide effective solutions to the daily problems populations encounter with the food system.

REFERENCES

Ajzen, I. 1991, 'The theory of planned behaviour' in *Organizational Behaviour and Human Decision Processes*, vol. 50, pp. 179–211.
Allen, M.W., Wilson, M., Ng, S.H. and Dunne, M. 2000, 'Values and beliefs of vegetarians and omnivores' in *Journal of Social Psychology*, vol. 140, no. 4, pp. 405–22.

Bandura, A. 1986, *Social Foundations of Thought and Action: A Social Cognitive Theory*, Prentice Hall, Englewood Cliffs, New Jersey.

Biener, L., Glanz, K., McLerran, D., Sorensen, G., Thompson, B., Basen-Engquist, K., Linnan, L. and Varnes, J. 1999, 'Impact of the Working Well Trial on the work-site smoking and nutrition environment' in *Health Education and Behavior*, vol. 26, no. 4, pp. 478–94.

Birch, L.L. 1999, 'Development of food preference' in *Annual Review of Nutrition*, vol. 19, pp. 41–62.

Cheadle, A., Psaty, B., Diehr, P., Koepsell, T., Wagner, E., Curry, S. and Kristal, A. 1995, 'Evaluating community-based nutrition programs: Comparing grocery store and individual-level survey measures of program impact' in *Preventive Medicine*, vol. 24, pp. 71–79.

Ciliska, D., Miles, E., O'Brien, M.A. and Turl, C. 2000, 'Effectiveness of community-based interventions to increase fruit and vegetable consumption' in *Journal of Society for Nutrition Education*, vol. 32, pp. 341–52.

Diamond, J. 1998, *Guns, Germs and Steel*, Vintage, Random House, London.

Dooris, M. 2005, 'Healthy settings: challenges to generating evidence of effectiveness' in *Health Promotion International*, vol. 21, pp. 55–65.

Fischler, C. 1980, 'Food habits, social change and the nature/culture dilemma' in *Social Science Information*, vol. 19, no. 6, pp. 937–53.

Foley, R.M. and Pollard, C.M. 1998, 'Food Cent$: Implementing and evaluating a nutrition education project focusing on value for money' in *Australian and New Zealand Journal of Public Health*, vol. 22, pp. 494–501.

French, S.A., Jeffrey, R.W., Story, M., Breitlow, K.K., Baxter, J.S., Hannan, P. and Snyder, M.P. 2001, 'Pricing and promotion effects on low-fat vending snack purchases: The CHIPS study' in *American Journal of Public Health*, vol. 91, pp. 112–17.

Furst, T., Connors, M., Bisogni, C.A., Sobal, J. and Falk, L.W. 1996, 'Food choice: A conceptual model of the process' in *Appetite*, vol. 23, no. 3, pp. 247–66.

Glasgow, R.E., Vogt, T.M., Boles, S.M. 1999, 'Evaluating the public health impact of health promotion interventions: The RE-AIM Framework' in *American Journal of Public Health*, vol. 89, pp. 1322–27.

Glass, T.A. and McAtee, M.J. 2006, 'Behavioral science at the crossroads in public health: Extending the horizons, envisioning the future' in *Social Science and Medicine*, vol. 62, pp. 1650–71.

Green, L. and Kreuter, M. 1991, 'Health promotion planning: An educational and environmental approach' (second edition), Mayfield Publishing Company, Mountain View, California.

Grunert, K.G., Brunso, K. and Bisp, S. 1997, 'Food-related lifestyle: Development of a cross-culturally valid instrument for market surveillance' in Kahle, L.R. and Chiagouris, L. (eds) 1997, *Values, Lifestyles and Psychographics*, Lawrence Erlbaum Associates, New Jersey, pp. 337–54.

Gussow, J.D. and Contento, I. 1984, 'Nutrition education in a changing world' in *World Review of Nutrition and Dietetics*, vol. 44, pp. 1–56.

Horwath, C.C. 1999, 'Applying the transtheoretical model to eating behaviour change: Challenges and opportunities' in *Nutrition Research Reviews*, vol. 12, pp. 281–317.

Janz, N.K. and Becker, M.N. 1984, 'The Health Belief Model: A decade later' in *Health Education Quarterly*, vol. 11, pp. 1–47.

Johnson, D.W. and Johnson, R. 1985, 'Nutrition education: A model for effectiveness; a synthesis of research' in *Journal of Nutrition Education*, vol. 17, no. 2, pp. S1–24.

Kent, L. and Worsley, A. 2005, 'A sentinel study of trends in coronary heart disease risk factors in Australia', proceedings of Nutrition Society of Australia, Melbourne, December.

Kuhn, T. 1962, *The Structure of Scientific Revolutions*, University of Chicago Press.

Lowe, C., Horne, P., Bowsery, M., Egerton, C. and Tapper, K. 2001, 'Increasing children's consumption of fruit and vegetables' in *Public Health Nutrition*, vol. 4, pp. 387–93.

McIntyre, E., Turnbull, D. and Hiller, J.E. 1999, 'Breastfeeding in public places' in *Journal of Human Lactation*, vol. 15, no. 2, pp. 131–35.

Moore, V. and Davies, M. 2001, 'Lifecycle nutrition and cardiovascular health' in *Asia Pacific Journal of Clinical Nutrition*, vol. 10, pp. 113–17.

Nutbeam, D. and Harris, E. 2003, *Theory in a Nutshell: A guide to health promotion theory* (second edition), McGraw Hill, Sydney.

Nutbeam, D. and St. Ledger, L. 1997, *Priorities for research into health promoting schools in Australia*, Australian Health Promoting Schools Association, University of Sydney.

Pollard, C., Lewis, J. and Miller, M. 2001, 'Start Right–Eat Right award scheme: Implementing food and nutrition policy in child care centers' in *Health Education & Behaviour*, vol. 28, no. 3, pp. 320–30.

Prochaska, J. and DiClemente, C. 1984, *The Transtheoretical approach: Crossing traditional boundaries of therapy*, Dow Jones-Irwin, Homewood, Illonois.

Puska, P., Salonen, J.T., Nissinen, A., Tuomilehto, J. and Vartianinen, E., Korhonen, H., Tanskanen, A., Rönnqvist, P., Koskela, K. and Huttunen, J. 1983, 'Change in risk factors for coronary heart disease during 10 years of a community intervention program (North Karelia project)' in *British Medical Journal*, vol. 267, pp. 1840–44.

Rose, G. 1995, 'Sick individuals and sick population' in *International Journal of Epidemiology*, vol. 14, pp. 32–38.

Shaddish, W.R., Cook, T. and Campbell, D.T. 2002, *Experimental and Quasi-Experimental Designs for Generalized Causal Inference*, Houghton Mifflin, New York.

Sorensen, G., Stoddard, A., Peterson, K., Cohen, N., Hunt, M.K., Stein, E., Palombo, R. and Lederman, R. 1999, 'Increasing fruit and vegetable consumption through worksites and families in the Treatwell 5-a-Day Study' in *American Journal of Public Health*, vol. 89, pp. 54–60.

Sorenson, G., Emmons, K., Hunt, M.K. and Johnson, D. 1998, 'Implications of the results of community intervention trials' in *Annual Review of Public Health*, vol. 19, pp. 379–416.

Story, M. and French, S. 2004, 'Food advertising and marketing directed at children and adolescents in the US' in *International Journal of Behavioural Nutrition and Physical Activity*, vol. 1, pp. 3, 1–17.

Swinburn, B., Egger, G. and Raza, F. 1999, 'Dissecting obesogenic environments: The development and application of a framework for identifying and prioritizing environmental interventions for obesity' in *Preventive Medicine*, vol. 29, pp. 563–70.

Tansey, G. and Worsley, A. 1995, *The food system: A user's guide*, Earthscan, London.

Tapper, K., Horne, P.J. and Lowe, C.F. 2003, 'Food dudes to the rescue' in *The Psychologist*, vol. 16, pp. 18–21.

Thompson, B., Coronado, G., Snipes, S.A. and Puschel, K. 2003, 'Methodologic advances and ongoing challenges in designing community-based health promotion programs' in *Annual Review of Public Health*, vol. 24, pp. 315–49.

van Herwerden, E., Cooper, C., Flanagan, C., Crawford, D. and Worsley, A. 2006, 'Food and activity in out of school hours care in Australia' in *Nutrition & Dietetics*, vol. 63, pp. 21–27.

Wass, A. 1994, *Promoting Health: The primary health care approach*, W.B. Saunders Bailliere Tindall, Sydney.

World Health Organization (WHO) 1986, *Ottawa Charter for Health Promotion*, First International Conference on Health Promotion, Ottawa, 21 November, WHO, Geneva.

Worsley, A. 2002a, 'Nutrition knowledge and food behaviour' in *Asia Pacific Journal of Clinical Nutrition*, vol. 11, pp. S579–85.

—— 2002b, 'Nutrition communication: Is a new approach needed?' in *Asia Pacific Journal of Clinical Nutrition*, vol. 11, pp. S6, S202–06.

—— 2006, 'Lay people's views of school food policy options: associations with confidence, personal values and demographics' in *Journal of Health Education: Theory and Practice* (online journal), doi.10.1093/her/cy1138.

Worsley, A. and Crawford, D. 2005, *Review of Children's Healthy Eating Interventions*, Department of Human Services Victoria, Melbourne.

Worsley, A. and Lea, E. 2003, 'Personal values and consumers' trust in sources of nutrition information' in *Ecology of Food and Nutrition*, vol. 42, pp. 129–51.

Worsley, A. and Skrzypiec, G. 1997, 'Teenage vegetarianism: Beauty or the beast?' in *Nutrition Research*, vol. 17, no. 3, pp. 391–404.

Worsley, A., Coonan, W. and Worsley, A.J. 1987, 'The first Body Owner's Programme: An integrated school-based physical and nutrition education programme' in *Health Promotion*, vol. 2, pp. 39–49.

18

Policy and politics

Mark Lawrence

Have you ever wondered why nutrition recommendations and actions might be made in one situation, yet in another seemingly identical situation nothing happens, or the recommendations and actions might be quite different? How are such recommendations and actions decided? Who decides? Where and when can they be influenced? Understanding the answers to these types of questions requires specialised knowledge and practical skills in policy and politics.

There is a diversity of definitions for the term 'policy'. At its simplest, policy is what governments choose to do or not to do (Dye, 2002). In this chapter, public health nutrition policy is defined as, 'a statement of values, beliefs and intentions towards shaping the food and nutrition system to achieve a public health nutrition outcome(s)'. Throughout this book, various principles, populations and priorities have been analysed in relation to public health nutrition. Public health nutrition policy provides the framework of values, beliefs and intentions for putting these analyses into practice.

This chapter is designed as a primer for public health nutrition policy practice. In the space available it is not possible to provide a detailed 'how to' guide for planning, implementing and evaluating policy activities. Instead, the aims are to provide the reader with an introduction to policy science theory and offer professional insights to assist with policy practice. These aims are pursued by adopting a critical analysis perspective, for example, encouraging the reader to ask 'how?' and 'why?' questions about policymaking and policy outcomes. The chapter starts with an examination of why public health nutrition policy is important and the policy setting where policy development takes place. Then the political underpinnings vital to understanding how and why policy is made are analysed. Finally, the professional skills of policy science research and advocacy that are important for applying this knowledge to policy practice are briefly reviewed.

Why is public health nutrition policy important?

Increasingly, governments, non-government organisations and the private sector are developing policies addressing issues as diverse as promoting food security in vulnerable communities through to restricting the availability of soft drinks in school canteens as a means to help prevent obesity. Public health nutrition policy is important because the issues it might address contribute to promoting:

- a nutritionally adequate and accessible food supply
- a safe food supply
- a dietary intake that is associated with reduced risk of diet-related chronic diseases.

In accordance with these important reasons, the cornerstones for public health nutrition policy are the reference standards for nutrient intakes and dietary goals and guidelines examined in chapter 3 of this book.

The human, social and economic costs of ignoring public health nutrition problems are substantial. The 2002 World Health Report documents that six of the top ten causes of poor health globally are food related (WHO 2002). In the United Kingdom it has been estimated that food-related ill health is responsible for about ten per cent of morbidity and mortality and the cost to the national health system is twice the amount attributable to car, train, and other accidents, and more than twice that attributable to smoking (Rayner & Scarborough 2005). The vast majority of the burden is attributable to unhealthy diets rather than to food-borne diseases. In Australia, the annual economic cost of diet-related chronic diseases is approximately $6 billion (NHMRC 2003).

Where is public health nutrition policy made?

There are many policy activities that can create the conditions and circumstances most conducive for achieving public health nutrition outcomes. In order to improve policy practice and outcomes we need to be aware of the institutional structures and management procedures where policy activities take place, that is, the policy setting. In this section the nature and scope of the setting for public health nutrition policy activities are examined within government primarily. This examination is structured around viewing the policy setting as being both inter-sectoral in nature and with a scope that operates across multiple levels of government.

The inter-sectoral nature of the policy setting

Typically, public health nutrition policy has been, and is, initiated and overseen by the health sector of government (Lawrence 1987). A key motivation for such activity is that it is the health sector within government that bears primary responsibility for addressing the burden of nutritional health problems in society. However, there is an inherent dilemma with this approach to policy practice. The health sector has limited capacity for exerting leverage over the food and nutrition system where many of the determinants of public health nutrition are located. Instead, responsibility for many of these determinants rests with non-health sectors within and outside government.

Government departments with significant influence over the food and nutri-tion system include agriculture (production and processing of food), trade (food import/export), transport (transport and storage of food), finance (taxes on food) and education (curriculum development and training). The non-government sectors that influence the food and nutrition system include consumer groups, farmers, food manufacturers, retailers, academia, media and marketers. This situation highlights the importance of an inter-sectoral approach to policy-making in which all sectors (public and private) associated with the food and nutrition system are engaged in a coherent fashion to promote public health nutrition outcomes.

In her comparative review of public health nutrition policy activities across twelve countries, Robertson (2006) identified that inter-sectoral collaboration was a vital ingredient for the successful implementation of policy. Without inter-sectoral collaboration, policy is non-sustainable and the goodwill that may be present in its development can rapidly dissipate and for this reason many well-intentioned policy documents have quickly become 'dust collectors' on authorities' and professionals' shelves.

In recognition of the inter-sectoral nature of jurisdictional responsibility for factors that influence health, the World Health Organization (WHO) proposed the 'building of healthy public policy' as the first strategy in its Ottawa Charter for Health Promotion (WHO 1986). Healthy public policy places responsibility on policymakers in all government sectors to be accountable for the health impact of their policy decisions and factor health benefits and costs into their policy deliberations. The coordination of inter-sectoral collaboration requires political will and leadership. Walt (1996) suggests that the level of political will for a policy issue often relates to where it sits in relation to a hierarchy of 'high politics' (macro policies such as major economic agendas) and 'low politics' (specific sectoral interests). For this reason, it would be highly desirable in the future to locate coordinating responsibility for public health nutrition policy at the central or cabinet level of government to achieve a whole-of-government commitment to the policy.

The multiple levels of government associated with the policy setting
Responsibilities for components of the food and nutrition system that impact on public health nutrition occur at several levels of governance. Broadly, there are four levels of government with powers that can be exerted to influence the conditions and circumstances that help determine public health nutrition: the local, state/regional, national, and international levels. A coordinated approach to policy development and implementation across all four levels of government is required to deliver complementary activities to promote public health nutrition. Selected examples of policy activities that may occur at each of these four government levels are listed below.

Local government
Local government policy activities might include town planning approvals for fast-food outlets and/or farmers' markets, campaigns and education activities to promote public health nutrition and inspecting compliance with safety regulations in food premises. In addition, locally-based institutions such as schools and nursing homes may develop their own policies directed at food service and education activities to promote the nutritional health of their students and/or residents and/or staff.

Local government provides the umbrella for food policy councils (and coalitions). Generally, the purpose of food policy councils is to identify and implement improvements in and access to the local food supply. The Penrith food policy council was described in chapter 15. Another successful example is the Toronto food policy council (TFPC), which has been operating since the early 1990s as a sub-committee of the Toronto Board of Health (see <http://www.toronto.ca/health/tfpc_index.htm>). The membership of the TPFC includes city councillors and representatives from consumer, business, farm, faith, and community development groups, who work on a diversity of projects ranging from agricultural land preservation and urban planning to food waste recovery and community gardens.

State/regional government

Government responsibilities at the state/regional level will vary from country to country depending upon the nature of overall governance arrangements. For example, in Australia when the former separate colonies were united at the beginning of the twentieth century to form the Commonwealth of Australia, the constitution specified a separation of powers between the commonwealth and the states. Generally, responsibility for key aspects of public health nutrition policy areas, such as health and education services, remained with state governments — many food service and nutrition education activities in schools reflect state and regional government policy programs.

National government

Generally, national governments are responsible for the regulatory regimes for food production, labelling, composition, advertising, transport, pricing and taxes and retail. Policy responsibilities also include the development and implementation of both reference standards for nutrient intakes, dietary goals and guidelines, and national food and nutrition monitoring and surveillance systems.

International governance

At the international level, the WHO has assumed a leadership role in public health nutrition policy with the launching of its Global Strategy on Diet, Physical Activity and Health (WHO 2004). In addition, the food and nutrition system is global in its scope and food trade is becoming a major component of the global economy. Various international agreements and administering bodies have been established with legal authority to manage this food trade and these have a strong bearing on food supply and access at national, state and local level. It is the World Trade Organization's (WTO) agreement on agriculture, agreement on technical barriers to trade and agreement on sanitary and phytosanitary measures (with its linkage to the Codex Alimentarius Commission) that are among the strongest influences on public health nutrition from the international level of governance (Lawrence 2005).

This analysis of the inter-sectoral nature and multiple levels of governance to the policy setting highlights the importance of pursuing activities that are collaborative and multi-faceted if we are to avoid fragmented and/or contradictory policies. However, this is no easy task to achieve in practice. Policy analysts frequently identify that policy outcomes represent a compromise of contested views among different sectors and levels of government. Case study 18.1 illustrates a fragmented and contested approach to public health nutrition policymaking.

CASE STUDY 18.1

THE CONTESTED NATURE OF POLICYMAKING

This case study outlines a debate associated firstly with the relationship between sugar and health and subsequently with the setting of a dietary target for sugar for the 2004 WHO Global Strategy on Diet, Physical Activity and Health (WHO 2004).

The joint Food and Agriculture Organization/World Health Organization (FAO/WHO) Expert Consultation on Carbohydrates in Human Nutrition was held in Rome in April 1997. The Report (FAO 1998), made a number of useful contributions, particularly in clarifying the classification of carbohydrates and their role in the maintenance of human health. Unfortunately these positive aspects have to a considerable extent been eclipsed by the debate which ensued regarding the extent to which sugar (sucrose) might be detrimental to human health.

The draft report (written by an FAO consultant) appeared on the FAO website prior to it being signed off by the members of the consultation. The wording with regard to sugar was somewhat ambiguous in this draft report. It was first cited by someone who had also acted as a consultant to FAO at a sugar producer's conference in Fiji, and then was widely quoted subsequently throughout the world as clearly exonerating sugar from any serious adverse effects on human health.

Some members of the consultation complained to the director general of FAO that their views had been misrepresented. Much discussion followed and the final text was modified somewhat prior to final publication of the report. The recommendations which related to sugar, as they appeared in the text, are as follows:

> There is no evidence of a direct involvement of sucrose, other sugars and starch in the etiology of lifestyle-related diseases. [However] excess energy intake in any form will cause body fat accumulation, so that excess consumption of low fat foods, while not as obesity-producing as excess consumption of high fat products, will lead to obesity if energy expenditure is not increased. Excessive intakes of sugar which compromise micronutrient density should be avoided.

While these statements are perhaps not as clear as they might have been, as is often the case with statements requiring agreement by a committee, they certainly cannot be regarded as exonerating sugar from all ill effects. The relevant sentences might perhaps have read:

> While sugars have not been directly implicated as a cause of coronary heart disease or diabetes, excessive intakes in sugary drinks, energy dense foods or in other added forms contribute to overweight and obesity by promoting energy intakes in excess of

requirements. As a cause of obesity they may indeed contribute to the chronic diseases associated with excess adiposity.

This was certainly the intention behind the discussions.

For several years after its appearance the report continued to be quoted as an authoritative reference by those wishing to argue against any recommendation relating to the restriction of sugars. The WHO Technical Report 916 based on an Expert Consultation on Diet, Nutrition and the Prevention of Chronic Diseases recommended a restriction of free sugars to no more than ten per cent total energy (WHO 2003). The governments of the United States and several other countries objected to this recommendations as well as the incorporation of advice to reduce free sugars into the WHO Global Strategy on Diet, Physical Activity and Health, citing lack of evidence and the conclusions of the Carbohydrates in Human Nutrition report.

It was the BBC's 'Panorama' television programme which first revealed the attempts by organisations associated with industries linked with production or consumption of sugar to influence the process of the consultation. Correspondence, presumably leaked from within FAO, revealed offers of financial support for the consultation and responses from officials assuring an outcome which would satisfy the sponsors. The revelations led to an inquiry within FAO, an assurance that processes would be put in place to avoid a recurrence, and an update of important issues relating to carbohydrates in human health was then undertaken under the auspices of WHO and FAO in July 2006.

Source: Jim Mann, personal communication

The relationship between sugar and health might appear to be a rather innocuous topic for analysing the contested nature of policymaking, however, Mann's description of events in this case study provides the following insights into the potential for a fragmented approach to policymaking in the food and nutrition system.

A lack of inter-sectoral collaboration during the policymaking process
There were contested sectoral interests at two levels: firstly between industries linked with production or consumption of sugar and the WHO, and secondly between different agencies (FAO and WHO) within the United Nations.

The disjointed nature of the relationship among different levels of government
Certain national governments, such as the United States, exerted substantial pressure on the international level of governance to have their view represented

in the development of the WHO Global Strategy on Diet, Physical Activity and Health; that is a policy document for all national governments. For more information on the political activities of the United States government in this policymaking episode, see chapter 9 and the relevant newsroom release from Center for Science in the Public Interest (2004).

The hidden nature of conflict

Much of the contested nature of this policy debate was hidden behind subtleties, conducted under the guise of scientific discourse, for example, debates over the use of terms such as 'sugar', 'sucrose' or 'free sugars', and wording such as 'moderate intake', or 'restrict intake'. A danger of such debates is ambiguity in the resulting policy document, which leaves citizens confused and with the perception that scientists and governments cannot agree among themselves about the preferred policy.

The politics of public health nutrition policy

Public health nutrition policy is political in the sense that various stakeholders will have different understandings and expectations for its purpose and recommendations. Moreover, many stakeholders have competing values, beliefs and interests towards how the food and nutrition system should be shaped to achieve policy objectives. According to Tansey (1994):

> . . . ensuring a well-nourished world is primarily a political and economic problem concerning power and control over a range of resources and the distribution of benefits arising from their use . . . The food system, in reality, is not driven by nutritional but market and competitive needs.

Leading food policy analysts observe that there are disputes, negotiations and compromises over how food-related policies are made (Cannon 1987; Nestle 2002; Lang & Heasman 2004). Invariably, policy affects different stakeholders in different ways, or as Lasswell (1936) observed, politics is about who gets what, when and how. The competition among stakeholders over public health nutrition policy is resolved through political processes. Therefore, as Coveney (2003) comments, if we want to better understand the relationship between food policy and public health, 'we would do well to focus less on food policies per se and more on the politics of food'.

Politics influences the way that stakeholders frame problems, identify where responsibility for a problem might rest and the preferred policy instruments to address a problem. Invariably, stakeholders attempt to influence the definition of problems, the interpretation of policy objectives and the setting of policy agendas in accordance with their values, beliefs and interests. For example, many people have differing views towards the best approach to improve the nutritional adequacy of children's diets. While some people believe that government should invest more resources in educating children to eat more fruit and vegetables, others believe that policy also should focus on social and equity considerations, including making the environmental circumstances, such as the price of particular foods, more conducive to healthy decisions (Caraher & Coveney 2004; Robertson et al. 2006).

The choice of policy instruments available to government is also a source of political debate. A government may decide to rely on the free market, the use of persuasion and/or the use of regulation to solve policy problems. These are not random decisions. Milio (1990) states policy instruments, or tools, have different political and economic costs. She refers to instruments such as education or campaigns as important but nonetheless 'soft' or politically weak instruments. Conversely, 'hard' policy instruments include economic instruments such as the introduction of taxes and price controls on energy dense foods and subsidising the cost of healthful foods (Goodman & Anise 2006).

Recently, there have been calls for government to use harder policy instruments such as the law and regulation as instruments of public health nutrition policy to fight obesity (Mello et al. 2006). For example, many practitioners believe that the advertising of soft drinks to children either on television or in sponsorship of sports activities is contributing to obesity and should be restricted (Nestle 2006). In their research analysing thirteen potential obesity prevention policy interventions, Haby and colleagues (2006) reported that the greatest health benefit is likely to be achieved by the reduction of television advertising of high fat and/or high sugar foods and drinks to children.

Generally governments are required to undertake policymaking within the context of dominant political ideologies as well as competing food-related agendas from both within and external to government. The existence of differing ideologies and competing agendas among stakeholders provides fertile ground for politics in public health nutrition policy. An example of the influence of ideology is the debate about individual responsibility for healthy eating versus governmental responsibility to intervene in the food and nutrition system to help make healthier choices easier choices. The influence of competing food-related agendas within government is clearly illustrated with the co-existence of support for trade in highly processed snack foods that are high in salt, fat and sugar, while at the same time promoting dietary guideline messages that encourage the consumption of core (or minimally processed) foods and sustainable production practices.

The different ways that public health nutrition issues can be framed, the point of responsibility attributed and the preferred policy instrument selected, is illustrated in Case study 18.2.

The case study illustrates the different:

- ways that stakeholders frame the policy problem of the obesity epidemic and in particular whether it is primarily due to a lack of physical activity or dietary imbalance
- views of stakeholders regarding who is responsible for solving the obesity epidemic, either: individuals, food manufacturers, parents, or government
- ideological views towards the preferred policy instrument to address the problem and in particular whether government should regulate food marketing and availability to children or instead if it should focus on providing education and encouraging parental discipline.

Professional practice skills

Public health nutrition policy practice involves more than simply obtaining evidence and translating it into the ideal policy option – there is a need for special competencies to participate in policy processes. It is for this reason that public health nutrition policymaking, as with all policymaking, is both an art and a science (Milio 1988). The aim of this section is to apply the insights gained from the critical analysis approach taken throughout this chapter to introduce selected professional skills for policy practice. In particular, the focus is placed on examining policy science research and advocacy skills for policy practice.

Policy science research
Bismarck is credited with having said that there are two things that one should avoid watching being made – sausages and public policy. In a sense with public health nutrition policy research you observe both! Bismarck was alluding to the unsightliness and deft processes that lead to these two products that are then intended for public 'consumption'.

It is because of, and not in spite of, Bismarck's tongue-in-cheek comment, that public health nutrition policy research can be fascinating. Frequently there are many rich and interesting issues to observe, to analyse and to explain. There are two distinct orientations within which policy research can be undertaken

---

CASE STUDY 18.2

THE OBESITY EPIDEMIC AND THE POLITICS OF RESPONSIBILITY

This case study consists of a series of excerpts taken directly from the transcript of a documentary screened on the Australian Broadcasting Corporation's (ABC) programme 'Four Corners'. The documentary was an investigation into the obesity epidemic among Australian children and posed the question: 'Do parents need government help to control what their children eat?' The key responses to this question from different stakeholders involved in the obesity policy debate are listed.

DICK WELLS, CEO, AUSTRALIAN FOOD AND GROCERY COUNCIL:
We have 60 000 to 100 000 products on the market and that have been responding in terms of the range of low-fat, low-salt, these sorts of things. The choice is there, it's a matter of an education process for people to help them make better choices about balance in life . . . We have a role to play in addressing this issue but it's a longer-term societal issue. I think the root cause is really a lack of activity and a decline in activity by children.

PROFESSOR BOYD SWINBURN, PRESIDENT, AUSTRALIAN SOCIETY FOR STUDY OF OBESITY:
The food industry, I think, responded, initially, like big corporations would – like we saw tobacco do, like the alcohol industry do when there's a perceived external threat around products that we're producing. Then they go into denial phase and they go into obstruction phase and they go into diversion phase – 'It's physical activity, it's nothing to do with eating.' And they go into, 'We don't know the answers', 'the scientists can't agree'.

DR ROSEMARY STANTON, NUTRITIONIST:
Everybody likes to say, 'Look, it's a lack of exercise' because there's no anti-exercise brigade.

TONY ABBOTT, HEALTH MINISTER:
No one is in charge of what goes into my mouth except me. No one is in charge of what goes into kids' mouths except their parents. It is up to parents more than anyone to take this matter in hand.

BEC, PARENT:
They always put it onto the parents, 'The parents have to do this and do that'. Well, we are, but if we're not being backed up by the person we asked to run our country, then who is going to back us up?

DR MICHAEL BOOTH, DIRECTOR, NSW CENTRE FOR OVERWEIGHT AND OBESITY:
The federal government has been absolutely adamant that they will do absolutely nothing about the marketing of unhealthy junk foods to our young people. They usually start any meeting not with 'Hello', but, 'Don't ask about regulating marketing, we're not going to do it'.

ARCHIVE FOOTAGE OF JOHN HOWARD [PRIME MINISTER]:
I think governments have to be very reluctant to willingly embracing the 'nanny state', Mr Speaker.

KAYE MEHTA, CHAIR, COALITION ON ADVERTISING TO CHILDREN:
TV is often used as a nanny. We often stick children in front of the telly when parents have to do jobs, and that is perfectly reasonable. If TV was a real nanny, it would be sacked.

TONY ABBOTT, HEALTH MINISTER:
If you don't like the advertising on television, switch it off, as simple as that, watch the ABC . . . if their parents are foolish enough to feed their kids on a diet of Coca-Cola and lollies, well, they should lift their game, and lift it urgently . . . if parents don't think Coco Pops are good for their kids there's a very simple solution—don't buy it.

KAYE MEHTA, CHAIR, COALITION ON ADVERTISING TO CHILDREN:
We have regulations that were set up to protect children. But they're protecting industry, you know, big, big industries that don't need protecting, you'd think.

TONY ABBOTT, HEALTH MINISTER:
I think that it's most unwise to allow yourself to become overweight, let alone obese, and I think that all of us should seriously consider exercising more . . . But in the end, if people are obese, it's because they're eating too much or they're exercising too little, and the answer is in the hands of those individuals.

DICK WELLS, CEO, AUSTRALIAN FOOD AND GROCERY COUNCIL:
It's consumers drive this. Consumers want it, consumers buy it. We'll keep producing different products to meet that need.

Source: Fullerton 2005 (reproduced with permission)

(Parsons 1995). Firstly, there is research that is undertaken to provide evidence to help inform policy development and/or analyse systems to identify strategic approaches to know where to intervene. This is research *for* policy. The second type of research is that undertaken to increase theoretical understandings of how and why policy is made, with the aim of improving processes and ultimately policy outcomes. This is research *of* or *about* policy.

Research for policy

The purpose of research for policy is to provide information about a problem that needs to be solved and the best ways of solving it; for example, using evidence-based practice to develop, implement and evaluate policies so that they are thus better informed than they would be otherwise. Professional practice skills in evidence-based practice and project management feature prominently throughout this book and especially in chapters 1, 2, and 14 to 16. Here, the application of these professional skills to research policy is illustrated with specific reference to the work of Collins (2005).

Collins has outlined a relatively simple eight-step framework to assist in the examination of a policy issue and examine the options available to tackle the issue using the following steps:

1. define the context
2. state the problem
3. search for evidence
4. consider different policy options
5. project the outcomes
6. apply evaluative criteria
7. weigh the outcomes
8. make the decision.

A practical application of findings from an analytical process of the type outlined in Collins' framework to guide practitioners through the development of a local public health nutrition policy is provided in the British Nutrition Foundation's publication *Establishing a Whole School Food Policy* (British Nutrition Foundation 2006).

Research of policy

The principle of public health nutrition policy decisions being informed by scientific evidence, with its implicit notion of rationality and freedom from ideology, has an inherent appeal (Niessen et al. 2000). However, there is a fundamental paradox confronting evidence-based practice for public health nutrition policy. On the one hand, there is a substantial investment both in conducting research to obtain data and in developing criteria for its appraisal so as to assemble what is now an historically unprecedented body of scientific evidence.

On the other hand, there is a lack of understanding among practitioners of how and why this scientific evidence is being, or can be, applied to public health policy (Ham et al. 1995). Prominent epidemiologists have noted that epidemiology has increasingly focused on technical and methodological sophistication to the possible neglect of its more practical application to public health (Susser & Susser 1996).

The purpose of undertaking research of policy is to increase theoretical understandings of the political nature of policy and policymaking processes. The practical relevance of such theoretical understandings is that they can help explain how a political system is wired in order to know which lever to pull (Goodin 1982). Also, they can help explain decision-making processes and thereby assist in improving the translation of evidence into policy. Given the role of policy as a fundamental determinant of health, some are calling for this research orientation to be recognised as a special discipline and field of practice within the discipline of political science. The provisional name, 'health politics, the political science of health', has been suggested (Bambra et al. 2005).

The political science literature provides many theories and models to help explain how policy is made. However, there are few firm theories in the sense of being able to demonstrate both explanatory and predictive capabilities (Sabatier 1999). In this section three of these firm and more common theories and models of the policymaking process are briefly introduced and illustrated with a public health nutrition example. The three selected theories and models are: the rational-linear model; Kingdon's agenda-setting model; and the advocacy coalition framework.

The rational-linear model

Since the 1950s, when Lasswell (1951) first enunciated the policy sciences as scientific disciplines, many theories of the policymaking process have been derivative of Laswell's rational-linear model to explaining the public policy process. Laswell and his peers viewed the policy sciences as focused on investigating and explaining policymaking as a process that occurs in a rational and linear sequence of stages, or components of a policy cycle. The sequence begins with problem identification and agenda setting and moves on to policy formulation, adoption, implementation, evaluation and then the process feeds back to either identify new problems or refine policy formulation and the policy sequence continues. In its most classical form, this model is exemplified by Anderson's 'sequential pattern of action' an adaptation of which is illustrated in Figure 18.1 (Anderson 1975).

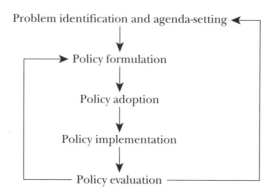

Figure 18.1 Key stages in the rational-linear model of the policymaking process

This relatively simple explanation of the policy process provides a convenient heuristic device around which many policy textbooks and courses have traditionally organised their representation of policy phenomena. The implicit assumption of policy theorists who subscribe to the rational-linear model of policymaking is that the use of evidence in decision-making involves systematic, policy relevant research being conducted by impartial scientists and then translated through a series of steps in a linear fashion to inform public policy. The development of public health nutrition policies to provide institutional feeding programmes based on nutrient reference standards is illustrative of the rational-linear stages model of policymaking.

However, the translation of the available evidence into policy practice often remains unfulfilled. For instance, why do so many scientists bemoan that their evidence is not used by decisionmakers and why do so many decisionmakers claim that scientists are not supplying policy relevant evidence? (Austin & Overholt 1988; Noack 2006). It is because of these types of questions that the rational-linear model of policymaking often is criticised as being an idealistic explanation for all policymaking circumstances. The model is challenged for assuming that research always is conducted rigorously, comprehensively, timely and then applied to policymaking in a consensual and accurate way.

Generally, public health nutrition policies are made in response to a problem. Irrespective of how serious the problem may be, public health nutrition policies do not arise of their own volition; they require individuals and groups of people to stimulate and then coordinate their development. The following two theories of policymaking propose explanations and predictions based around the actions of individuals and groups of people, and thereby capture a political dimension to the process.

Kingdon's agenda-setting model

Kingdon (1995) investigated case studies of policymaking in the United States to analyse how issues come to be issues, how they come to the attention of policy-makers, how agendas are set and why ideas have their time. He proposed his agenda-setting model of policy change in which policymaking is viewed as the product of opportunistic activity by policy entrepreneurs, such as advocates or bureaucrats. Kingdon invokes the metaphor of the existence of three streams (the 'problem' stream, the 'policy' stream consisting of specialists who formulate policy solutions, and the 'political' stream that sets the governmental agenda and determines the allocation of resources) as the components of policymaking. At strategic times, the three streams come together and it is when this occurs that policymaking happens. A representation of Kingdon's model is shown in Figure 18.2.

Advocacy coalition framework

A well-developed theory to explain the emergence of and changes in public policy is the advocacy coalition framework (ACF) proposed by Sabatier and Jenkins-Smith (1993) and depicted in Figure 18.3. The ACF explains policy change as the product of competition between two or more advocacy coalitions. An advocacy coalition is formed with the coming together of individual policy actors who share a common belief system and who seek to manipulate the rules of various governmental institutions to achieve their core beliefs. Scientific evidence is perceived to influence policy through the beliefs of advocacy

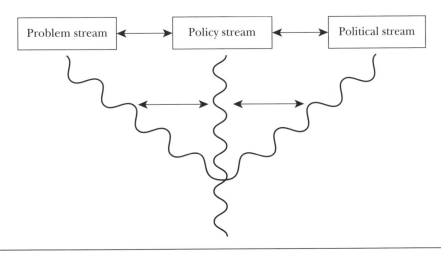

Figure 18.2 A simplified version of Kingdon's model of policy change

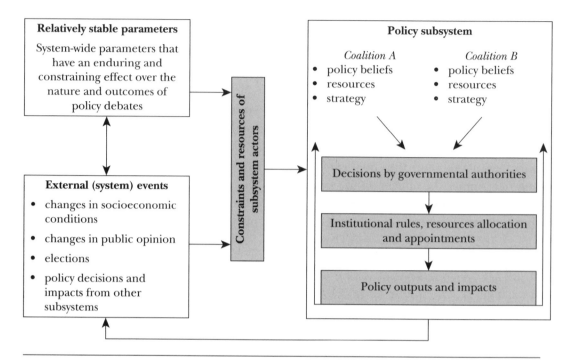

Figure 18.3 A simplified version of the advocacy coalition framework

Source: Adapted from Sabatier and Jenkins-Smith, 1993

coalitions who are able to sponsor research and accept or reject data based on how it aligns with their core beliefs. Policy change is explained as an outcome of fluctuations in the dominant belief systems within a given policy subsystem, here the food subsystem, over time.

These fluctuations are a function of three sets of processes:

1. the interaction of competing advocacy coalitions within a policy subsystem
2. changes external to the subsystem, such as changes in socioeconomic conditions, changes in governance and decisions from other policy subsystems
3. the effects of stable system parameters such as basic social structure and constitutional rules – on the constraints and resources of various actors.

Sabatier and Jenkins-Smith's ACF theory offers insights into how and why scientific evidence is used in the public health nutrition policymaking process. They challenge the implicit assumption that the interpretation and application of scientific evidence arises as an independent component in the policy process. Instead, these policy analysts view public health nutrition policy as the outcome of competition among stakeholders regarding contested values, beliefs and interests relating to public health and how evidence is collected, analysed and interpreted. This theory has a particular resonance with the public health nutrition policy debate associated with the marketing of food to children (see Case study 18.2). In many countries, advocacy coalitions have been formed to represent interests either for or against issues such as the banning of certain food advertising to children.

Advocacy

The importance of advocacy as a core skill within the public health nutritionists' 'toolbox' has been stressed in several chapters in this book, and in chapters 9 and 15 in particular. Advocacy has variously been described as a 'strategy', a 'process', or a 'calling', with the purpose of speaking out for an issue, belief or cause.

Advocacy skills are important for professional practice because policy-making is an inherently political process. Whose values, beliefs and interests prevail, or are obscured, in policy outcomes is determined largely by advocacy battles among stakeholders during the policymaking process. As McAlister and colleagues (1991) comment:

> Democracy, as we know it, proceeds through compromises between conflicting public, private, collective, and individual interests. Thus modern history abounds in irony, not the least being the way in which private corporations, public institutions, communication media, and clinical professions absorb vast resources in contrary activities influencing the health of human populations.

Traditionally, advocacy to influence policymaking has not been included as a core training competency for nutritionists. Nor is it a competency for which everyone is suited. Practitioners may feel uncomfortable about engaging in an activity that can involve selling a position, and possibly entering into adversarial debates. Also it rarely is a straightforward process and there are challenges. For example, Yeatman (2002) explains the challenges for public health organisations and individuals to be familiar with the technical and dynamic nature of the food regulatory system if they are to undertake advocacy in this important policy setting environment.

The importance of advocacy as a core public health nutrition policy skill is now receiving increasing attention. It is experiences gained from advocacy in the area of tobacco control that is providing many valuable lessons for public health nutrition advocacy (Yach et al. 2005). As an increasing number of public health advocacy activities are implemented, analysed and reported, undertakings of effective advocacy strategies continues to evolve. Three well-documented analyses of strategic approaches to public health advocacy are Chapman (2004), Galer-Unti and colleagues (2004) and Catford (2006).

There are two particular purposes for which advocacy might be considered in a public health nutrition setting. Firstly, advocacy associated with promoting the public health nutrition workforce and agenda in general. Secondly, advocacy associated with promoting a public health nutrition perspective towards a specific policy topic such as whether television advertising of soft drinks and confectionary to children should be restricted. In Case study 18.3 that follows we consider an advocacy episode from the first perspective.

CASE STUDY 18.3

LEADERSHIP AND ADVOCACY FOR BUILDING WORKFORCE CAPACITY

Queensland Health is the state government department responsible for delivering public health services to around four million people living in Australia's second-largest state, Queensland. Historically, Queensland Health employed fewer nutrition and dietetic staff per capita than other states, and few community nutritionists. The total workforce in 2001 consisted of 123 full-time nutrition positions, mostly hospital-based. However between 2002/3 and 2005/6, Queensland Health committed an additional A $9.6 million of recurrent funding towards improved nutrition and physical activity, with a focus on primary prevention of chronic diseases. This investment included recruitment of 93 new staff across the state (including public health nutritionists, community nutritionists, indigenous nutrition workers, physical activity promotion officers, project officers). Funding also supported a five-year commitment to social marketing of fruit and vegetables, social marketing of breastfeeding, and a healthy food supply strategy for schools.

This investment is the result of the work of many Queensland Health staff over more than a decade. The 1990s saw the emergence of indigenous health as a major issue both nationally and in Queensland (Epidemiology and Health Information Branch 1994). The first public health nutritionist was employed in north Queensland in 1992 and highlighted the poor nutrition and inadequate food supply of Aboriginal and Torres Strait Islander people living in rural and remote Queensland (Leonard et al. 1995). This position provided a model of what public health nutrition specialists could achieve and created an impetus for subsequent investment. In 1994, Queensland Health funded the University of Queensland to develop the Queensland Aboriginal and Torres Strait Islander Food and Nutrition Strategy (QATSIFNS), which identified nutrition as a key determinant of the poor health outcomes of indigenous Queenslanders, and advocated for the development of an indigenous-focused nutrition workforce.

The Australian Institute of Health and Welfare (AIHW) estimated the cost of preventable diet-related disease in Australia and Queensland Health epidemiologists applied this to Queensland (Epidemiology and Health Information Branch 1997). A working paper drew heavily on this work to advocate for the establishment of a Queensland workforce to address primary prevention of these conditions (Health Advancement Branch 1995).'

Funding to advance indigenous health was secured in 1998, to implement the recommendations of the QATSIFNS, including the creation of public health nutritionist positions in the newly created branch Public Health Services. A critical mass of public health nutritionists, including a senior nutritionist within the Queensland Health corporate office, was now able to influence senior decisionmakers through briefings, presentations and funding submissions to advocate for the expansion of the nutrition workforce. Submissions used an evidence-based approach focussed on the burden of disease and health costs associated with poor nutrition.

The development of a state nutrition strategy in response to *Eat Well Australia* (SIGNAL 2001) was identified as a key priority for the nutrition workforce. In 2001 Queensland Health funded the Queensland Public Health Forum (QPHF) to develop *Eat Well Queensland: Smart Eating for a Healthier State*, which was launched by the Queensland Premier in 2002 and endorsed by the eighteen-member organisations of the QPHF, including Queensland Health. *Eat Well Queensland* summarised the evidence on the nutrition-related burden of disease, effectiveness of interventions, potential health gain, priority population groups and key issues to be addressed.

Subsequent funding submissions from the nutrition team identified the investment in workforce required to implement the recommendations of *Eat Well Queensland*. Key enablers for this investment have included:

- advocacy emphasised the urgency of the problem and focused on evidence for health outcomes associated with nutrition, physical activity and obesity rather than on discipline-specific benchmarking
- some senior Queensland Health administrators recognised and championed the prevention agenda including the role of nutrition in indigenous health

- the appointment of a principal public health nutritionist within the Queensland Health corporate office enabled strong and effective advocacy
- a supportive policy context included strategies previously mentioned, and *Smart State: Health 2020*, in which the Queensland government recognised the challenges facing the health system due to population growth, the ageing population and the obesity epidemic
- recognition of the obesity epidemic in the popular press from around 2003 meant that this was an 'idea whose time has come'; however, constant advocacy is required to reinforce the role of nutrition and physical activity interventions as the means to prevent obesity
- the development of an agreement on a joint work plan between the chief executives of the health and education ministries enabled the two departments to work together to develop a policy approach to school food supply
- the ministers of health and education and the premier all took a personal interest the issue of nutrition and established a cross-government working group in 2004 to develop an action plan to promote healthy weight in children and young people.

The process resembled a building-block approach, with each step building on previous steps (sometimes the foundations get forgotten in the glow from subsequent achievements). The advocates displayed strong leadership and were themselves the beneficiaries of previous leaders.

Source: Christina Stubbs (personal communication)

This case study illustrates the following five key components for creating political will, as suggested by Catford (2006):

1. *issue* — strategic research was undertaken to demonstrate that an increased workforce capacity would enable a perceived problem to be addressed
2. *source* — advocates demonstrated their own credibility and status, for example, alliances were forged to maximise the impact of the advocacy
3. *benefits* — the focus of the advocacy was on providing solutions for decision-makers, rather than adding more problems
4. *timing* — the advocacy occurred in the mid-term period of the election cycle with a view to placing the issue on the political agenda in time for achieving investment in the third-year budget and thereby inclusion in forward commitments. It took time and repetition to get the message across
5. *methods* — advocates worked on building supportive and constructive relationships with decisionmakers.

Challenges for professional practice

Here, two common challenges for professional practice in policy and politics, namely capacity constraints and implications for professional roles and responsibilities, are considered.

Capacity constraints

The political process rarely takes place on a level playing field. Invariably, there exists differential capacity among stakeholders to participate in and influence policy processes. Those with greatest capacity in terms of factors such as resources, workforce numbers and links with decisionmakers, are best placed to influence processes and ultimately shape policy outcomes to support their particular views.

Differences in capacity to participate in public health nutrition policy-making have been reported at various levels of governance ranging from local to international food and nutrition policy settings. In their study of decision-making for local food and nutrition policy, Pelletier and colleagues (2003) report that within local communities the difference in capacity (they refer to power) between disenfranchised people and powerful individuals is critical in explaining processes and outcomes. They identify that capacity differences are exercised through three means:

1. the forms and patterns of participation in decisionmaking
2. institutional agenda setting
3. the ability of powerful groups to frame social and political issues through defining the causes and solutions to identified problems.

Similar capacity constraints have been observed at the international level. For instance, difficulties have been experienced with negotiations around WTO agreements and barriers presented to individual member countries to implement policy strategies to tackle the rising obesity epidemic. Australia, New Zealand and the United States export to Pacific Island countries (PICs) poor nutritional quality food products such as mutton flaps that are rarely consumed in their domestic markets. Many PICs are compromised in their ability to restrict the import of such products for fear of transgressing on commitments made in signing up to WTO agreements and the potential for economic retaliation from more powerful member countries (Lawrence 2005). Paradoxically, PICs are among the most economically vulnerable countries in the world and potentially have the opportunity to negotiate special and differential provisions when signing onto the WTO agreements. The shame here is that many PICs have not taken advantage of these provisions because they were lacking in the legal expertise to be aware of their existence and/or how to exploit them (Hughes & Lawrence 2005).

There are opportunities to address capacity differentials. Internationally, some steps are being taken by UN agencies to address challenges confronting vulnerable countries in participating in policymaking settings and having their public health nutrition concerns addressed (FAO 2006). At the local level there are many examples of individuals and groups joining together to form alliances around common interests to share ideas and resources and strengthen their capacity to participate in policymaking. Here the role of the public health nutritionist might be to facilitate such activities by helping to identify opportunities and bring groups together. For example, the Parent's Jury (see chapters 9 and 15) that was established by parents and public health nutritionists first in the United Kingdom, then in Australia is active in drawing attention to practices that they argue are misleading and calling for stronger government policy to protect public health nutrition. In 2005, the Parents Jury in Australia, announced that Kellogg's Coco Pops had 'won' its inaugural Smoke and Mirrors award for food advertising (Parents Jury 2005). The Parents Jury expressed concern that the advertisement used a popular children's television identity to promote the product as one with high nutritional value (based on its high level of nutrient fortification), while failing to mention that it contained over 36 per cent added sugar.

Professional roles and responsibilities

Participating in political activities can be an especially vexed professional role and responsibility for public health nutritionists. By definition, policy captures values and intentions and as such public health nutritionists wishing to participate in policy practice need to continually reflect on their own values and intentions. Of course there are varying degrees of engagement with political activities and some may be more acceptable to employers than others. Sometimes an outcome to promote or protect public health nutrition cannot be achieved by means other than by engaging in some form of political lobbying or related activity.

A challenge for public health nutritionists is to balance their role as a professional employed by an organisation with being an advocate for a public health nutrition issue (or vice versa). For example, knowledge that a policy decision is being made on poor evidence or as a result of especially inappropriate lobbying can raise ethical and professional dilemmas. Often individuals most informed and aware of a contentious issue are least able to act on the information as they may be perceived as being too closely aligned or too passionate about the issue to provide an objective, scientific analysis in their workplace. Some professionals might argue that in such circumstances it is better to work for change from within and avoid potential confrontation from acting on such information which might lead to a career-limiting outcome. Other professionals might adopt the view that they believe they should make a stand and use their knowledge and insights to challenge the policy process.

Conclusion

A basic understanding of what policy is and how and why it is made is an essential competency requirement for public health nutrition professionals. Central to the critical analysis perspective presented in this chapter is the premise that the making of public health nutrition policy frequently involves a struggle among stakeholders to achieve a policy outcome that is consistent with their values, beliefs and interests. In other words, evidence-based practice certainly is fundamental, but policymaking is a complex political process, as well as an analytical problem-solving exercise. Ultimately, public health nutrition policy takes on meaning in the context of power and processes that shape the interpretation of competing views among stakeholders towards food and health. Nevertheless, improved processes that are democratic and transparent and policy outcomes that promote public health nutrition are the objectives for which to strive with professional policy practice.

An inherent danger of a critical analysis approach of the type presented in this chapter is that the reader may become too cynical towards policy. They might ask, 'how can you apply rational analysis to an inherently irrational process?' Similarly, if motivations, processes and outcomes are predetermined by power and networks, then the reader might ask, 'is the cause of the independent public health nutritionist armed with expert knowledge inevitably stultified in the policy process?' This chapter has attempted to avoid creating these potential scenarios by empowering the reader in three ways. Firstly, by promoting critical awareness of the food and nutrition policy setting, secondly, by providing a brief review of the political underpinnings inherent in policymaking, and thirdly, by introducing the core skills of policy science research and advocacy for professional practice.

References

Anderson, J. 1975, *Public Policy-Making*, New York, Praeger.

Austin, J. and Overholt, C. 1988, 'Nutrition policy: Building the bridge between science and politics' in *Annual Review of Nutrition*, vol. 8, pp. 1–20.

Bambra, C., Fox, D. and Scott-Samuel, A. 2005, 'Towards a politics of health' in *Health Promotion International*, vol. 20, no. 2, pp. 187–93.

British Nutrition Foundation 2006, 'Establishing a Whole School Food Policy', cited at <http://www.nutrition.org.uk/upload/wholeschoolfoodpolicy.pdf> on 27 November.

Cannon, G. 1987, *The Politics of Food*, Century Hutchinson, London.

Caraher, M. and Coveney, J. 2004, 'Public health nutrition and food policy' in *Public Health Nutrition*, vol. 7, no. 5, pp. 591–98.

Catford, J. 2006, 'Creating political will: Moving from the science to the art of health promotion' in *Health Promotion International*, vol. 21, no. 1, pp. 1–4.

Centre for Science in the Public Interest 2004, 'Bush administration trying to bury WHO obesity report', CSPI Newsroom, cited at <http://www.cspinet.org> on 7 August, 2006.

Chapman, S. 2004, 'Advocacy for public health: A primer' in *Journal of Epidemiology and Community Health*, vol. 58, pp. 361–65.

Collins, T. 2005, 'Health policy analysis: A simple tool for policy makers' in *Public Health*, vol. 119, pp. 192–96.

Coveney, J. 2003, 'Why food policy is critical to public health' in *Critical Public Health*, vol. 13, no. 2, pp. 99–105.

Dye, T. 2002, *Understanding public policy* (tenth edition), Prentice Hall, New Jersey.

Epidemiology and Health Information Branch 1994, 'Causes of excess deaths in Aboriginal and Torres Strait Islander populations', information circular no. 26, Queensland Health, Brisbane.

—— 1997, 'Queensland hospital costs attributable to inappropriate diet', information circular no. 44, Queensland Health, Brisbane.

Food and Agriculture Organization (FAO) 1998, 'Carbohydrates in human nutrition', Report of the Joint FAO/WHO Expert Consultation, FAO Food and Nutrition Paper 66, FAO, Rome.

Food and Agriculture Organization (FAO) and World Health Organization (WHO) 2006, 'Enhancing developing country participation in FAO/WHO scientific advice activities', Report of a Joint FAO/WHO Meeting in Belgrade, Serbia and Montenegro, 12–15 December, FAO, Rome, 2006.

Fullerton, T. 2005, 'Generation O: The obesity epidemic and the politics of responsibility' on Australian Broadcasting Corporation's 'Four Corners', 17 October, cited on http://www.abc.net.au/4corners/content/2005/s1484310.htm> on 27 November 2006.

Galer-Unti, R.A., Tappe, M.K. and Lachenmayr, S. 2004, 'Advocacy 101: Getting started in Health Education Advocacy' in *Health Promotion Practice*, vol. 5, no. 3, pp. 280–88.

Goodin, R. 1982, *Political theory and public policy*, University of Chicago Press, Chicago.

Goodman, C. and Anise, A. 2006, 'What is known about the effectiveness of economic instruments to reduce consumption of foods high in saturated fats and other energy dense foods for preventing and treating obesity?', Health Evidence Network Report, WHO Regional Office for Europe, Copenhagen, cited at <http://www.euro.who.int/document/e88909.pdf> on 13 July.

Haby, M., Vos, T., Carter, R., Moodie, M., Markwick, A., Magnus, A., Tay-Teo, K-S. and Swinburn, B. 2006, 'A new approach to assessing the health benefit from obesity interventions in children and adolescents: The assessing cost-effectiveness in obestity project' in *International Journal of Obesity*, vol. 30, no. 10, pp. 1463–75.

Ham, C., Hunter, D.J. and Robinson, R. 1995, 'Evidence based policymaking: Research must inform health policy as well as medical care' in *British Medical Journal*, vol. 310, pp. 71–72.

Hughes, R. and Lawrence, M. 2005, 'Globalisation, food and health in Pacific Island countries' in *Asia Pacific Journal of Clinical Nutrition*, vol. 14, no. 4, pp. 298–306.

Kingdon, J.W. 1995, *Agendas, Alternatives, and Public Policies* (second edition), HarperCollins College Publishers, New York.

Lang, T. and Heasman, M. 2004, *Food Wars: The global battle for mouths, minds and markets*, Earthscan, London.

Lasswell, H. 1936, *Politics: Who gets what, when, how*, McGraw-Hill, New York.

—— 1951, 'The policy orientation' in Lerner, D. and Lasswell, H. (eds) 1951, *The Policy Sciences*, Stanford University Press, California, pp. 3–15.

Lawrence, M. 1987, 'Making healthier choices easier choices: The Victorian Food and Nutrition Project' in *Journal of Food and Nutrition*, vol. 44, no. 2, pp. 57–59.

—— 2005, 'The potential of food regulation as a policy instrument for obesity prevention in developing countries' in Crawford, D. and Jeffery, R.W. 2005, *Obesity prevention and Public Health*, Oxford University Press, Oxford.

Leonard, D., Beilin, R. and Moran, M. 1995, 'Which way kaikai blo umi? Food and nutrition in the Torres Strait' in *Australian Journal of Public Health*, vol. 19, no. 6, pp. 589–95.

McAlister, A., Puska, P., Orlandi, M., Bye, L. and Zbylot, P. 1991, 'Behaviour modification: Principles and illustrations' in Holland, W., Detels, R. and Knox, G. (eds) 1991, *Oxford Textbook of Public Health*, pp. 3–16.

Mello, M.M., Studdert, D.M. and Brennan, T.A. 2006, 'Obesity: The new frontier of public health law' in *New England Journal of Medicine*, vol. 354, no. 24, pp. 2601–10.

Milio, N. 1988, 'Making public policy: Developing the science by learning the art; An ecological framework for policy studies' in *Health Promotion*, vol. 2, no. 3, pp. 263–74.

—— 1990, *Nutrition Policy for Food-rich Countries: A strategic analysis*, The Johns Hopkins University Press, Baltimore and London.

National Health and Medical Research Council (NHMRC) 2003, *Dietary Guidelines for Australians Adults*, Commonwealth of Australia, Canberra.

Nestle, M. 2002, *Food Politics: How the food industry influences nutrition and health*, University California Press, London.

—— 2006, 'Food marketing and childhood obesity: A matter of policy' in *New England Journal of Medicine*, vol. 354, no. 24, pp. 2527–29.

Niessen, L.W., Grijseels, E.W.M. and Rutten, R.F.H. 2000, 'The evidence-based approach in health policy and health care delivery' in *Social Science and Medicine*, vol. 51, pp. 859–69.

Noack, R.H. 2006, 'President's column: How can we reduce the knowledge gap between public health research and policy/practice?' in *European Journal of Public Health*, vol. 16, no. 3, pp. 336–38.

Parents Jury, The, 2005, 'Junk food ads slammed by Parents Jury', cited at <http://www.parentsjury.org.au/downloads/2005_Awards_ announcement_media_release.pdf> on 27 November 2006.

Parsons, W. 1995, *Public Policy: An introduction to the theory and practice of policy analysis*, Edward Elgar, Aldershot.

Pelletier, D., McCullum, C., Kraak, V. and Asher, K. 2003, 'Participation, power and beliefs shape local food and nutrition policy' in *Journal of Nutrition*, vol. 133, pp. S301–04.

Rayner, M. and Scarborough, P. 2005, 'The burden of food related ill health in the UK' in *Journal Epidemiology Community Health*, vol. 59, pp. 1054–57.

Robertson, A. 2006, *Comparison of nutrition policy implementation in Scotland with twelve countries: An international expert commentary for the Scottish Diet Action Plan Review*, Suhr's University College, Copenhagen.

Robertson, A., Brunner, E. and Sheiham, A. 2006, 'Food is a political issue' in Marmot, M. and Wilkinson, R.G. (eds) 2006, *Social determinants of health*, (second edition), Oxford, Oxford University Press, pp. 172–95.

Sabatier, P.A. (ed.) 1999, *Theories of the policy process*, Westview Press, Boulder, Colorado.

Sabatier, P.A. and Jenkins-Smith, H.C. 1993, *Policy change and learning: An advocacy coalition approach*, Westview Press, Boulder, Colorado.

Steele, J. 1995, 'Health gain in Queensland: the contribution of food and nutrition action', Health Advancement Branch, Queensland Health, Brisbane.

Strategic Intergovernmental Alliance (SIGNAL) 2001, *Eat Well Australia: An agenda for action for public health nutrition 2001–2010*, National Public Health Partnership, Canberra.

Susser, M. and Susser, E. 1996, 'Choosing a future for epidemiology II: From black box to Chinese boxes and eco-epidemiology' in *American Journal of Public Health*, vol. 86, no. 5, pp. 674–77.

Tansey, G. 1994, 'From words to action' in *Ecology of Food and Nutrition*, vol. 32, pp. 45–50.

Walt, G. 1996, *Health Policy: An introduction to process and power*, Zed Books, London, pp. 4–9.

World Health Organization (WHO) 1986, *Ottawa Charter for Health Promotion*, First International Conference on Health Promotion, Ottawa, 21 November, WHO, Geneva.

—— 2002, *The World Health Report 2002: Reducing risks, promoting healthy life*, WHO, Geneva.

—— 2003, *Technical Report 916 based on an Expert Consultation on Diet, Nutrition and the Prevention of Chronic Diseases*. WHO, Geneva.

—— 2004, *Global Strategy Diet, Physical Activity and Health*, WHO, Geneva.

Yach, D., McKee, M., Lopez, A.D., and Novotny, T. 2005, 'Improving diet and physical activity: 12 lessons from controlling tobacco smoking' in *British Medical Journal*, vol. 330, pp. 898–900.

Yeatman, H. 2002, 'Australia's food regulations: Challenges for public health advocacy' in *Australian and New Zealand Journal of Public Health*, vol. 26, no. 5, pp. 515–17.

Acknowledgements

One of the joys of editing a book of this type is the opportunity it provides to work and share ideas with colleagues whom we respect so highly. We acknowledge all the hard-working authors and referees for writing such enlightening chapters and reviews. We strove to prepare a coherent and integrated reference book that was greater than simply being the sum of its chapter parts. In this regard we have much gratitude to the overseers of each book section — Agneta Yngve, Simone French, Barrie Margetts and Roger Hughes. We asked these international leaders in public health nutrition to adopt a role akin to that of a chairperson at a conference plenary session. For their generosity in reviewing the chapters in each of their 'sessions' and providing us with many critical suggestions we thank them.

The success of a reference book this substantial would not be possible without the assistance of many dedicated people. In particular, Anita Lawrence provided invaluable expert advice and continual encouragement throughout the book's conception and preparation. Several colleagues assisted us with accessing reference materials — we are especially indebted to Lluis Serra-Majem, Keyou Ge, Toulla Hoskins, Sandra Ribas and Maria Daniel Vax de Almeida. In addition, we want to acknowledge Tim Lang, Barbara Smith and Rosemary Stanton whose commitment to public health nutrition was an inspiration in the planning of the book. Also, Sharon Melder provided patient assistance with editorial administration. Finally, we thank Elizabeth Weiss, Joanne Holliman and Pedro Almeida and everyone at Allen & Unwin for their warm support and material help throughout the book's preparation and production.

Index

Page numbers in *italics* refer to figures. An 'n' after a page number indicates a reference to an endnote.

[478]